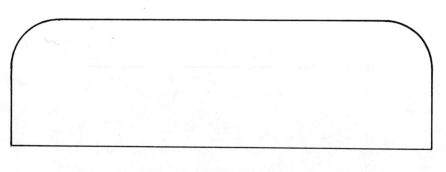

Food Allergies
and
Adverse Reactions

Contributors

John A. Anderson, MD
Head, Division of Allergy and Clinical Immunology
Department of Medicine
Henry Ford Hospital
Detroit, Michigan

Kathleen C. Barnes, BS, MA
Doctoral Student
Department of Anthropology
University of Florida
Gainesville, Florida

Paul L. Doering, MS
Professor of Pharmacy Practice
College of Pharmacy
University of Florida
Gainesville, Florida

Leslie Sue Lieberman, PhD
Associate Professor of Anthropology and Pediatrics
Departments of Anthropology and Pediatrics
University of Florida
Gainesville, Florida

Victoria Olejer, MS, RD
Nutritionist
Asthma Allergy Clinic
Shreveport, Louisiana

Judy E. Perkin, DrPH, RD
Program Director and Associate Professor
Clinical & Community Dietetics
College of Health Related Professions
University of Florida
Gainesville, Florida

Steve L. Taylor, PhD
Professor and Head
Department of Food Science and Technology
University of Nebraska
Food Processing Center
Lincoln, Nebraska

Food Allergies and Adverse Reactions

Judy E. Perkin, DrPH, RD

Program Director of Clinical and Community Dietetics
University of Florida
Gainesville, Florida

AN ASPEN PUBLICATION®
Aspen Publishers, Inc.
Gaithersburg, Maryland
1990

Library of Congress Cataloging-in-Publication Data

Perkin, Judy E.
Food allergies and adverse reactions / Judy E. Perkin.
p. cm.
Includes bibliographical references and index.
ISBN: 0-8342-0170-4
1. Food allergy. I. Title.
RC596.P37 1990
616.97'5—dc20
90-684
CIP

Aspen Publishers, Inc., is not affiliated with the American
Society of Parenteral and Enteral Nutrition

The authors have made every effort to ensure the accuracy of the information
herein, particularly with regard to drug selection and dose. However, appropriate
information sources should be consulted, especially for new or unfamiliar drugs
or procedures. It is the responsibility of every practitioner to evaluate the
appropriateness of a particular opinion in the context of actual clinical situations
and with due consideration to new developments. Authors, editors, and the
publisher cannot be held responsible for any typographical or other errors found
in this book.

Editorial Services: Ruth Bloom

Library of Congress Catalog Card Number: 90-684
ISBN: 0-8342-0170-4

Printed in the United States of America

1 2 3 4 5

This book is dedicated to the memory of

James C. (Jim) Rose, MS, RD.

Jim was both a mentor and friend. Jim aided in providing me with opportunities to publish and followed through with encouragement. Jim was a significant force in the lives of many of us in the dietetics community. I hope in some small way this volume speaks positively to his influence.

Table of Contents

Preface xi

Acknowledgments xiii

Chapter 1—Food Allergy or Sensitivity Terminology,
Physiologic Bases, and Scope of the Clinical Problem ...   1
John A. Anderson

Introduction 1
Terminology Concerning Reactions to Food
and Food Additives 3
Immune Basis of Food Allergy Reactions 3
Type I Allergic Reaction 5
Mechanisms Known or Suspected To Be Responsible
for Food Intolerance Reactions 7
Clinical Manifestations of Adverse Food Reactions 9
Diagnoses, Management, and Prevention of Adverse
Reactions to Food 10

Chapter 2—Diagnosis of Food Allergy 15
Part I: The Physician's Perspective 15
John A. Anderson

Introduction 15
Presenting History of Food Reactions 16
Immunologic Tests Used in the Diagnosis
of Food Allergy 19
Screening *In Vitro* Allergy Assays 21
Immediate-Reacting IgE Skin Test 22
In Vitro IgE Food Allergen-Specific Assays 24
Other Immunologic Tests of Value in the Diagnosis
of Food Allergy 27

vii

Unproven and Unapproved "Allergy" Tests Used
in the Diagnosis of Suspected Food Allergy   27

Part II: The Dietitian's Perspective...................................   *30*
Victoria Olejer

Introduction..   30
Food Challenges   43

**Chapter 3—Major Food Allergens and Principles of
Dietary Management** **51**
Judy E. Perkin

Introduction..   51
Major Food Allergens   52
Principles of Dietary Management....................................   62
Summary   63

Chapter 4—Drug Therapy of Food Allergies **69**
Paul L. Doering

Introduction..   69
Epinephrine and Other Adrenergics................................   69
Oral Cromolyn   71
Antihistamines   73
Corticosteroids   76
Summary   78

**Chapter 5—Maternal Influences on the Development of Food
Allergy in the Infant** **81**
July E. Perkin

Prenatal Sensitization..   81
Breastfeeding and Atopic Disease   83
Diet Modification during Pregnancy and Lactation:
Strategies To Prevent Allergy   106
Summary and Implications for Dietetic Practice   109

Chapter 6—Managing Food Allergies in Infants and Toddlers **117**
Victoria Olejer

Management of Food Allergies in Infants......................   122
Management of Food Allergies in Toddlers and
Older Children   123
Recommendations for Enhancing Patient
Compliance   124

Chapter 7—Adverse Reactions to Food Additives and Other Food Constituents **129**
Judy E. Perkin

    Introduction 129
    Aspartame 129
    Sulfites 134
    Other Food Additives 140
    Food Contaminants 140
    Naturally Occurring Food or Beverage
        Constituents 145
    Conclusion 160

Chapter 8—Adverse Food Reactions: Relationship to Arthritis and Migraine **171**
Judy E. Perkin

    Arthritis and Other Disorders of Connective and
        Joint Tissue 171
    Migraine 181
    Conclusion 184

Chapter 9—Food Allergies and Related Adverse Reactions to Foods: A Food Science Perspective **189**
Steve L. Taylor

    The Nature and Chemistry of the Offending
        Substances in Foods 189
    Effect of Processing and Preparation 192
    Construction of Safe and Effective Avoidance Diets 196
    Conclusion 201

Chapter 10—Food Allergies and Adverse Food Reactions: An Anthropological Perspective **207**
Leslie Sue Lieberman and Kathleen C. Barnes

    A Biocultural Perspective on Food Allergies
        and Intolerances 207
    Gluten Sensitivity (Celiac Disease): Sensitivity to
        Cereal Grains 211
    Lactose Intolerance: An Example of Biocultural
        Adaptations 212
    Adverse Reactions to Food Additives: Chinese
        Restaurant Syndrome As an Example 220
    Food Habits and Allergies 221
    Summary 229

Chapter 11—Controversies in Food Allergy and Adverse
Reactions 233
Judy E. Perkin

    Clinical Ecology 233
    Candidiasis Hypersensitivity 235
    Food and Behavior 236
    Vitamin Supplementation.. 239
    Conclusion 240

Appendix A—General Guidelines for Management of Cow's
Milk Allergy 243

Appendix B—General Guidelines for Management of Soy
Allergy 249

Appendix C—General Guidelines for Management of Egg
Allergy 253

Appendix D—General Guidelines for Management of Wheat
Allergy 257

Appendix E—General Guidelines for Management of Corn
Allergy 259

Appendix F—Examples of Recipe Sources for the Allergic
Individual 261

Appendix G—Examples of Products Containing Aspartame 263

Appendix H—Examples of Products Containing Sulfites 267

Appendix I—Examples of Products Containing Tartrazine
(FD&C Yellow No. 5) 269

Appendix J—Examples of Products Containing Benzoates 273

Appendix K—Lactose Content of Common Food Items 275

Index 277

Preface

Dietitians and other nutrition professionals are becoming increasingly involved in the treatment of food allergies and adverse food reactions. Prevention of these problems is also a focus.

This book is an attempt to speak to dietitians and others with a nutrition focus about current allergy or adverse food reaction practice and research. Although some general dietary guidelines are found in the Appendixes and are present in the text, this book does not attempt a diet manual or recipe book approach to the subject. Excellent examples of these approaches are referenced in the text, and readers are referred to these sources. Other texts in the area offer an in-depth perspective from a medical viewpoint (diagnosis and symptoms) or approach the general public. This book is a guide written from a dietetics perspective. It is hoped this work will fill a need of the nutrition community.

Judy E. Perkin, DrPH, RD
September 1990

Acknowledgments

This book is a product of the work of many. Both to those who worked on this volume and those who inspired us, I say thank you. Many of the authors have not only made contributions of chapters, but have provided help and advice with regard to other sections as well.

In addition to the major contributors to this volume, I would like to thank all of the authors and publishing concerns who granted permission to reprint works. These permissions have made significant contributions to our text.

This book could not have been produced without excellent technical and secretarial support. Homer Bates, PhD, CPA, is to be thanked for his many hours of technical assistance with product ingredient inventories. Thanks for secretarial support goes to Barbara Brand (Gator Typing Services), Donna Simpson, and Theresa Haefner.

Janet Coggan, Robert Lockwood, and the Health Science Center Library staff of the University of Florida deserve recognition for their help with references.

I would like to thank Faye Dong, PhD, RD, Henry Bone, MD, Mike Brown, and Diane Dimperio, MA, RD. Their help in the conceptual stages of this work was invaluable. Finally, thanks is offered to Richard Gutekunst, PhD, Dean of the College of Health Related Professions, University of Florida, for his moral support in this endeavor.

Chapter 1

Food Allergy or Sensitivity Terminology, Physiologic Bases, and Scope of the Clinical Problem

John A. Anderson

INTRODUCTION

Hippocrates (460–370 BC) recognized that cow's milk could cause gastric upset and urticaria. Since this ancient time, food "allergy" has become clearly recognized by the medical community worldwide.[1] The true prevalence today of food allergy is unknown. Food reactions are often suspected. These reactions, however, frequently go unproven. The mother's perception of bad reactions occurring in her newborn infant during the first year of life has ranged between 20% and 28%.[2,3] In most of these studies, adverse reactions were due to fruit. Many of these reactions were due to the organic acids (rash) or the fruit sugar (diarrhea). True persistent adverse reactions to food in infants, proven by the method of double-blind placebo-controlled food challenge (DBPCFC), have been assessed at 3%.[3,4]

The natural history of proven food reactions that involve immune mechanisms (food allergy) to food such as chicken eggs or cow's milk protein is that by 2 to 3 years of age most allergic children would be expected to clinically tolerate that food.[5] Other food allergies acquired in childhood or in later life to foods such as peanuts, fish, crustacean seafoods (ie, shrimp), or tree nuts may last for a lifetime.

Adverse reactions (sensitivities) can be broken down into two types: (1) true food allergies or hypersensitivities, which are reactions involving immune mechanisms to food protein, and (2) other reactions, which are called food intolerances (see Table 1-1).[6] Allergy probably accounts for less than 20% of all food reactions. The vast majority of true food allergic reactions occur in children. Most of these true food allergic reactions resemble allergic reactions due to other substances such as penicillin drugs or honeybee stings. In patients with gastrointestinal complaints, however, it is often difficult to clearly tell a food allergy from a food intolerance. It is sometimes difficult to

1

Table 1-1   Common Terminology Concerning Adverse Reactions to Foods and Food Additives

Adverse Reaction to a Food or Food Additive
The general term applied to an abnormal response attributed to an exposure to a food or food additive. (Synonymous with food sensitivity.)

Food Allergy
An adverse food or food additive reaction caused by, or influenced by, an immunological mechanism. (Synonymous with food hypersensitivity.)

Food Intolerance
An abnormal physiologic response with exposure to a food or a food additive in which the mechanism is unknown or is not immunologic in nature.

Food Anaphylaxis and Anaphylactoid Reactions
Anaphylaxis is a classic allergic reaction that is mediated by immunologic activity of IgE antibodies. It involves mast cells or basophils and the release or formation of chemical mediators. Anaphylactoid reactions resemble anaphylaxis, clinically, and result from nonimmunologic release or formation of chemical mediators.

Food Idiosyncrasy
A food intolerance reaction, resembling an allergy, that may involve individuals who are generally prediagnosed such as those who lack specific enzymes needed to digest certain food components.

Food Toxicity or Poisoning
A food intolerance reaction, involving either contamination of foods with microorganisms or parasites or release of chemical mediators either directly or because of food contamination.

Pharmacologic Food Reaction
A food intolerance reaction that is drug-like.

Metabolic Food Reaction
An adverse food reaction that results in a metabolic change in the host recipient.

---

determine whether a food (or a food additive) has anything at all to do with the concerns of the patient.

Immunologic tests, as well as other tests, have only a limited value in the diagnosis of adverse reactions to food or food additives. Diet avoidance, followed by specific food or food additive challenge, is an important diagnostic tool.[7] Although this method of evaluation does not establish the mechanism of the reaction, it does confirm objectively that a specific food or food additive is the cause of a specific clinical sign or symptom. Once a specific food or food additive has been identified as causing an adverse reaction, avoidance of that food or food additive is the principal way to manage the problem. Should acute symptoms occur, however, due to a food or food additive exposure (i.e., anaphylaxis or anaphylactoid reaction), these should be treated promptly. Injectable aqueous epinephrine is the drug choice for this emergency situation. This drug can also be used in an autoinjector device for emergency treatment of an inadvertent food allergy exposure (ie, EpiPen®). The possible use of a prophylactic diet program in mothers and children, designed to lessen or prevent food allergy signs and symptoms in the newborn, as well as to lessen the chance of respiratory allergy later in life, has been debated for a number of years.[1] Recent well-controlled studies have demonstrated that although it may be possible to lessen the degree of food allergy signs and symptoms in the newborn, such a dietary program is difficult to adhere to strictly.[8] Also, by 2 years of age, the patients in these studies were found to have no different degree of respiratory allergy signs and symptoms whether on or off the dietary prevention program.[9]

TERMINOLOGY CONCERNING REACTIONS TO FOOD AND FOOD ADDITIVES

Many misunderstandings have occurred as a result of investigators calling the same thing by different names. The term "food allergy" is overused and often used to identify an overall reaction, when it is not. Allergy specialists use this term to describe only those events involving immune mechanisms— usually one involving IgE antibodies (a so-called type I immune reaction) (see Tables 1-2 and 1-3). The laity, as well as some physicians, have used this term to describe all bad or adverse reactions to food. A better general term than the term allergy is "an adverse reaction to food or food additive."

Food intolerance is a term that best fits all nonimmune reactions to food or food additives. In many of these reactions, the exact mechanisms are unknown. This includes food idiosyncratic reactions and food anaphylactoid reactions (the latter of which resemble allergy), as well as food toxic and poisoning reactions, pharmacologic food reactions, and food additive reactions that affect body metabolism. Table 1-1 defines these terms in simple language.[6]

IMMUNE BASIS OF FOOD ALLERGY REACTIONS

Gell and Coombs have classified all immune reactions into four types: Types I, II, III, and IV (see Table 1-3).[10] As shown in Table 1-3, type I through III reactions involve antibodies, whereas type IV reaction is exclusively a cell-mediated event.

Type I reactions involve the IgE antibody class. A few allergy-like clinical reactions have allegedly been related to IgG_4 antigen-specific antibodies (one of the four subclasses of immunoglobulin G).[11]

Table 1-2   The Type I Allergic Reaction

Stage	Description
1st	Familial Predisposition: To make IgE allergen-specific antibodies—Atopy.
2nd	Sensitization and Fixation: Specific allergen exposure, sensitization to form IgE allergen-specific antibodies followed by mast cell (or basophil effector cells) fixation.
3rd	An-Ab Interaction, Mediator Release/ Formation: Re-exposure to specific allergen, allergen + IgE antibody interaction followed by both preformed chemical mediator release from mast cells (or basophils) or activation of other mediator pathways outside the effector cells.
4th	Immune Inflammation: Influx of leukocytes and monocytes. Release of other chemical mediators from all types of cells, plus tissue reactive substances from eosinophils. Release of cytokine histamine releasing factor (HRF) to promote nonspecific reactivity.
5th	Clinical Reactions: (1) Early phase—within minutes to hours an allergic reaction occurs, including vasodilation, smooth muscle contraction, and hyperglandulin secretion. (2) Late phase—in one third to one half of all cases, in 6 to 12 hours a late inflammatory reaction occurs that is characterized by eosinophil (and other leukocytes and monocytes) infiltration—tissue damage and other mediator release (from all cells). (3) Prolonged phase—clinical hyperreactivity induced by nonspecific chemical mediator release, following nonallergic stimuli and modified by HRF.

Table 1-3   Classification of Immune Reaction[10]

Type	Description
I	IgE-Mediated Reactions Involving immune release of chemical mediators from mast cells (basophils)
II	Antitissue Antibody Reactions Involving IgG, M, or A antibodies against solid organs
III	Immune-Complex Reactions Involving circulating antibodies, usually IgG or IgM, and antigen combinations that activate complement, which in turn is involved in tissue injury
IV	Cell-Mediated Reactions Involving delayed-onset lymphocyte tissue infiltrates directed against tissue antigens

Type II Gell and Coombs immune reactions relate to the formation of antibodies against tissue antigens. This type of reaction does not occur in allergic reactions to food or food additives.

Type III reactions involve circulating immune complexes—IgG or IgM antibodies, plus the antigen they are directed to combine with to form complexes and in turn activate the complement cascade. This activated complement contributes to the tissue damage. Some immune reactions involving food proteins may involve a type III reaction. A well-studied classic example of this is the cow's milk-induced syndrome with pulmonary disease (Heiner's syndrome).[1,12]

Type IV, or cell-mediated immune reaction, involves so-called delayed hypersensitivity. The classic example of this type of reaction is the TB skin test reaction in humans. Delayed (in onset) adverse reaction to ingested food or food additives may be due to a number of mechanisms, some of which may be immune in nature such as type I IgE-mediated reactions.[13] Type IV, cell-mediated reactions in the case of foods have often been suspected, but usually these reactions have not been well documented.[14] In gluten enteropathy (celiac disease), both a toxic reaction to wheat protein (food intolerance) and a type IV cell-mediated immune reaction (food allergy) are involved.[1]

TYPE I ALLERGIC REACTION

Table 1-2 outlines the five stages of the type I (IgE-mediated) allergic reaction that may occur in immune reactions to food proteins. The first stage involves a familial predisposition to make excessive antibodies to various food allergens of the IgE class. Individuals are not born with a specific allergy—they are born with the potential to develop allergy. This tendency is inherited through families and is called atopy. The exact mode of transmission of this tendency varies with families and is not classified as dominant or recessive in the strict genetic sense.

However, children born in families in which both parents are atopic are very prone to be allergic. The specific clinical manifestation of allergy (ie, atopic dermatitis or asthma) also tends to run in families. The development of an allergy to a specific food depends on the frequency of exposure to that food, as well as to other factors such as the "allergenicity" of that food. (Some foods are more likely to cause allergy than others, eg, cow's milk, eggs, peanuts, fish, and shrimp compared to rice, lamb, squash, and pineapple.)

The second stage of the type I allergic reaction involves sensitization of the allergic individual to the specific allergen. After exposure to the allergen, IgE allergen-specific antibodies are manufactured by B cells on tissue surfaces in the human (skin, gastrointestinal tract, and, in some cases, the mucosal surfaces of the sinopulmonary tract). Antibody production is followed by fixation of the IgE allergen-specific antibody to the surfaces of tissue mast cells that are also on the tissue surfaces (see Fig. 1-1). Mast cells and basophils (which are similar) are the effecter cells of allergic reactions. They contain not only preformed chemical mediators (P.C.M.) in packets, ready to be released from the cell, but also the ability, in the case of the mast cell membrane, to stimulate the activation of the arachidonic acid pathway in surrounding tissues, so other chemical mediators are generated (G.C.M.). The best known P.C.M. is histamine, and examples of G.C.M. are the prostaglandins and leukotrienes. Basophils differ from mast cells because they circulate in the bloodstream, but they share the ability to fix with IgE antibodies and release P.C.M.s with mast cells . They are important in the IgE late phase reaction.

The third stage of the type I allergic reaction involves first the re-exposure of the human to the specific food protein allergen. This is followed by the stimulation of two molecules of allergen-specific antibodies that are fixed to the tissue mast cell effecter cell surface, which in turn causes the release of G.C.M. and the formation of P.C.M. (see Fig. 1-1).

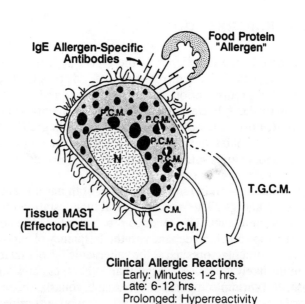

Figure 1-1   The Type 1 Allergic Reaction. C.M.: Mast cell membrane; N: Mast cell nucleus; P.C.M.: Preformed chemical mediators; T.G.C.M.: Tissue-generated chemical mediators.

The fourth stage involves the influx of other cells into the area of reaction. These cells are often attracted to these sites by mediators released by the mast cell or basophil. These cells (leukocytes, monocytes, eosinophils), in turn, release other chemical mediators. Some, like the eosinophils, contain toxic proteins that can damage tissues. This is called immune inflammation. Only a small amount of specific allergen re-exposure is necessary to produce a maximum release of chemical mediators. This differs from the typical dose-response relationship found in other immune reactions.

The fifth stage involves the clinical manifestations of the allergic reactions to food protein. Most of these clinical reactions occur within minutes to a few hours after exposure. An example of such a reaction is an anaphylactic reaction to a food like peanuts, which results in urticaria and shock. With a proven allergic reaction, it has been recognized that following a vigorous immediate reaction, in as many as a third of the cases, a second or dual late-phase reaction occurs. This second reaction peak is also the result of an IgE-mediated immune event and probably occurs in food allergy reactions more often than previously recognized. Second-phase reactions do occur with other types of allergic reaction.[13] There is growing evidence that IgE reactions to food in atopic dermatitis may involve this late-phase IgE reactivity.[15]

It is now recognized that mast cells and basophils that are actively "sensitized" with IgE, directed against food allergens, are prone to release mediators (P.C.M.) nonspecifically because of nonallergic factors. This process is modulated by the cytokine histamine releasing factor (HRF).[16] Thus, a clinical state of "prolonged hyperactivity" exists in this situation.

MECHANISMS KNOWN OR SUSPECTED TO BE RESPONSIBLE FOR FOOD INTOLERANCE REACTIONS

Most adverse reactions to food and food additives are due to nonimmunologic mechanisms. Where the mechanism is obvious, probably food contamination or poisoning with microorganisms or parasites is the most common nonimmune mechanism worldwide accounting for adverse food reaction. Food toxicity can be caused by natural toxic agents in food, eg, the ingestion of the poisonous plant foxglove, *Digitalis purpurea,* which contains the drug digitoxin. Adverse reactions can also occur because of natural pharmacologic agents found in food. Examples are the vasoactive amines, tyramine (in cheese), phenylethylamine (in chocolate), and caffeine (coffee and tea). These types of reactions can also be called pharmacologic reactions to food.

Toxic food reactions can cause direct chemical-mediator release from the mast cell (bypassing the immune reaction as described under type I IgE allergic reactions). A rash caused by the ingestion of strawberries is a common food toxic (nonallergic) example of this type of adverse reaction. Histamine, which causes the rash and itching, can be released from the mast cell (or basophil) upon direct contact of the strawberry food allergen.

Some of these nonimmunologically mediated food intolerance reactions are called anaphylactoid reactions, because they look like food anaphylaxis.[17] This type of reaction invariably involves nonimmune release or formation of chemical mediators. One of the more striking adverse reactions of this type is due to histamine poisoning, secondary to the ingestion of scombroid fish (tuna or mackerel) or mahimahi. In this type of fish reaction, contamination with *Proteus morganii* or *Klebsiella pneumoniae* (usually due to inadequate preservation) results in decarboxylation of histidine in the fish tissue to yield large quantities of histamine. These large quantities of histamine cause a clinical reaction.

One of the most common genetically inherited food intolerances worldwide is primary lactose intolerance that results from bowel wall lactase deficiency (a food idiosyncratic reaction). The intestinal enzyme, lactase, is necessary for the metabolism of lactose sugar found in cow's milk. The lack of this enzyme results in fermentation of lactose sugar to lactic acid and an osmotic effect in the bowel, causing symptoms of bloating, cramps, flatulence, and, on occasion, diarrhea. Certain population groups manifest this deficiency in greater frequency. Primary lactose intolerance usually first manifests itself from three to nine years of age. A significant viral or bacterial gastroenteritis, however, may bring on the condition at an earlier age. Secondary lactose intolerance is a temporary condition following any diarrhea in normal infants and is usually not a problem after two weeks.

Proven adverse reactions to food additives are generally considered to be food intolerances. Examples include tartrazine (FD&C yellow #5), which is thought to exacerbate asthma in a few aspirin-sensitive individuals and rarely causes hives or shock. Tartrazine and other colors may also be responsible for a pharmacologic food reaction by exacerbating hyperactivity in a small number of patients with the attention deficit syndrome with hyperkinesis.[17,18] Consumption of monosodium L-glutamate, related to the so-called Chinese restaurant syndrome, may cause headache, facial flush, palpitation, and occasionally chest pain. Sulfites may cause exacerbation of severe asthma and rarely urticaria and shock.

Other reactions suspected of being related to diet that have unclear mechanisms include infant colic, relieved by infant formula change, and migraine headaches, exacerbated by specific foods other than those foods containing vasoactive amines.[19,20] In both of these conditions, there is very little evidence immune reactions to food—food allergy—play a role in etiology. In the infant colic syndrome, many cases improve spontaneously, and parental counseling on how to deal with a crying infant usually helps.[21] In migraine headaches, IgE-mediated food allergy has been shown not to be related in most cases.[20] In a single study, however, a few atopic patients were shown to have migraines triggered by specific foods identified by IgE-mediated skin tests.[22] In another study involving a small number of adults with migraine proven to be related to either egg, corn, or wheat on DBPCFC, the headaches correlated with chemical-mediator release or formation, but not with allergy.[23] It has long been suspected, but not often proven, that the naturally occurring chemical agents in food such as tyramine (cheese and chocolate), histamine (red wine), and caffeine (coffee, tea, or cola) may trigger migraine headaches.[18]

CLINICAL MANIFESTATIONS OF ADVERSE
FOOD REACTIONS

The signs and symptoms of proven adverse reactions to food and food additives are varied. Most commonly the skin (eg, urticaria, eczema), followed by the gastrointestinal tract (eg, diarrhea, vomiting), is affected. Less commonly, the respiratory system is involved. Most immune reactions involve type I (IgE-mediated) allergy, and food-related events appear similar to all other types of allergic reactions. The most classic of this type of reaction is anaphylaxis, which is a multisystem reaction. Anaphylactoid food reactions appear as a "look-alike" to anaphylaxis. The clinical manifestations are the result of chemical-mediator release without IgE antibody involvement.

Anaphylaxis is an acute multisystem allergic reaction to an allergen, such as food, that can develop within minutes to a few hours after exposure to that allergen. This condition is characterized by both mild and more severe (systemic) signs and symptoms. The milder reactions include generalized skin itching and/or erythema, urticaria (hives), and occasionally angioedema (swelling of the face, particularly ears, mouth parts, and around the eyes, as well as the hands or feet or genitalia). More serious systemic reactions include hay fever-like symptoms (sneezing, runny nose, and itching, swelling, redness of the eyes), asthma-like symptoms (wheezing, coughing, respiratory distress), as well as possible vascular shock, gastrointestinal vomiting and diarrhea, uterine cramping, and possibly progressing to cardiovascular collapse and death.

Nasal or other respiratory manifestations of adverse food reactions are uncommon. When the respiratory problems do occur, they are usually found in children (eg, nasal rhinitis or asthma after the ingestion of cow's milk). Another immune reaction example with pulmonary involvement is type III reactions to cow's milk in Heiner's syndrome.

Most proven nonimmune intolerance food reactions such as poisoning or toxicity do not appear or look like true allergies. Some food intolerances, however, may be confused with allergy. These include anaphylactoid reactions (eg, rash to strawberries), exacerbation of asthma by sulfite preservatives (SO_2), and GI bloating or loose stools from lactose sugar fermentation (lactose intolerance).

Many common somatic, behavioral, and neurologic complaints have been attributed to food allergy.[24] These include headaches, muscle aches, fatigue, "tension-fatigue," arthritis or arthralgia, mental lapses, seizures, and bizarre behavior. In the total allergy syndrome, the patient is allegedly incapacitated by adverse reaction not only to food, but water and natural and other chemical pollutants in the air and home and work place.[25,26] Little evidence exists to prove a relationship between a given food and the alleged food exposure and the alleged immune (ie, allergic) reactions in these patients.[26] Psychologic problems are common in this group of patients.[25]

DIAGNOSES, MANAGEMENT, AND PREVENTION OF ADVERSE REACTIONS TO FOOD

The diagnosis of an adverse reaction to food is based on reasonable assumption after taking an adequate history, supportive evidence based on diet manipulation, and possible *in vitro-in vivo* test information.[7] Often patients suspect that food or food additives are the root cause of their complaints when, in fact, there are other explanations for their illnesses. It is up to the physician to determine if there is any reasonable assumption that diet may play a role in illness. When a relationship between a food or food additive and illness is suspected, then supportive information may be sought. In the case of a severe life-threatening reaction (such as systemic anaphylaxis), the potential offending agent may often be clearly identified in the history by the timing of the event. In this situation, the only confirmatory information that may be required is an *in vitro* assay for IgE-specific food antibody so a presumptive diagnosis of food allergy can be made.

In other cases of suspected adverse reaction to food or food additives, dietary elimination followed by food or food additive challenge is commonly done. The gold standard for this type of evaluation is the DBPCFC.[4] Often, however, the clinical problem can be unraveled by the use of single- or multiple-food eliminations, followed by open challenge. It should be noted, however, that these dietary manipulations, even if correlative, do not identify the mechanism of the food reaction.[27]

In the case of food allergy reactions, which are mostly IgE-mediated, *in vivo* epicutaneous skin testing or *in vitro* food IgE-specific antibody testing can be helpful. In a patient population where food allergy reactions are relatively common (eg, children with atopic dermatitis), positive skin test to the most frequently prevalent food allergens may correlate with actual proven sensitivity (DBPCFC results) about 50% of the time.[28] If the skin test is negative to these foods in this population, it usually indicates the patient does not have a food allergy to these allergens. In other patient populations (eg, adults) in whom food allergies are not frequent and especially when the suspected food rarely causes food allergies, the correlation between a positive food skin test reaction and actual proven sensitivity is very low—much less than 50%.[29] In this latter situation, however, a negative food test generally still rules out a specific food allergy.

Under the best circumstances, a positive specific food allergy skin test only puts the physician in the ball park. Only an open or controlled dietary challenge with a specific food can prove the relationship one way or the other. On the other hand, the skin test is an excellent screening test for patients who are suspected of reacting to a food on the basis of an IgE immune reaction.[4] In the case of atopic dermatitis, the IgE skin test (or IgE *in vitro* assay) has been found to be more reliable[28] than the history in screening patients for specific food challenge.

The *in vitro* allergy assay can also be used to test for specific food allergens. This test, however, is not generally as sensitive under the best conditions as the epicutaneous skin test (prick, scratch, puncture).[29] It may be useful, however, in the evaluation of systemic anaphylaxis and local anaphylaxis (the so-called oral allergy or fruit-vegetable allergy syndrome).[29] It should be noted, however, that all *in vitro* allergy assays are not the same—some are valuable only as screening tests.[30]

Most other immune-type tests are not helpful in the evaluation of food reactions. An exception is the cow's milk precipitants test in the rare infants suspected of having Heiner's syndrome.[12] Many other tests of unproven value have been used in the evaluation of the patient allegedly having adverse reactions to food or food additives. These tests have been considered as experimental at best.[31]

Once a specific food has been identified as causing an adverse reaction, it should be avoided, if at all possible. An inadvertent food exposure, especially in the case of a life-threatening event (eg, peanut anaphylaxis), is a problem. In this situation, some protection for the emergency situation is afforded with the patient carrying a preloaded epinephrine self-injector device (ie, EpiPen® or EpiPen Jr.®).[32]

Prophylactic manipulation in the pregnant or nursing mother and/or the potentially allergic infant is difficult.[8] Such programs may reduce food allergy in the infant during the first year of life, but apparently have no effect on the long-term atopic disease.[9]

REFERENCES

1. Anderson JA, Sogn DD. *Adverse Reactions to Foods.* Bethesda, MD: National Institutes of Health; 1984. NIH Publication No. 84-2442, pp 2–3, 58–61, 64–67, 103–121, 175–189.

2. Foucard T. Developmental aspects of food sensitivity in childhood. *Nutr Rev.* 1984; 42:98–104.

3. Bock SA. Prospective appraisal of complaints of adverse reaction to foods in children during the first three years of life. *Pediatrics.* 1987; 79(5):683–688.

4. Bock SA, Sampson HA, Atkins FM, et al. Double-blind placebo-controlled food challenge (DBPCFC) as an office procedure: a manual. *J Allergy Clin Immunol.* 1988; 82(6):986–997.

5. Bock SA. The natural history of adverse reactions to foods. *NE Allergy Proc.* 1986; 7:504–510.

6. Anderson JA. The establishment of common language concerning adverse reactions to foods and food additives. *J Allergy Clin Immunol.* 1986; 78(1):140–144.

7. Bock SA. Evaluation of patients with adverse reactions to foods. In: Bierman CW, Pearlman DS, eds. *Allergic Diseases from Infancy to Adulthood.* 2nd ed. Philadelphia: WB Saunders, 1988: 359–366.

8. Zeiger RS, Heller S, Mellon M, O'Connor R, Hamburger RN. Effectiveness of dietary manipulation in the prevention of food allergy in infants. *J Allergy Clin Immunol.* 1986; 78(2):224–238.

9. Zeiger RS, Heller S, Mellon M, O'Connor R, Hamburger RN, Schultz M. Effect of combined maternal and infant food allergen avoidance or development of atopy. *J Allergy Clin Immunol.* 1989; 83(1):240. Abstract.

10. Coombs RRA, Gell PGH. Classification of allergic reactions responsible for clinical hypersensitivity and disease. In: Coombs RRA, Gell PGH, eds. *Clinical Aspects of Immunology.* Oxford, England: Blackwell Scientific Publication Ltd; 1975:761–781.

11. Parish WE. Detection of reaginic and short-term sensitizing anaphylactic or anaphylactoid antibodies to milk in sera of allergic and normal persons. *Clin Allergy.* 1971; 1:369–380.

12. Heiner DC, Sears JW, Kniker WT. Multiple precipitins to cow's milk in chronic respiratory disease: a syndrome including poor growth, gastrointestinal symptoms, evidence of allergy, iron deficiency anemia, and pulmonary hemosiderosis. *Am J Dis Child.* 1962; 103:634–654.

13. Heiner DC, Wilson JF. Delayed immunologic food reactions. *NER Allergy Proc.* 1986; 7:520–526.

14. Minor JD, Tolber SG, Frick OL. Leukocyte inhibition factor in delayed-onset food allergy. *J Allergy Clin Immunol.* 1980; 66(4):314–321.

15. Broadbent JB, Sampson HA. Food hypersensitivity and atopic dermatitis. *Pediatr Clin North Am.* 1988; 35(5):1115–1130.

16. Sampson HA, Broadbent KR, Bernhisel-Broadbent J. Spontaneous release of histamine from basophils and histamine-releasing factor in patients with atopic dermatitis and food hypersensitivity. *N Engl J Med.* 1989, 321(4):228–232.

17. Anderson JA. Non-immunologically-mediated food sensitivity. *Nutr Rev.* 1984; 42:109–116.

18. Feingold BF. Food additives and child development. *Hosp Pract.* 1973;8(10):11–21. Editorial.

19. Hewson P, Oberklaid F, Menahem S. Infant colic, distress and crying. *Clin Pediatr.* 1987; 26(2):69–76.

Terminology, Physiologic Bases, and Scope of the Problem   13

20. Egger J, Wilson J, Carter CM, et al. Is migraine food allergy?—double-blind controlled trial of oligoantigenic diet treatment. *Lancet.* 1983; 2:865–869.

21. Taubman B. Parental counseling compared with elimination of cow's milk or soy milk protein for the treatment of infant colic syndrome: a randomized trial. *Pediatrics* 1988; 81(6):756–761.

22. Mansfield LE, Vaughan TR, Waller SF, Haverly RW, Ting S. Food allergy and adult migraine: double-blind and mediator conformation of an allergic etiology. *Ann Allergy.* 1985; 55:126–129.

23. Olson G, Vaughan T, Ledoux R, et al. Food induced migraine: search for immunologic mechanisms. *J Allergy Clin Immunol.* 1989; 83(1):238. Abstract.

24. Easton JG, Kaplan MS. Controversial concepts and practices in allergy. In: Bierman CW, Pearlman DS, eds. *Allergic Diseases from Infancy to Adulthood.* 2nd ed. Philadelphia: WB Saunders Co; 1988: 735–747.

25. Brodsky CM. Allergic to everything—A medical subculture. *Psychosomatics* 1983;24:731–742.

26. Terr AI. Environmental illnesses—A clinical review of 50 cases. *Arch Intern Med.* 1986; 146:145–149.

27. Mahan LK, Furukawa CT. General nutritional considerations and diet for adverse food reactions. In: Bierman CW, Pearlman DS, eds. *Allergic Diseases from Infancy to Adulthood.* 2nd ed. Philadelphia: WB Saunders Co; 1988: 367–376.

28. Sampson HA, Albergo R. Comparison of results of skin tests, RAST and double-blind, placebo-controlled food challenges in children with atopic dermatitis. *J Allergy Clin Immunol.* 1984; 74(1):26–33.

29. Ortolani C, Ispano M, Pastorello EA, Ansaloni R, Magri GC. Comparison of results of skin prick tests (with fresh foods and commercial food extracts) and RAST in 100 patients with oral allergy syndrome. *J Allergy Clin Immunol.* 1989; 83(3):683–690.

30. Ownby DR. Allergy testing: In vivo versus in vitro. *Pediatr Clin North Am.* 1988; 35(5):995–1009.

31. Shapiro GG, Anderson J. Commentary: controversial techniques in allergy. *Pediatrics.* 1988; 82(6):935–937.

32. Yunginger J, Squillace D, Jones R, Helm R. Fatal anaphylactic reactions induced by peanuts. *Allergy Proc.* 1989; 10:249–253.

Chapter 2

Diagnosis of Food Allergy

Part I: The Physician's Perspective

John A. Anderson

INTRODUCTION

When a diagnosis of food allergy is being considered, it is well to remember less than 20% of all adverse reactions to food are immunologic in nature (food allergy) and only one-half to one-third of all those adverse reactions thought to be allergic in nature can be proven by double-blind placebo-controlled food challenge (DBPCFC).[1,2] True food allergy is more of a problem when dealing with infants and children.[3] Food allergy as a cause of a set of signs and symptoms in adults should be less of a consideration. An exception would be in cases of food anaphylaxis (including acute urticaria), where the signs and symptoms in adults are usually clearly temporally related (within minutes to hours) to the ingestion of specific foods—especially those foods known to be likely causes of food anaphylaxis. Most immunologic tests have limited value in the diagnosis of adverse reactions to food. In proven allergies to foods, however, where IgE reactions are most common, the classic epicutaneous skin test (prick, scratch, or puncture) is a useful screening tool.[2] A positive skin test puts the physician investigating the problem in the ball park, whereas a negative reaction to this type of skin testing correlates almost 100% with the probability that a patient would not react in a properly controlled DBPCFC.[4] *In vitro* IgE food antibody assays are also helpful, like the epicutaneous skin tests, but are generally less sensitive.

Patients can be put on specialized diets that are generally free of those foods to which most people are felt to be allergic and then, at a later date, can be challenged with specific foods to prove (or disprove) the suspected relationship between a set of signs and symptoms and the ingestion of that food.[5] In the case of a patient suspected of having food anaphylaxis, however—especially when systemic symptoms have occurred that may be life-threatening in nature—food challenges are usually not advisable. Challenging a patient under these conditions might be dangerous, with the likelihood of precipitating another, perhaps more serious, episode of life-threatening systemic anaphylaxis. In this situation, IgE food antibodies are usually quite elevated in the bloodstream, especially within two weeks to six months of the episode. Thus, in this situation, an *in vitro* IgE food assay (though usually not as sensitive as the IgE epicutaneous skin test) should be positive, providing of course the case involved is true food anaphylaxis. Because this *in vitro* test is safer than the skin test, it is the method of choice for investigating patients with this condition. If the IgE *in vitro* food assay is positive, then a presumptive diagnosis of food allergy can be made and a recommendation can be made to avoid the food.

It is not unusual for patients, or the parents of patients, to suspect common medical complaints may be related to diet.[6] Such complaints may include maladies that are not usually associated with allergies such as headache, arthritis, generalized fatigue, behavioral problems, mental fuzziness, learning disorders, and, in the child, colic, recurrent abdominal pain, enuresis, and hyperactivity. Although there is usually little proof diet has anything to do with these medical maladies and almost no proof food allergy may be involved, some physicians claim there are relationships between diet and/or food allergy with these conditions.[7] In order to attempt to prove a relationship between a patient's diet and a food allergy, valid immunologic tests are misused or tests of unproven validity are tried.[6,7]

PRESENTING HISTORY OF FOOD REACTIONS

The four important aspects of taking a history from a patient presenting with complaints suspected of being caused by an adverse reaction to food include (1) a description of the symptoms, (2) the timing of the onset and the duration of those symptoms, (3) the frequency of the occurrence of those symptoms, and (4) the circumstances under which the food exposure occurred (including the quantity of food involved and other foods that might be involved) (see Table 2-1).[8]

Description of the Food Reaction

Most allergic food reactions occur in individuals who are generally allergic (eg, have atopic dermatitis, hay fever, or asthma) or who have allergic

Table 2-1 Diagnosis of the Patient Suspected of Having Food Allergy

I. Presenting History of Food Reaction
   A. Description
   B. Timing
   C. Frequency of Occurrence
   D. Circumstances under Which the Reaction Occurred
II. Differential Diagnosis of Food Allergy
III. Immunologic Tests
   A. Allergy Screening Test
   B. Allergy (IgE) Food Skin Tests
   C. IgE Food Allergen-Specific *In Vitro* Test
   D. Other Immunologic Tests
IV. Unproven and Unapproved Allergy Tests
V. Diet Elimination and Food Challenges

---

families. An exception may be adults who have systemic anaphylaxis to single foods. Although not proven, it may be analogous to patients anaphylactically sensitive to other single allergens such as penicillin.[9] In the case of penicillin, hypersensitivity allergy is as common in the nonatopic (nonallergic) population as in the atopic population.

Most true allergic food reactions are IgE-mediated and look like allergic reactions to other allergens. In studies of infants with proven food allergies, most symptoms involve either the skin (eg, urticaria or atopic dermatitis) or gastrointestinal tract (eg, diarrhea).[10,11] Respiratory symptoms, except as a component of anaphylaxis, are relatively uncommon, but remain a possible consideration in early childhood.[4,11]

Some food intolerance reactions may be confused with allergies. Examples include gas, bloating, and loose stools after cow's milk ingestion, which might be due to lactose intolerance. Other examples are anaphylactoid reactions (eg, rash to strawberries or components of wine) due to direct chemical-mediator release[3] (see Chapter 1 text, Table 1-1, and Fig. 1-1).

Timing of the Food Reaction

Adverse reactions to food can generally be divided into reactions that occur within minutes to one hour after eating (or food exposure)—immediate food reactions, and reactions that occur hours to days later—delayed food reactions.[12] In the case of immediate food reactions (eg, urticaria occurring within one hour after eating shrimp in a restaurant), IgE pathogenesis is usually involved in a temporal relationship with eating a food. This close temporal relationship helps pin down the diagnosis.

IgE may be involved in delayed food reactions also. An example is the so-called IgE late-phase reaction, resulting in an atopic dermatitis flare-up due to specific food sensitivity (see Fig. 1-1).

An example of another delayed food reaction due to an immune pathogenesis (but not IgE) is that of IgE milk antibody and milk complex reactions in Heiner's syndrome. Cell-mediated immune reactions are typically delayed in timing. Although there is some evidence that points to the existence of cell-mediated immune reactions, this evidence is spotty[13] (see text in Chapter 1, Table 1-3). Gastrointestinal digestion of food and the possible subsequent formation of new food allergens could delay the clinical manifestation of such reactions. Studies, however, have shown that patients allergic to an experimental protein digest of food were also allergic to the whole food (eg, milk, proteins).[3]

Frequency of Occurrence of Food Reactions

The more frequently the suspected set of symptoms occurs in relationship to the ingestion or exposure to a specific food, the more likely the association, especially if it occurs three times.[8] In the case of intermittent acute urticaria (with complete recovery in between times), often a diary is the only way to narrow the field of possible food-symptom associations. In some proven food-induced allergic reactions, however, the perceived history of specific food-induced reactivity is poorly correlated with the actual food reaction. An example of this situation is food-induced flares in atopic dermatitis.[4] In this situation, the results of food allergy skin testing or *in vitro* assays are more valuable because they are more reliable than the history.

Circumstances under Which the Food Exposure Occurred

Some food reactions occur upon direct exposure to the raw food. Examples include rash on the face after exposure to tomatoes and oranges in infants (probably due to the organic acid). Another example is pruritus or swelling of the mouth parts after exposure to melons or bananas (USA), apples, potatoes, or hazel nuts (Scandinavia), or apples, pears, cherries, or other fruits and vegetables (Italy). These reactions occur in patients highly allergic to ragweed, tree, and tree-grass pollen, respectively.[14,15]

Some reactions to food occur only after a large quantity of food has been ingested. These reactions, if proven to be related to diet, are typically delayed in onset. Some food reactions occur only when eaten in association with other foodstuff such as the ingestion of alcohol. (Alcohol is known to increase absorption of foods across mucosal membranes.) Acute urticaria occurs more frequently when the patient has an inflamed bowel such as the child with acute viral gastroenteritis. Reactions to rapidly absorbed abnormal macroparticles of food could be responsible.[3] Urticaria and shock have been associated with the ingestion of specific foods (eg, celery or shrimp) followed by running: the so-called exercise-induced anaphylaxis syndrome.[16]

The grouping of foods into biologic relationships has been cited as important when considering the possibility of a reaction to one food after the ingestion of another.[3] The clinical importance of such relationships within food families, however, may not be as important as previously believed. In the pea (legume) family, for instance, the peanut is recognized as a very important allergen that can be associated with severe systemic symptoms and anaphylaxis and even death.[17] In a series of patients with immunologic evidence of allergy to one or more legumes, there was no more risk of clinical allergy on DBPCFC if the patient was IgE skin-test positive to two or more legumes than to one legume.[18] In fact, only 2 of 69 patients (3%) reacted to another legume on challenge. Reactivity (both by skin test and clinical challenge) to peanuts far exceeded reactivity to other legumes. As allergy is investigated in regard to other food groups, the risk of clinical reactivity may differ significantly from the immunologic sensitivity, despite the documented presence of major cross-reacting allergens within different food types of the same biologic family.[3]

Differential Diagnosis of Food Allergy

Patients or parents of patients may suspect that a set of symptoms is related to food. When physicians are considering the presenting history from a patient or a report of patient symptoms from the parent of a patient, they must consider (1) food intolerances, (2) factors that may be related to the process of eating but unrelated to specific food, and (3) problems that are only assumed to be related to food, general diet, or the process of eating. With these ideas in mind, a differential diagnosis of other medical problems can be constructed for consideration (see Table 2-2).[2,3,12]

IMMUNOLOGIC TESTS USED IN THE DIAGNOSIS OF FOOD ALLERGY

Most of the standard immunologic tests are either of no value or have limited value when diagnosing food allergy. There is no one immunologic test that confirms the existence of clinical reactivity to a specific food—only direct

Table 2-2   Differential Diagnosis of Food Allergy

I. Food Intolerances
   (Nonimmunologically Mediated Adverse Food Reactions)
   A. Food Additive Reactions
      1. Colors (dyes), eg, yellow #5 or tartrazine
      2. Flavor enhancers, eg, monosodium glutamate
      3. Preservatives
         a) Butylated hydroxyanisole (BHA) and butylated hydroxytoluene (BHT)
         b) Nitrites and nitrates
         c) Sodium benzoate
         d) Sulfiting agents
   B. Anaphylactoid Reactions (Mediators—Release Anaphylaxis-Like)
      1. Histamine-releasing foods (eg, strawberries, wine)
      2. Histamine poisoning (eg, tuna and mackerel fish)
   C. Chemical Contamination of Foods
      1. Antibiotic
      2. Heavy metals
      3. Pesticides
   D. Enzyme Deficiencies (Inherited and Acquired)
      1. Galactosemia
      2. Glucose-6-Phosphate dehydrogenase deficiency
      3. Lactase deficiency (primary and secondary)
   E. Infectious Agents
      1. Bacterial (eg, *E. coli, Salmonella, Shigella*)
      2. Parasites (i.e., *Amoeba, Giardia,* trichinosis)
      3. Viruses (eg, enterovirus, hepatitis)
   F. Insect Parts
   G. Molds
   H. Pharmacologic Agents (Endogenous or Exogenous)
      1. Alcohol
      2. Caffeine and theobromine
      3. Dopamine and norepinephrine
      4. Hallucinogenic alkaloids
      5. Histamine
      6. Phenylethylamine
      7. Serotonin
      8. Tryptamine and tyramine
   I. Toxins
      1. Bacterial (eg, botulism, staphylococcal)
      2. Mushroom toxins
      3. Mycotoxins (aflatoxins)
      4. Seafoods and fish
         a) histamine poisoning (scombroid fish: tuna, mackerel)
         b) Saxitoxin (shellfish)
         c) Ciguatera poisoning (grouper, snapper fish)

continues

Table 2-2 continued

II. **Factors That May Be Related to Eating but Unrelated to Foods**
   A. AIDS and Other Immunodeficiencies
   B. Collagen Vascular Diseases
   C. Endocrine Disorders
   D. Gastrointestinal Diseases
      1. Infantile colic
      2. Cystic fibrosis
      3. Gall bladder disease
      4. Peptic ulcer
      5. Hiatal hernia
      6. Intestinal obstruction
   E. Malignancy
III. **Problems Assumed but Unproven To Be Related to Foods, Diet, or the Process of Eating**
   A. Arthritis
   B. Behavioral Abnormalities
   C. Enuresis
   D. Fatigue
   E. Hyperactivity
   F. Learning Disabilities
   G. Headache
   H. Mental Haziness
   I. Other Psychological Reactions

---

challenge under controlled conditions can confirm clinical reactivity (regardless of the cause, immunologic or nonimmunologic in nature).[19] The immunologic tests that are of some value include (1) screening tests for general atopy (allergic tendency), (2) allergy (IgE) immediate-reacting epicutaneous skin test (prick, scratch, or puncture), (3) IgE food-allergen specific *in vitro* assays, and (4) other specific immunologic tests (such as cow's milk precipitants used to diagnose Heiner's syndrome or possible food-specific cell-mediated assays used to assess delayed food reactions).

SCREENING *IN VITRO* ALLERGY ASSAYS

Because most patients who have true allergies to food are generally allergic or have allergic family members, screening tests for atopy (allergic tendency) have some value. The results of a good allergy history and specific allergy skin testing or *in vitro* tests are very helpful in making this determination.

However, short of this complete allergy workup, the existence of screening tests may be valuable. Two tests are often used for this purpose: (1) total serum IgE levels (total IgE) compared to normal levels for age and (2) the examination of the nasal secretion for eosinophils (nasal Eos).[20] Another *in vitro* screening test is the multiantigen (triple) radioallergosorbent (RAST) test (multi-RAST).

The predictive values of positive tests for total IgE (greater than two standard deviations for age in matched normals), nasal Eos (greater than 5%), and multi-RAST (ragweed-grass-mite) are 86%, 91%, and 98%, respectively. However, the predictive values of negative tests for total IgE, nasal Eos, or multi-RAST are only 33%, 60%, and 46%, respectively.[20] Thus, these tests are helpful in the diagnosis of general allergy (atopy) only if they are positive. If they are negative, there is still a reasonable chance that the patient may be generally allergic.

IMMEDIATE-REACTING IgE SKIN TEST

Food allergen-specific skin testing can be done by two methods: (1) the epicutaneous skin test (prick, scratch, or puncture) and (2) the interdermal skin test.[21] In the epicutaneous skin test, a drop of food extract (usually 1:10 or 1:20 weight by volume) in glycerol is placed on the skin surface, followed by pricking, scratching, or puncturing through the drop (and the skin) with a needle or scarifier. This test is read at 20 minutes. The wheal and flare reaction is compared to a histamine control on a 0-4+ scale. This epicutaneous skin test, in the evaluation of food allergy, is the *in vivo* test of choice.[4,8,12]

The intradermal skin test, which is done by injecting a small amount of 1:1000 weight by volume food allergen intradermally (0.02 cc) and then reading the wheal and flare reactions at 20 minutes, is too sensitive. Positive reactions using this latter method are too often associated with nonspecific reactions (false positives) and do not correlate with clinical food allergy reactivity.[21] The value of the epicutaneous food skin test has been evaluated as a predictor of clinical specific food sensitivity in a group of atopic dermatitis children using the DBPCFC technique (see Table 2-3).[4] If the combined results of skin tests in DBPCFC reactions to the six most common foods these children are sensitive to (egg, peanut, cow's milk, wheat, soy, and fish) are taken under consideration, it can be seen that the epicutaneous skin test is a valuable screening tool for the patient suspected of having IgE-mediated food allergy. The epicutaneous food skin test, under these conditions, is of special value if it is negative because close to 100% of the time it correlates with the probability of a negative food challenge to that food.[19]

Table 2-3 Value of Allergy (IgE) Skin Test or *In Vitro* Assay in the Diagnosis of Food Allergy

Situation	Results of Tests	Prevalence of Specific Food Sensitivity and Population*	Likelihood of DBPCFC Results (Clinical Sensitivity)
1	Negative Skin Test or Negative *In Vitro* Test	High or Low	82–100% Negative
2	Positive Skin Test	High	Up to 48% Positive
3	Positive *In Vitro* Test	High	Up to 33% Positive
4	Positive Skin Test or *In Vitro* Test	Low	3% or Less Positive

*Prevalence of Specific Food Sensitivity: High 37.5%; Low 1%. Based on data in Sampson and Albergo, *J Allergy Clin Immunol.* 1984; 74:26–33.

On the other hand, the presence of a positive epicutaneous food skin test is not diagnostic of clinical food allergy. When the prevalence of this specific food sensitivity is high (such as in the case of egg allergy in atopic dermatitis patients at 37.5% reactivity), then the presence of a positive skin test at least places the physician in the ball park.[4] History alone is a poor predictor of specific food sensitivity in these patients.[22] Specific food challenge can be used to confirm clinical sensitivity. (It would be expected that about 50% of the time, a patient with a positive skin test would also be positive as determined by DBPCFC.)

It is indicated in Table 2-3, however, if the prevalence of a specific food sensitivity in the general population is low (eg, an adult, especially one who was generally not allergic), then the likelihood of a positive epicutaneous food skin test being clinically significant is very low, i.e. less than 3% (if the patient has undergone DBPCFC to that food). The allergy IgE-mediated skin test is only as reliable as the allergens used. Comparative studies of commercially available food allergens in the United States have shown a considerable variation between the different food allergens and allergen lots of the same food allergen from three different commercial sources.[23] In the case of patients who react to fruits and vegetables with pruritus and swelling of the mouth parts upon eating, the use of freshly prepared fruit or vegetable juices in the skin test may be superior to the use of commercial food allergens.[24] In some cases, food allergen-specific IgE *in vitro* assays were found to be better than skin testing using commercial food allergens.

IN VITRO IgE FOOD ALLERGEN-SPECIFIC ASSAYS

In vitro IgE allergen-specific assays were developed in the late 1960s by Wide, Bennich, and Johansson, following the discovery of human IgE—the so-called allergic antibody class. With the availability of large quantities of purified IgE, antibodies (antihuman IgE) could be produced in another species (eg, rabbits). The first test using this new technology was the radioallergosorbent test (RAST) (see Fig. 2-1).[25] The first step requires coupling the allergen (eg, cow's milk protein) to a solid support (eg, a paper disk).[26] When this disk is placed in a test tube with patient serum, the coupling of antibodies directed against milk or that were anti-cow's milk in nature (this includes IgE, M, A, or E class) occurs. After washing, the third step is the addition of radio-labeled ($_{125}$I) rabbit antihuman IgE antibodies. These antibodies will attach themselves only to the IgE antimilk antibodies (which in turn are coupled to the cow's milk protein on the paper disk). Then the amount of radioactivity can be measured, and thus the amount of cow's milk–allergen–anti-IgE cow's milk antibody can be quantitated.

As shown in Fig. 2-2, the second type of IgE *in vitro* assay is called the enzyme-linked immunosorbent assay (ELISA).[26] This is a more recent type of test, but is just like the RAST test except for two factors. First, allergen is usually coupled to the inner surface of small plastic wells (into which the patient's serum and other ingredients of the test are placed). The second, and more important, difference is the final quantitative factor. In the RAST system, the amount of radioactivity from $_{125}$I-labeled antihuman IgE is measured. In the ELISA system, an enzyme coupled to the antihuman IgE denatures a substrate, which either changes color or becomes fluorescent. Then the amount of color or fluorescence can be measured.

This new system is becoming increasingly popular, because radio labeling is no longer necessary (which is expensive) and gamma counters are not required (which are slow and expensive).[26] This new type of allergen-specific IgE assay is as sensitive as the RAST and has been adaptive to a variety of screening allergy assays.

The *in vitro* IgE food allergen-specific assays can be used in the same way as the IgE food allergen-specific immediate-reacting epicutaneous skin test (see Table 2-3). The *in vitro* IgE assay is less sensitive, however, than the epicutaneous skin test.[21,23,26] The *in vitro* assay uses the same commercial food extracts.[23] The *in vitro* tests may not be standardized, and there can be a great

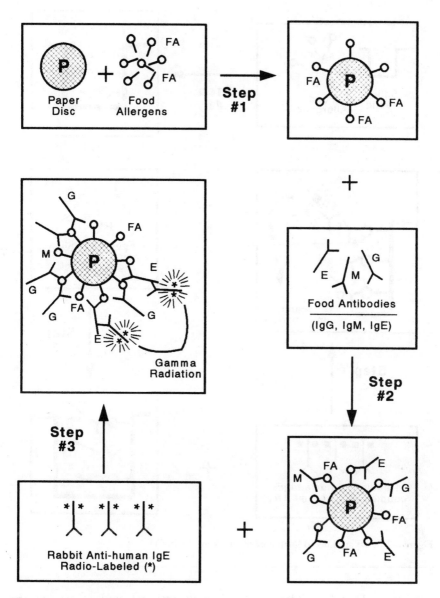

Figure 2-1 Radioallergosorbent Test (RAST)

deal of commercial laboratory variability.[26] On an individual food test basis, the *in vitro* tests are often more expensive.[26]

If the epicutaneous skin test is negative, the *in vitro* assay can be expected to be negative as long as the skin test is done under properly controlled

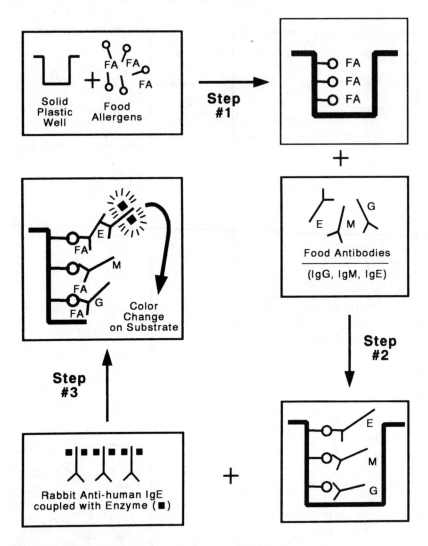

Figure 2-2   Enzyme-Linked Immunosorbent Assay (ELISA)

conditions. Therefore, it is not valuable to do both tests under these circumstances. The reverse, however, is not true. If the *in vitro* test is negative, the epicutaneous skin test may be positive. The *in vitro* test system is preferred in the following situations: (1) systemic anaphylaxis, (2) extensive dermatitis on the patient, (3) dermographism in the patient, and (4) antihistamine use by the patient which can block the skin test reaction.

OTHER IMMUNOLOGIC TESTS OF VALUE IN THE DIAGNOSIS OF FOOD ALLERGY

Most of the conditions in which non-IgE food-related immune reactions have been considered seem to fall into the general category of delayed (in timing) reactions.[12,13] If immune mechanisms are involved, they are usually classified as Gell and Coombs type III—immune complex reactions—or type IV cell-mediated reactions (see Chapter 1, Table 1-3 and text). The only recognized proven IgE type III immune food reaction is cow's milk-induced syndrome with pulmonary disease (Heiner's syndrome). In this condition, serum cow's milk precipitants are associated with the signs and symptoms of the disease. The milk-precipitant test, which measures high levels of IgG-milk antibody, is performed by a gel diffusion technique in which the cow's milk antigen allergens are placed in one well of Ochterlony agar gel plate and the patient's serum in another well. After an overnight incubation at room temperature, precipitant bands are seen in the gel between the wells as the milk allergen and milk antibody diffuse from each of the plate wells.

Tests of cell-mediated immunity (Gell and Coombs type IV) reactions have been used in an attempt to identify an immune reaction in patients with late-onset reactions due to food (delayed clinical reactions).[27] These tests, which include lymphocyte transformation and the measurement of lymphokines, are usually research tools.[13]

UNPROVEN AND UNAPPROVED "ALLERGY" TESTS USED IN THE DIAGNOSIS OF SUSPECTED FOOD ALLERGY

Historically, the term "allergy" refers to an altered response. In this sense then almost any reaction might be identified as an allergy, even if those reactions bear little or no resemblance to an immune response or a type I IgE-mediated allergic reaction[1,6] (see Chapter 1, Table 1-1 and text). Because eating foods is a daily event, it should not seem unusual that common medical complaints patients might have could be attributed to food and diet, not just those complaints having a recognized etiology. Some of these complaints share common characteristics.

1. They involve a large portion of the population.
2. They are symptoms, not diseases.
3. They have many trigger factors.
4. They have no one proven pathogenesis.
5. Rarely is there one single standardized test to objectively and conveniently prove (or disprove) the existence of the condition.

Symptoms or conditions such as headache, myalgia, hyperactivity, fatigue, behavioral abnormalities, learning disorders, mental fuzziness, depression, restlessness, confusion, colic, and enuresis fall into this category.

Occasionally, these complaints are attributed to food allergy in its broadest historical sense, an altered response. In an attempt to prove an altered response or allergy to either a diet or specific food, several tests have evolved through the years and have been promoted as valuable by a few physicians who believe food and diet can cause these conditions or complaints, many times through a dysfunction of the immune system.[6,8,28] Unfortunately, the tests are called allergy tests but fortunately no immune abnormality is likely to be proven by these tests.

All of these so-called allergy tests can be classified as unproven and unapproved.[29] None of them has satisfied a proper evaluation trial to be acceptable as safe and efficacious. The tests that have been falsely promoted as helpful in the diagnosis of food allergy include the following:

1. *The Leukocytoxic Food Test:* The leukopenic index was introduced in 1934. In this clinical test, the total white cell count (WBC) was believed to fall following oral challenge with a specific food in the patient. Black introduced the leukocytoxic *in vitro* test in 1956, and it was refined by Bryan and Bryan in 1960 (and now frequently bears their names). The technique is based on the theory that the addition of a specific food allergen to a microscopic slide on which there is a drop of fresh WBC and fresh plasma from the patient will result in the alteration or destruction of the WBCs. Results of many controlled studies have failed to show that this type of testing is efficacious.[6,7,28,29] In 1985, the US Food and Drug Administration (FDA) ruled this test as unproven and further ruled against marketing cytoxic testing kits.[30]

2. *Intracutaneous and Subcutaneous Food Provocation and Neutralization Testing:* This type of clinical testing was first introduced by Lee in 1961 and refined by Rinkel in 1964. In one variety of the technique, successive five-fold dilutions of food extract are injected intradermally in minute doses (usually 0.01 cc) to an endpoint (the dose which produces a wheal 2 mm in diameter or produces subjective symptoms). When using the subcutaneous technique, serial doses of 0.05 cc are injected subcutaneously. In the case of both techniques, attempts are made first to neutralize the provoked subjective symptom by further injections (intracutaneously or subcutaneously) of weaker dilutions of the same food allergen. If this is unsuccessful, then stronger dilutions are injected in order to attempt to neutralize the reaction. If the neutralizing weaker dose worsens the symptoms, still weaker doses are used.[28,29]

   Currently there is no immunologic rationale for this procedure. Most controlled trials (all involving food allergens) have failed to show any correlation between clinical symptoms and allergen injections.[7] In spite of these facts, this type of testing is still practiced today.

3. *Sublingual Provocation and Neutralization:* In 1941 Hansel described a method for coseasonal treatment of hay fever, involving drops of ragweed extract under the tongue. In 1964, Dickey and Pfeiffer expanded on this concept to the diagnosis and treatment of food allergy. According to the technique usually used, diluted food extracts are administered by dropper (eg, three drops of 1:10 weight by volume) sublingually. If the symptoms appear within 20 minutes, a diagnosis of food allergy is established. Once this has occurred, a more dilute solution of food extract is applied under the tongue in order to neutralize these subjective symptoms. If this is successful, this latter dose can be used routinely by the patients who cannot (or do not wish to) avoid the offensive food. The proponents of the use of this test theorized that the sublingual administration of the allergen allows for unaltered and direct absorption. Supposedly, this type of absorption leads to a desensitization process for that specific food allergen.

In spite of these theories, the immunologic basis for this technique has never been proven. No studies involving food allergen have proven its efficacy in controlled trials.[31] One study, however, involving allergic rhinitis patients, has shown that house dust mite extracts administered sublingually at the neutralizing dose over a 2-week period relieved nasal symptoms.[32] At this stage, this diagnostic (and treatment) technique should be considered experimental and not be routinely administered as a clinical test (or treatment).

4. *Food-Specific IgG Antibodies and Immune Complex In Vitro Assays:* In an effort to explain immune changes in patients with apparent delayed (in timing) onset food reactions, investigators have turned to assays involving the measurement of IgG antibodies and IgG-immune complexes to specific foods.[28] These tests have become more popular in recent years, as support for the leukocytoxic food test has waned. In spite of this popularity, there is little or no justification for the use of such tests in the diagnosis of suspected food allergy.[33] IgG antibodies to food (eg, bovine gammaglobulin) can be detected in 70% of normal individuals. IgG-immune complexes can be routinely found in normal individuals, and many studies have shown no differences in the type or amount of food-immune complexes generated between healthy and sick patients, even with delayed clinical reactions.[28]

5. *Tests of Immune Functions To Support a Clinical Ecology Diagnosis:* In 1950, Randolph and Rollins first reported on patients allergic to foods (beet sugar—sucrose) and food chemical additives (monosodium glutamate of beet origin) that resulted in multiple symptoms, atypical of the

usual allergic reaction.[34] Later Randolph developed a new concept: clinical ecology, in which patients who suffered from multiple typical complaints reacted to things in their environment such as foods, food chemical additives, and chemicals in the atmosphere.[35] The claims of factors in the environment that can affect the patients adversely has recently been extended to a common fungus (*Candida albicans*) hypersensitivity by Crook, as popularized in his book "The Yeast Connection."[36] Some of these patients have become psychologically incapacitated because of the belief they were allergic to everything—the so-called 20th century syndrome.[37] One of the major explanations for this reaction is that patients with this condition develop an abnormal immune response, so-called immune dysfunction.

Practitioners who believe in clinical ecology theories routinely use the unapproved and unproven diagnostic test techniques such as the leukocytoxic testing, provocation and neutralization procedures, and IgG-immune complex assays. They also use a number of routine immune function tests, such as lymphocyte counts, assays of T and B cells, measures of T suppressor cells, immunoglobulin determination, and autoimmune tests.

An extensive analysis of 50 consecutive patients with a clinical ecology diagnosis supposedly caused by environmental chemicals and/or foods, who had been worked up by practitioners of the clinical ecology beliefs, demonstrated that no evidence of abnormal immune response could be found in any of the patients. All immune tests fell within the range of normal patients.[35] The clinical ecology concepts, advanced first by Randolph in the 1950s and 1960s, are still promoted by some physicians 30 and 40 years later, in spite of the fact that the theories have never been adequately validated.[7,28,31,35]

Part II: The Dietitian's Perspective
Victoria Olejer

INTRODUCTION

Due to the enormity of the task, little is known of the overall incidence of adverse food reactions in the general population. Food intolerance is believed to far outnumber true allergic reactions, but the affirmation of this belief awaits confirmation. Instead, attention has focused on the prevalence of food allergy in the general pediatric population with particular emphasis placed on the incidence of cow's milk allergy (CMA). Based on studies in the

United States, Canada, Great Britain, and the Scandinavian countries, estimates of CMA vary but are thought to fall in the range of 0.3-7.5%, with the incidence decreasing with increasing age.[38-44] Not surprisingly, the incidence for CMA is much higher in allergic children, approaching, for example, 30-59% in children with atopic dermatitis referred to tertiary health care centers.[45-47] Allergy to hen's eggs is estimated to occur in approximately 0.5% of the general pediatric population, increasing to approximately 5% in atopic children.[48]

In an impressive effort to examine the incidence of adverse food reactions in a normal pediatric population, 480 previously unselected, consecutively born infants were followed prospectively from birth to 3 years of age.[49] Of the 133/480 (28%) children suspected by either parents or physicians of experiencing adverse food reactions, only 8% could be confirmed by elimination and oral provocative food challenge, pointing to the relatively high frequency with which foods are thought to result in symptoms in this age group. More conservative estimates place the incidence of adverse food reactions between 4-6% in infants and between 1-2% in children.[50]

While experts disagree concerning the exact incidence of food allergy, few contest the difficulty involved in diagnosing and managing this malady. Until accurate laboratory tests possessing reliable clinical correlations are developed, clinicians must continue to rely on repeated trials of elimination and challenge, with the obvious exception of systemic anaphylaxis, to substantiate the removal of individual foods from the diet.

Despite the lack of standardization of commercially available food extracts, skin testing remains the most accessible diagnostic tool for evaluating the presence of food-specific IgE. The popularity and utility behind the use of skin testing as an aid in identifying potentially sensitizing foods rest largely in the strength of its negative predictive indices.[4,23,51] Nonetheless, negative skin test results do not rule out the presence of an IgE-mediated food response.[52] Likewise, positive skin test results do not confirm the presence of a clinically relevant allergic response to the food in question,[52] but provide a basis for additional investigation. Intradermal skin testing, as compared to prick-puncture skin testing, does not improve on the sensitivity of the test procedure, results in a higher frequency of false-positives, and risks the occurrence of systemic anaphylaxis in exquisitely sensitive individuals.[51] Radioallergosorbent tests (RAST) using a patient's serum also do not add to the predictive accuracy of the test, contribute substantially to the cost, and are best reserved for the occasional patient with pronounced dermatographism, extensive eczematous or urticarial skin lesions, or a history of suspected or confirmed anaphylaxis to foods.[50]

The diagnostic process in food allergy, regardless of the age of the patient, always begins with a careful medical history and physical examination aimed first at removing from consideration serious medical considerations or disease processes that may mimic a food allergy and, secondly, at distinguishing immunologically mediated reactions (eg, food allergy or hypersensitivity) from nonimmunologically mediated reactions (eg, food intolerance). When possible, detailed information should be obtained from the primary caregiver(s), which in some cases may include grandparents, aunts, older siblings, etc., regarding a description of symptoms, including the time of onset following ingestion and the duration; quantity of food required to elicit symptoms; form of the food or method of preparation most often associated with symptoms; number of times the reaction has been observed to occur, including the date of the most recent reaction; complexity of the diet with respect to the introduction of solid foods; and attempted remedies. Despite the critical nature of this information in designing both the elimination and challenge schemes, the reader is cautioned regarding the notoriously poor predictive capacity of the clinical history in diagnosing food allergy. Reports of even relatively recent and convincing adverse reactions following the consumption of specific foods are confirmed in less than half of the cases.[4,22,53-54]

Additionally, the physical examination should be directed toward identifying objective signs supporting the description of symptoms, particularly as they apply to the gastrointestinal, cutaneous, and respiratory systems. Any history of rapidly worsening serial reactions or life-threatening reactions to foods involving angioedema, laryngeal edema, wheezing, or hypotension should be duly noted in the medical record. These families should be instructed in the proper procedures to be taken in an emergency. Two frequently used emergency devices, available by prescription only, include the EpiPen® Jr. Autoinjector (Center Laboratories, Port Washington, NY 11050) and the Ana-Kit® Insect Sting Treatment Kit (Hollister-Stier Laboratories, Spokane, WA 99207). When used as directed, these devices may provide valuable time to transport the child experiencing a severe reaction where appropriate emergency care may be given.

Elimination Diets and Diet-Symptom Diaries

As a convenient starting place, elimination diets have traditionally eliminated foods or families of foods that have repeatedly been observed to produce adverse reactions in sensitized individuals. In infants, cow's milk, soy, and wheat immediately come to mind due to their high level of allergenicity and frequent presence in infant's diets in the form of proprietary formulas and teething aids. Potato, tomato, peas, beans, sweet potato, apple, banana, peach, beef, pork, chicken, and the remaining cereals (rice, barley, oat, rye) are less frequently implicated in this age group, but can also be troublesome due to the frequency with which they appear in infant diets. Sensitivities to such potent food allergens as egg, peanut, the true nuts (almond, pecan, walnut, cashew, etc.), citrus fruits (lemon, lime, orange, grapefruit, etc.), cocoa, crustaceans (crab, crayfish, lobster, prawn, shrimp), and the bony fish are seldom encountered in the first year of life due to their relative absence from the diet, but represent particularly potent allergens for the older child. Indeed, milk, egg, peanut, and soy account for approximately 80-90% of the food allergic reactions diagnosed in the first few years of life.[46,49,51,55] There is no universally safe food.

The prospect for widespread cross-reactivity occurring among individual members of the many taxonomic food families represented by foods[56] appears to be less of a reality than originally suspected,[47,57-59] making generalizations regarding their utility in the diagnosis and management of food allergy somewhat questionable. *In vitro* studies identifying common allergenic determinants among members of individual food families, in particular, legumes, the true nuts, bony fish, crustaceans, and mollusks, should not automatically be interpreted as reflecting an *in vivo* sensitivity.[59] Food allergic reactions appear to be highly specific, even among members of the same species (as demonstrated by allergens that are species specific for shrimp).[60] This is despite the fairly common occurrence of *in vitro* cross-reactivity among foods with a shared taxonomic relationship. While these findings are most encouraging, a continued cautious approach with respect to the potential for cross-reactivity, albeit rare, appears prudent and is best assessed on a case-by-case basis, employing appropriately administered food challenges to once again substantiate the removal of a food from the diet.

Very helpful in the initial workup of the young child with suspected food allergies is the completion of a 1 to 2 week baseline diet and symptom diaries (see Fig. 2-3). In these diaries, caregivers are instructed to record the times of all feedings, meals, or snacks; amount of formula and actual foods consumed; dosage and types of medications taken, including vitamin and mineral supplements; and a description of symptoms, noting time of occurrence, duration, and severity. Due to their lack of maturity and poor communication skills, very young children present a more challenging assessment picture than older children and adults who are better able to localize and communicate pain and discomfort. Clinicians must instead rely on the very visual symptoms of rhinorrhea, nasal congestion, wheeze, cough, chest congestion, vomiting, diarrhea, constipation, eczema, xerosis, erythema, and scratching as an indicator of pruritus. Subjective complaints such as irritability and sleeplessness often occur with the former symptoms, but are more difficult to grade objectively.

By indicating the amounts of formula and/or foods consumed, the diet may be assessed for nutritional adequacy. Many of the signs and symptoms of

Patient's name: _____   Baseline/elimination/reintroduction

DIET DIARY: Record the times of your meals/snacks/beverages and exactly what you ate. Be specific.
Include brand names and the names of restaurants where you ate. You may also want to
include the weather conditions, work-shifts, vacations, shopping excursions, parties, etc.

Date	/ /	/ /	/ /	/ /	/ /	/ /

Figure 2-3 Diet Diary

malnutrition have mistakenly been ascribed to a food allergy. Baseline diet diaries have the added advantage of forcing parents to more carefully examine the diet of their infant or child and, based on these records, may provide the practitioner with sufficient information to recommend only minor dietary changes as opposed to complicated elimination regimens. For example, certain foods will occasionally result in symptoms suggestive of food allergy based on an inherent irritant or pharmacologic activity. Prunes, most legumes, and the cruciferous vegetables (eg, broccoli, cabbage, cauliflower, mustard, turnip, etc.) are notorious for producing gastroenteric complaints. Additionally, infants and small children especially fond of fruit and fruit juices who present with a history of frequent loose stools accompanied by bloating and abdominal pain may be consuming excessive amounts of sorbitol, a naturally occurring sugar alcohol that is poorly absorbed in the intestinal tract of small children. Sorbitol is present in large amounts in pears, in small amounts in apples, and is a frequent ingredient in sugar-free candies and chewing gums.

Methylxanthines present in coffee, tea, cocoa, and colas can result in nervousness, excitability, tremor, and tachycardia in excessive amounts. It is not unusual for older infants and small children to consume pharmacologic amounts of these compounds in the form of ice tea and carbonated beverages given even in the form of frequent sips of a parent's or older sibling's drink.

Occasionally parents will innocently assert that their infant is consuming no other food by mouth but breast milk or formula. Following careful questioning, though, mention will be made that in addition to the breast milk or formula, the infant may also be receiving small amounts of numerous other foods, usually in the form of small handouts or snacks, particularly if multiple caregivers are involved. Even small amounts of such complex food mixtures as cookies, ice cream, or macaroni and cheese may be sufficient to sensitize susceptible infants.

If sufficient information exists in a child's medical or dietary history to justify the use of an elimination diet, the degree of elimination to be exercised must be determined next. This can vary from the simple elimination of one or two key foods, such as cow's milk or soy in the formula-fed infant, to the complete removal of all native foods through the feeding of a hypoallergenic, cow's milk casein hydrolysate-based infant formula or, possibly, in very rare situations a chemically defined, elemental diet. Important criteria to consider when assessing the necessary degree of elimination include the severity of the child's symptoms; the number of potentially unsafe foods suggested by the medical and dietary histories; the availability of affordable alternative infant formulas or foods; and the family's level of commitment and ability to comply with a potentially rigorous elimination diet (a cursory examination of the baseline diet and symptom diaries frequently provides some insight into this assessment).

The goal of any elimination diet should be to achieve as asymptomatic a state as possible while also providing optimal nutrition. Gross malnutrition, often in the form of protein-calorie malnutrition, is not uncommon in this very vulnerable age group.[61-63] The length of time required to become symptom-free will vary from child to child, depending on the type and severity of symptoms. Ideally, elimination diets should be of sufficient duration to cover the range of variability in symptom occurrence and severity reported in the baseline symptom diary. Seven to 14 days is generally sufficient, but longer periods may occasionally be required. In highly atopic infants and small children, possible coexisting inhalant sensitivities to perennial allergens such as mold, house dust, mites, and cat and dog hair may further complicate the diagnosis.

Infant and Child Dietary Manipulations: From Diagnosis to Therapy

Infants are quite possibly the most rewarding population of food-allergic patients to work with due to the simplicity of their diets and the relative immaturity of their senses of smell and taste. This lack of sophistication permits the clinician to make rather drastic dietary changes with relatively little fuss from the infant. In exclusively formula-fed infants, a simple formula change using a different protein, carbohydrate, or fat source may be all that is necessary to either rule out or confirm a food sensitivity. A natural progression of formula changes might include cow's milk, soy protein, cow's milk casein hydrolysate [Nutramigen®, Mead Johnson Nutritional Division, Mead Johnson & Company, Evansville, IN 47721; Alimentum®, Ross Laboratories, Columbus, OH 43216], and chemically defined elemental diets [Neocate® (Infant Elemental Diet), Scientific Hospital Supplies, Inc., Gaithersburg, MD 20877); Criticare HN,® Mead Johnson Nutritional Division; Tolerex® (formerly Standard Vivonex), Norwich Eaton Pharmaceuticals, Inc., Norwich, NY 13815].

Much discussion has surrounded the role of soybean-based formulas in the diagnosis and management of CMA.[42,64-69] Soy-based formulas are not without their advocates and represent a first line of defense for infants with presumed CMA in many institutions.[67] They are readily available, convenient, and comparable in cost to standard milk-based formulas. In high allergic risk or seriously ill infants, it may be expeditious to proceed directly from a milk-based formula to one containing casein hydrolysates in light of the documented 15-50% incidence of soy protein allergy in cow's milk allergic infants,[42,64,65] and the greater likelihood of inducing soy sensitivity in infants in whom gut damage has occurred. In mild-to-moderate cases of suspected CMA, the expense of using casein hydrolysates must be weighed against the presumed benefits of skipping over the more moderately priced soy-based formulas, because the cost can be prohibitive for even moderate-income families. A possible coexisting or newly developed soy-protein allergy should be entertained when an infant's allergic symptoms are not significantly improved within 3 to 5 days of initiating a formula change from cow's milk to soy. Alternatively, temporary use of a casein-hydrolysate formula to promote symptom relief and recovery of the gastrointestinal tract, followed by the careful introduction of a soy-based formula, may well be the most cost-effective approach. Fortunately, casein hydrolysates are available through the WIC Program (Supplemental Food Program for Women, Infants, and Children, USDA) to qualifying infants of low-income families who are at nutritional risk when the need is substantiated by a physician.

Milk contains two major classes of protein: caseins, which are precipitated by acid and form the basis of most cheeses; and whey proteins, which result in a small curd. The whey proteins in breast milk differ greatly from the whey proteins of cow's milk.[68] Breast milk whey consists predominantly of α-lactalbumin, while β-lactoglobulin is the major whey protein of cow's milk. Goat's milk is occasionally considered as an alternative for cow's milk, but is unsuitable on two accounts. Goat's milk contains clinically significant cross-reactive β-lactoglobulin with cow's milk and is reported to cause allergic symptoms in up to 80% of infants previously diagnosed with CMA.[70] Goat's milk is also deficient in folic acid,[71] further rendering it unsuitable for infants without appropriate supplementation.

Table 2-4 illustrates the many hypoallergenic formulas commercially available for pediatric use. Not surprisingly, they vary considerably in their cost, availability, palatability, osmolality, and efficacy. Breast milk remains the ideal feeding choice for infants, but is not always a viable alternative and may, indeed, be a source of antigenic stimulation in a subset of high allergic risk infants. It is well established that exquisitely sensitive, exclusively breastfed infants may become sensitized to foods the mother is consuming and passively transferring to the infant via her breast milk.[72-75] As a result, it may be necessary for the mothers of these infants to adhere to individualized elimination diets (with appropriate supplementation) before maximum symptom relief may be achieved in the child.

There have been numerous additions in recent years to the hypoallergenic marketplace (eg, Alimentum®, Carnation Good Start®, Neocate®, Elemental 028®, and Peptamen®), presenting the clinician with what is often a confusing array of choices. Nutramigen® has overwhelmingly been the protein-hydrolysate formula of choice, due to approximately 50 years of accumulated experience in infants with sensitivities to intact proteins, but the utility of the remaining formulas should not be overlooked. The moderately high carbohydrate content of both Nutramigen® and Pregestimil®, which may aggravate

Table 2-4 Hypoallergenic Formulas—General Characteristics

| Formula | Caloric Distribution (%) | | | Nutrient Sources | | | kcal/oz | Osmolality (mOsmol/kg H_2O) |
	Pro	CHO	Fat	Protein	Carbohydrate	Fat		
I. Breast Milk	7.0	38.0	55.0	Whey, Casein	Lactose	Human Fat	22	300
II. Protein Hydrolysates								
A. Nutramigen[a]	11.0	54.0	35.0	Casein Hydrolysate	Glucose Polymers	Corn Oil	20	320
B. Pregestimil[a]	11.0	41.0	48.0	Casein Hydrolysate	Glucose Polymers	MCT Oil (60%), Corn Oil (20%), High Oleic Saffl. Oil (10%)	20	320
C. Alimentum[b]	11.0	41.0	48.0	Casein Hydrolysate	Sucrose, Tapioca, Starch	MCT (50%), Saffl. Oil (40%), Soy Oil (10%)	20	370
D. Carnation Good Start[c] (not currently marketed as hypoallergenic)	9.8	44.2	46.0	Whey Hydrolysate, Whey Protein Isolate	Lactose (70%), Maltodextrin	Palm Oil (60%), Saffl. Oil (22%), Coconut Oil (18%)	20	265
III. Elemental Formulas								
A. Neocate[d]	11.4	44.3	44.3	Crystalline Amino Acids	Maltodextrin	Pork Fat, Beef Fat, Peanut Oil, Coconut Oil	24	320

B. Elemental 028[d]	9.7	75.7	14.5	Crystalline Amino Acids	Sucrose, Maltodextrin	Arachis Oil (Refined Peanut Oil)	30	450
C. Criticare HN[a]	14.2	83.1	2.7	Casein Hydrolysate	Maltodextrin, Cornstarch	Saffl. Oil	30	650
D. Tolerex[e]	8.2	90.5	1.3	Crystalline Amino Acids	Glucose Polymers	Saffl. Oil	30	550
E. Peptamen[c]	16.0	51.0	33.0	Whey Hydrolysate	Maltodextrin, Starch	MCT (70%), Sunfl. Oil (30%)	30	260

[a]Mead Johnson Nutritional Division, Evansville, IN 47721.
[b]Ross Laboratories, Columbus, OH 43216.
[c]Clintec Nutrition Company, Deerfield, IL 60015.
[d]Scientific Hospital Supplies, Inc., Gaithersburg, MD 20877.
[e]Norwich Eaton Pharmaceuticals, Inc., Norwich, NY 13815.

Note: Content of formulas should be confirmed with manufacturers as product formulations change.

Editor's Note: As of March 1989, the product now known as Carnation Good Start® removed the term "hypoallergenic" from its front label. The product label currently states, "The protein in Good Start® is specially processed to be well tolerated by your baby. *Caution:* If you suspect your baby is allergic to milk, use only under a doctor's supervision."

an underlying acquired carbohydrate malabsorption secondary to severe diarrhea, is counterbalanced by the fact that these formulas are sucrose- and lactose-free. Sucrose and, particularly, lactose intolerance can occur as a result of severe, protracted diarrhea, regardless of the precipitating cause. Both Pregestimil® and Alimentum® contain medium-chain triglycerides (MCT) in a blend with other oils to prevent an essential fatty acid deficiency. MCTs are more readily hydrolyzed and absorbed than triglycerides from long-chain fatty acids and are indicated in conditions of impaired fat absorption. Ingestion of large amounts of MCT may produce abdominal distention, cramping, nausea, or diarrhea due to the hypertonic load resulting from the rapid hydrolysis of MCT to free fatty acids and glycerol.[76]

Carnation Good Start®, a whey protein hydrolysate, represents a break from the long-standing casein-hydrolysate tradition due to the presumed increased allergenic potential of whey protein over caseins. Chandra and colleagues[69] reported a significantly decreased incidence of atopic manifestations (eg, eczema, wheeze, rhinitis or otitis, gastrointestinal, colic) in high allergic risk infants followed prospectively from birth to age 6 months on Carnation Good Start,® as compared to infants consuming either a cow's milk or soy-based formula or breastfed infants whose mothers were consuming unrestricted diets. While there may be a specific population of infants who would benefit from the reduced allergic capacity, cost, and improved taste of this formula over the more tried casein hydrolysates, it would be premature at this time, in the opinion of the author, to make any broad-based recommendations regarding the use of Carnation Good Start® in the diagnosis and management of infants with allergies to intact food proteins based on the very limited amount of research conducted this far.* Whey protein hydrolysates have in fact been associated with adverse reactions as discussed in Chapter 3.

Very rarely, infants may be encountered who do not tolerate casein hydrolysates but recover on a chemically defined, elemental diet presumably due to the further reduced allergic load of simple amino acids or differences in carbohydrate content. When considering using elemental diets, an understanding of the limitations associated with their use in a pediatric population is critical.[67] Most adult-oriented enteral feedings are formulated to provide 30 kcal/oz (1 kcal/ml). Infant formulas, on the other hand, are formulated to provide 20 kcal/oz. Formulas providing up to 24 kcal/oz (0.8 kcal/ml) are generally well tolerated by most infants.[76] When the caloric density exceeds 24 kcal/oz, the resulting high osmolality and renal solute load may present added stresses for infants with excessive water losses, malabsorption, or restricted fluid intake.[76] These infants should be closely monitored for signs of dehydration and other complications. The essential fatty acid content of Tolerex® (formerly, Standard Vivonex®) is inadequate for infants and very

---

*Editor's Note: Use of wheat protein hydrolysates to reduce allergic potential or treat allergy cannot be recommended based on current evidence.[77]

young children, because linoleic acid provides only approximately 1% of the total calories versus a minimum of 2.7% recommended by the Committee on Nutrition of the American Academy of Pediatrics[78] and the Infant Formula Act of 1980.[79] Neocate® represents the first elemental formula designed with infants in mind. It has only recently been introduced into this country from Great Britain and experience with it is, therefore, quite limited. Availability is, unfortunately, a problem with this formula because it must be shipped by UPS directly to the consumer or physician's office. Neocate® and Peptamen® represent the only isotonic elemental formulas currently available. Due to the hypertonic nature (osmolality greater than 400 mOsm/kg H_2O) of the remaining elemental formulas, their high carbohydrate content, and frequent very low fat content, these diets should be viewed only as temporary diets of last resort. Infants consuming a chemically defined elemental diet should be weaned to a more nutritionally complete casein-hydrolysate formula as soon as they are stabilized. Interaction with a registered dietitian or health care worker trained in the use of elemental diets for the diagnosis of adverse food reactions is very helpful in avoiding complications and improving compliance.

Abrupt formula changes in older infants are occasionally met with considerable resistance. This may be greatly lessened by gradually titrating the new formula into the old formula in ever increasing amounts over a period of several days to a week or until a 100% solution of the new formula is being consumed. The addition of a vanilla flavor packet (Norwich Eaton Pharmaceuticals, Inc., Norwich, NY 13815) to each 8-oz feeding of new formula may facilitate the switch but will increase the osmolality by 45 mOsm/kg H_2O per packet used.

Infants with a long-term history of suspected food sensitivities consuming a mixed diet of breast milk or formula plus solid foods and infants in whom symptoms suggestive of food sensitization did not appear until after solid foods were introduced can both be managed in a similar fashion. The goal in each situation is to remove as many potential food allergens as possible from the diet, while also providing optimal nutrition. This is accomplished by removing all solid foods from the diet, and returning the infant, when possible, exclusively to either breast milk or a casein-hydrolysate formula. Discretion should be used with infants who are older than six months of age, who are consuming more than one quart of formula per day, who have doubled their birth weight, or who are anemic. Due to their increased nutrient needs, these infants are best managed on a case-by-case basis with attention given to both developmental and nutritional implications.

As infants mature, so do their palates. They tire very quickly of diets consisting solely of breast milk or formula. It becomes increasingly difficult, not to mention inappropriate, to return them to breast milk or casein hydrolysates exclusively. These infants, particularly those nine months of age and older, are best managed, in the author's experience, by using a strict rotary elimination diet supplemented with appropriate amounts of breast milk or casein hydrolysates. Foods reputed to be highly sensitizing (eg, cow's milk, egg, legumes, wheat, citrus fruits, cocoa, etc.) are temporarily removed from the diet. Any food that results in a positive RAST or prick-puncture skin test (ie, wheal size 3 mm greater than the negative control) will also be eliminated from the diet, in addition to foods suspected by the child's family of causing a response. In order to carry out these directives correctly, families must be educated regarding the fairly ubiquitous presence of derivatives of such foods as milk, egg, soy, corn, and wheat in commercially prepared foods and staple items and cautioned repeatedly to read all food and drug labels. It is important not to exceed the capacity of a family to carry out an elimination diet by requiring the elimination of vast numbers of foods when, for example, there may be limited access to alternative foods or significant time constraints imposed on two working parents. Foods to be eliminated and challenged in situations such as these are best prioritized and then carried out in stages, addressing the most likely food offenders first. The remaining presumed safe foods in the diet are then arranged in a rotary pattern of varying length with three to four days being the average. While rotary elimination diets are considered controversial and of little or no benefit during the management phase, the diversity imposed by rotary elimination diets during the brief diagnostic phase has a two-fold purpose: (1) the provision, albeit mandatory, of a degree of variety necessary for optimal nutritional and patient compliance; (2) as a means of possibly recognizing the presence of any remaining sensitizing foods in the elimination pattern. Diet diaries kept during the elimination period serve as an important tool not only for assessing compliance, but for identifying the possible presence of any additional food triggers.

Partial or complete symptom relief occurring during the elimination phase strongly suggests that the child's symptoms were triggered by one or more of the eliminated foods. The diagnosis becomes definitive when a challenge with adequate amounts of suspect food reproduces some or all of the child's symptoms.

If the infant or small child does not achieve a measurable degree of improvement within one to two weeks on an elimination diet, several explanations are possible. Most obvious is the possibility that no food sensitivities exist. Other important considerations include the possibility of poor dietary compliance, either willful or unintentional; the continued presence of unrecognized offending foods in the elimination pattern; the presence of symptoms resulting from intercurrent infections or other disease processes occurring during the elimination period. Lengthening the elimination period is much preferred over incorrectly making a diagnosis that food sensitivities do not exist in children whose elimination diets have been interfered with by external circumstances.

FOOD CHALLENGES

Eliminated foods may be reintroduced into the diet of children in either an open or blinded format, depending on the number of incriminated foods, the age of the patient, and the perceived level of physician and family bias. In an open, oral provocative food challenge, both the observer (physician, nurse, dietitian, etc.) and the patient or patient's family are aware of the food's identity. Blinded food challenges, on the other hand, interject an element of mystery into the proceedings that many patients or patients' families find fascinating. Blinded food challenges may be single-blind, where only the patient is unaware of the food's identity, or double-blind, where both the patient and the observer are left unaware. Placebo foods may additionally be randomly included in the challenge sequence to further remove bias and are considered necessary when a patient's symptoms are largely subjective in nature (eg, hyperactivity, irritability, headache, etc.).

Double-blind, placebo-controlled food challenges (DBPCFC) are universally considered the gold standard for the accurate diagnosis of an adverse food reaction. In infants and very small children, it is arguably unnecessary to blind the challenge food, except possibly in very precocious youngsters. With this population of patients, it is occasionally more important to hide the food's identity from the patient's family. Challenge vehicles used to mask a food's identity in very young children include applesauce, pudding, milk shakes, orange juice, and on occasion, an elemental diet because of its superior capacity to mask strong flavors. It should go without saying that all carrier foods should be documented safe foods beyond a shadow of a doubt. Opaque capsules, a frequently used challenge vehicle in older children and adults, are contraindicated in infants and small children who are too young to swallow them. Nose clamps, a blindfold, and repeated ice water chasers complete the blinding process.

It is important to give some thought to the potentially diverse tastes and textures of the particular food(s) a patient is scheduled to be challenged to when selecting the identity of the carrier food and the placebo. Some foods are better at masking certain flavors and textures than others. For example, a young child who is to be challenged to egg and wheat will invariably be able to detect the textural differences between the two foods if similarly textured placebos are not also included in the challenge scheme. It is, therefore, not surprising that desiccated foodstuffs are the preferred form of challenge food for blinded challenges in light of the decreased volume displacement and textural characteristics inherent in them. Desiccated foods are widely available from camping supply stores.

Open challenges are not without their place in the reintroduction period and may be suitable for challenging foods that the history suggests result in only mild reactions, but to which the patient skin tested negatively, assuming the skin tests are a reliable indicator of IgE sensitization in these particular patients.[4,19] Open challenges may be carried out in the home of the reliable patient, but are preferably conducted in an office setting if there is even a remote chance of a severe reaction occurring.[19] For a comprehensive review of the indications for open vs blinded food challenges, in addition to the provision of helpful forms, the reader is referred to Sampson[4] and Bock et al.[19]

Regardless of the type of challenge format selected or the number of foods to be challenged, some general guidelines apply. The purest possible form of the food should be used for challenging purposes. It should contain as few other ingredients as possible and be only minimally processed. It should not contain derivatives of foods not yet challenged or previously shown to be poorly tolerated. Sample size is an extremely important consideration when challenging with potentially sensitizing foods. Until proven otherwise, it must be assumed that every child is exquisitely sensitive to each food eliminated from the diet. To avoid causing a severe reaction, always initiate the challenge with a very small portion size, gradually titrating up the amount of challenged food consumed until a serving size equal to or exceeding a meal-sized portion is consumed. If a reaction occurs at any time during the challenging of a food, no further testing of that food should be permitted and the patient's symptoms treated accordingly. Symptoms resulting from a previous positive food challenge must have completely resolved before proceeding to the next food in the challenge sequence; a 24-hour symptom-free period is preferred. No food that resulted in an especially severe or life-threatening response should be rechallenged without careful consideration of the risks and dangers involved and without immediate access to properly equipped treatment rooms staffed with personnel skilled in performing cardiopulmonary resuscitation.[80] If qualified emergency care is not available, challenges of this nature are best avoided.

A challenge format employed by the author for young children is summarized below.

1. Since optimal nutrition is based on maximum variety in the diet, no food should be eliminated unless it is absolutely necessary.
2. Each challenge food is returned to the diet for a period of three consecutive days in the following manner:

Day 1:	Breakfast:	1/16 of a portion
	10:00 AM:	1/8 of a portion
	Noon:	1/4 of a portion
	2:00 PM:	1/2 of a portion
	4:00 PM:	1 whole portion

Dinner:	1 whole portion
HS:	2 whole portions

Days 2 and 3: Consume at least 2-3 portions of challenge food per day.

3. "Portions" represent a serving size considered to be a meal-sized portion and have largely been taken from diabetic exchange lists so the amount of protein, carbohydrate, and fat contributed by various members of individual food groupings would be approximately the same.

4. Open oral challenges resulting in a positive reaction should be repeated to confirm the reaction. DBPCFCs represent the gold standard and should be employed in equivocal challenges when bias is suspected.

The preceding format is condensed into a 4-hour block when used for a blinded challenge or an open challenge conducted in an office setting.

In summary, no food challenge is without risks. Patients must be duly educated regarding the possible consequences of a severe reaction, as well as the benefits of learning that a previously suspected food is actually well tolerated. Fortunately, the prognosis for food allergy for very young patients is very optimistic.

REFERENCES

1. Anderson JA. The establishment of common language concerning adverse reactions to foods and food additives. *J Allergy Clin Immunol.* 1986; 78(1):140–144.

2. Anderson JA. The pediatrician's guide to food allergy. *Henry Ford Hosp Med J.* 1988; 36:198–203.

3. Anderson JA. Adverse reactions to food. In: Bierman CW, Pearlman DS, eds. *Allergic Diseases from Infancy to Adulthood.* 2nd ed. Philadelphia: WB Saunders; 1988: 130–140.

4. Sampson HA, Albergo R. Comparison of results of skin tests, RAST, and double-blind, placebo-controlled food challenges in children with atopic dermatitis. *J Allergy Clin Immunol.* 1984; 74:26–33.

5. Mahan LK, Furukawa CT. General nutritional considerations and diet for adverse food reactions. In: Bierman CW, Pearlman DS, eds. *Allergic Diseases from Infancy to Adulthood.* Philadelphia: WB Saunders; 1988: 367–376.

6. Anderson JA. Unproven and unapproved methods of diagnosis and treatment. In: Breneman JC, ed. *Handbook of Food Allergies.* New York: Marcel Dekker, Inc; 1987: 211–231.

7. Shapiro GG, Anderson JA. Commentary: Controversial techniques in allergy. *Pediatrics.* 1988; 82:935–937.

8. Bock SA. Evaluation of patients with adverse reactions to food. In: Bierman CW, Pearlman DS, eds. *Allergic Diseases from Infancy to Adulthood.* Philadelphia: WB Saunders; 1988: 359–366.

9. Levine BB. Immunologic tests for hypersensitivity reactions to drugs. In: Rose NR, Friedman H, eds. *Manual of Clinical Immunology.* Washington, DC: American Society for Microbiology; 1976: 637–641.

10. Foucard T. Developmental aspects of food sensitivity in childhood. *Nutr Rev.* 1984; 42:98–104.

11. Bock SA. Prospective appraisal of complaints of adverse reactions to foods in children during the first three years of life. *Pediatrics.* 1987; 79(5):683–688.

12. Metcalfe DD. A current practical approach to the diagnosis of suspected adverse reactions to food. *NER Allergy Proc.* 1987; 8:22–26.

13. Heiner DC, Wilson JF. Delayed immunologic food reactions. *NER Allergy Proc.* 1986; 7:520–526.

14. Enberg RN, McCullough J, Ownby DR. Antibody responses in watermelon sensitivity. *J Allergy Clin Immunol.* 1988; 82:795–800.

15. Moller C. Effects of pollen immunotherapy on food hypersensitivity in children with birth pollinosis. *Ann Allergy.* 1989; 62:343–345.

16. Kidd JM III, Cohen SH, Sosman AJ, Fink JN. Food dependent exercise-induced anaphylaxis. *J Allergy Clin Immunol.* 1983; 71:407–411.

17. Yunginger J, Squillace D, Jones R, Helm R. Fatal anaphylactic reactions induced by peanuts. *Allergy Proc.* 1989; 10:249–253.

18. Bernhisel-Broadbent J, Sampson HA, Atkins FM, et al. Cross-allergenicity in the legume botanical family in children with food hypersensitivity. *J Allergy Clin Immunol.* 1989; 83:435–440.

19. Bock SA, Sampson HA, Atkins FM, et al. Double-blind placebo-controlled food challenge (DBPCFC) as office procedure: A manual. *J Allergy Clin Immunol.* 1988; 82:986–997.

20. Ownby DR, Anderson JA, Jacobson GL, Homburger HA. Development and comparative evaluation of a multi-antigen RAST as a screening test for inhalant allergy. *J Allergy Clin Immunol.* 1984; 73:466–472.

21. Bousquet J. In vivo methods for study of allergy: Skin tests, technique, and interpretation. In: Reed C, Ellis E, Adkinson NF Jr, Yunginger J, eds. *Allergy Principles and Practice.* St. Louis: CV Mosby; 1988: 419–436.

22. Sampson HA. Role of immediate food hypersensitivity in the pathogenesis of atopic dermatitis. *J Allergy Clin Immunol.* 1983; 71:473–480.

23. Sampson HA. Comparative study of commercial food antigen extracts for the diagnosis of food hypersensitivity. *J Allergy Clin Immunol.* 1988; 82:718–726.

24. Ortolani C, Ispano M, Pastorello EA, Ansaloni R, Margi G. Comparison of results of skin prick test (with fresh food and commercial food extracts) and RAST in 100 patients with the oral allergy syndrome. *J Allergy Clin Immunol.* 1989; 83(3):683–690.

25. Wide L, Bennich H, Johansson SGO. Diagnosis of allergy by an in vitro test for allergen antibodies. *Lancet.* 1967; 2:1105–1107.

26. Ownby DR: Allergy testing: In vivo vs. in vitro. *Pediatr Clin North Am.* 1988: 35(5):995–1009.

27. Minor JD, Tolber SG, Frick OL. Leukocyte inhibition factor (LIF) in delayed-onset food allergy. *J Allergy Clin Immunol.* 1980; 66:314–321.

28. Easton JG, Kaplan MS. Controversial concepts in practices in allergy. In: Bierman CW, Pearlman DS, eds. *Allergic Diseases from Infancy to Adulthood.* 2nd ed. Philadelphia: WB Saunders; 1988: 735–747.

29. Van Metro TE Jr. Unproven procedures for diagnosis and treatment of food allergy. *NER Allergy Proc.* 1987; 8:17–21.

30. *FDA Compliance Policy Guide 7124.27 Devices.* Washington, DC: US Food and Drug Administration; March 1985; ch. 24.

31. AMA, Council on Scientific Affairs. In vivo diagnostic testing in immunotherapy for allergy, report I, part II of allergy panel. *JAMA.* 1987; 258:1505–1508.

32. Scadding, GK, Brostoff J. Low dose sublingual therapy in patients with allergic rhinitis due to house dust mite. *Clin Allergy.* 1986; 16: 483–491.

33. AMA, Council on Scientific Affairs. In vitro testing for allergy, report II of the allergy panel. *JAMA.* 1987; 258(12):1639–1643.

34. Randolph TG, Rollins JP. Beet sensitivity: allergic reactions for the ingestion of beet sugar (sucrose) and monosodium glutamate of beet origin. *J Lab Clin Med.* 1950; 36:407–415.

35. Terr AI. Environmental illnesses—A clinical review of 50 cases. *Arch Intern Med.* 1986; 146:145–149.

36. Crook WG. *The Yeast Connection—A Medical Breakthrough,* 2nd ed. Jackson, TN: Professional Books; 1984.

37. Brodsky CM. Allergic to everything—A medical subculture. *Psychosomatics.* 1983; 24:731–742.

38. Collins-Williams C. The incidence of milk allergy in pediatric practice. *J Pediatr.* 1956; 48:39–47.

39. Bachman KD, Dees SC. Milk allergy, II: Observations on incidence and symptoms of allergy to milk in allergic infants. *Pediatrics.* 1957; 20:400–407.

40. Goldman AS, Anderson DW, Sellers WA, Saperstein S, Kniker WT, Halpern SR. Milk allergy, I: Oral challenge with milk and isolated milk proteins in allergic children. *Pediatrics.* 1963; 32:425–443.

41. Freier S, Kletter B. Milk allergy in infants and young children. *Clin Pediatr.* 1970; 9:449–454.

42. Gerrard JW, MacKenzie JWA, Goluboff N, Garson JZ, Maningas CS. Cow's milk allergy: Prevalence and manifestations in an unselected series of newborns. *Acta Paediatr Scand.* 1973; 243(suppl):1–21.

43. Jakobsson I, Lindberg T. A prospective study of cow's milk protein intolerance in Swedish infants. *Acta Paediatr Scand.* 1979; 68:853–859.

44. Stintzing G, Zetterstrom R. Cow's milk allergy, incidence and pathogenetic role of early exposure to cow's milk formula. *Acta Paediatr. Scand.* 1979; 68:383–387.

45. Bachman KD, Dees SC. Milk allergy, I: Observations on incidence and symptoms in "well" babies. *Pediatrics.* 1957; 20:393–399.

46. Sampson HA. The role of "allergy" in atopic dermatitis. *Clin Rev Allergy.* 1986; 4:125–138.

47. Burks AW, Mallory SB, Williams LW, Sherrill MA. Atopic dermatitis: clinical relevance of food hypersensitivity reactions. *J Pediatr.* 1988; 113:447–451.

48. Ratner B, Untracht S. Egg allergy in children. *Am J Dis Child.* 1952; 83:309.

49. Bock SA. Prospective appraisal of complaints of adverse reactions to foods in children during the first three years of life. *Pediatrics.* 1987; 79:683–688.

50. Sampson HA. Food hypersensitivity. In: Grant JA, ed. *Insights in Allergy.* St. Louis: CV Mosby Company, 1986.

51. Bock SA, Lee W-Y, Remigio L, Holst A, May CD. Appraisal of skin tests with food extracts for diagnosis of food hypersensitivity. *Clin Allergy.* 1978; 8:559–564.

52. Foucard T. Development of food allergies with special reference to cow's milk allergy. *Pediatrics.* 1985; 75(suppl): 177–181.

53. May CD. Objective clinical and laboratory studies of immediate reactions to foods in asthmatic children. *J Allergy Clin Immunol.* 1976; 58:500–515.

54. Bock SA, Lee W-Y, Remigio LK, May, CD.: Studies of hypersensitivities reactions to foods in infants and children. *J Allergy Clin Immunol.* 1978; 62:327–334.

55. Eggleston PA. Prospective studies in the natural history of food allergy. *Ann Allergy.* 1987; 59(5):179–182.

56. NIAID Task Force Report. *Adverse Reactions to Foods.* Bethesda, MD: National Institutes of Health; 1984. NIH Publication No. 84-2442; 17–25.

57. Sampson HA, McCaskill CM. Food hypersensitivity in atopic dermatitis: evaluation of 113 patients. *J Pediatr.* 1985; 107:669–675.

58. Sachs MI, O'Connell EJ. Cross-reactivity of foods—mechanisms and clinical significance. *Ann Allergy.* 1988; 61:36–40.

59. Bernhisel-Broadbent JB, Sampson HA. Cross-allergenicity in the legume botanical family in children with food hypersensitivity. *J Allergy Clin Immunol.* 1989; 83:435–440.

60. Morgan JE, O'Neil CE, Daul CB, Lehrer SB. Species-specific shrimp allergens: RAST and RAST-inhibition studies. *J Allergy Clin Immunol.* 1989; 83:1112–1117.

61. Lloyd-Still JD. Chronic diarrhea of childhood and the misuse of elimination diets. *J Pediatr.* 1979; 95(1):10–13.

62. Sinatra FR, Merritt RJ. Iatrogenic kwashiorkor in infants. *Am J Dis Child.* 1981; 135:21–23.

63. David TJ, Waddington E, Stanton RHJ. Nutritional hazards of elimination diets in children with atopic eczema. *Arch Dis Child.* 1984; 59:323–325.

64. Kjellman N-IM, Johansson SGO. Soy versus cow's milk in infants with a biparental history of atopic disease: development of atopic disease and immunoglobulins from birth to 4 years of age. *Clin Allergy.* 1979; 9:347–358.

65. Perkkio M, Savilahti E, Kuitunen P. Morphometric and immunohistochemical study of jejunal biopsies from children with intestinal soy allergy. *Eur J Pediatr.* 1981; 137:63–69.

66. Savilahti E, Verkasolo M. Intestinal cow's milk allergy: pathogenesis and clinical presentation. *Clin Rev Allergy.* 1984; 2:7–23.

67. Brady MS, Richard KA, Fitzgerald JF, Lemons JA. Specialized formulas and feedings for infants with malabsorption or formula intolerance. *J Am Diet Assoc.* 1986; 86:191–200.

68. Benkov KJ, LeLeiko NS. A rational approach to infant formulas. *Pediatr Ann.* 1987; 16:225–230.

69. Chandra RK, Singh G, Shridhara B. Effect of feeding whey hydrolysate, soy and conventional cow milk formulas on incidence of atopic disease in high risk infants. *Ann Allergy.* 1989; 63:102–106.

70. Juntunen K, Backman A. Goat's milk—a substitute for cow's milk? *Proceedings of the 2nd International Symposium on Immunological and Clinical Problems of Food Allergy,* Milan, Italy, Oct. 25–26, 1982.

71. Maksimak M, Winter HS. The infant at nutritional risk: cow's milk sensitivity and lactose intolerance. In: Howard RB, Winter HS, eds. *Nutrition and Feeding of Infants and Toddlers.* Boston: Little Brown & Co; 1984: 245–250.

72. Matsumura T, Kuroume T, Oguri M, et al. Egg sensitivity and eczematous manifestations in breast-fed newborns with particular reference to intrauterine sensitization. *Ann Allergy.* 1975; 35:221–229.

73. Kilshaw PJ, Cant AJ. The passage of maternal dietary proteins into human breast milk. *Int Arch Allergy Appl Immunol.* 1984; 75:8–15.

74. Cant AJ, Marsden RA, Kilshaw PJ. Egg and cow's milk hypersensitivity in exclusively breast fed infants with eczema and detection of egg protein in breast milk. *Br Med J.* 1985; 291:932–935.

75. Cavagni G, Paganelli R, Caffarelli C, et al. Passage of food antigens into circulation of breast-fed infants with atopic dermatitis. *Ann Allergy.* 1988; 61:361–365.

76. Wilson SE, Dietz WH, Grand RJ. An algorithm for pediatric enteral alimentation. *Pediatr Ann.* 1987; 16:233–240.

77. Businco L, Cantani A, Longhi A, et al. Anaphylactic reactions to a cow's milk whey protein hydrolysate (Alpha-Ré, Nestlé) in infants with cow's milk allergy. *Ann Allergy.* 1989;62:333–335.

78. Committee on Nutrition, American Academy of Pediatrics. Commentary on breastfeeding and infant formulas, including proposed standards for formulas. *Pediatrics.* 1976; 57:278–285.

79. United States Congress. Infant Formula Act of 1980. Public Law 96-359, September 26, 1980.

80. Bock SA. Natural history of severe reactions to foods in young children. *J Pediatr.* 1985; 107:676–680.

Major Food Allergens and Principles of Dietary Management

Judy E. Perkin

INTRODUCTION

Food allergens identified to date are predominantly proteins, although some may be polysaccharides.[1,2] To serve as an antigen (or allergen) a food molecule must have the capacity to initiate the production of IgE. In order to affect such production, it is believed a food allergen must be of appropriate size and shape to bridge two IgE molecules on a mast cell's surface. Such bridging is thought to be required for histamine release. Molecular weights ranging from 10,000 to 70,000 daltons are common for food allergens.[1] Food molecules too small to serve as antigens in their own right may still be involved in stimulating an immune response by linking with a carrier molecule, such as a protein in body tissue. These small food molecules are known as haptens.[2]

The complexity of the surface of a food molecule is important in determining its capability to produce IgE. Food molecules with more complex surfaces seem to be more likely to elicit an allergic response.[1] It is also important to remember antibodies are produced in response to a specific antigen surface characteristic.[2] The effects of food processing and preparation on the ability of food proteins to be allergenic are discussed in Chapter 9.

There is inquiry about the existence of allergen cross-reactivity. (Cross-reactivity is a phenomenon by which allergy may exist to more than one food within a food family group.) Some believe this phenomenon to be rare[3] or as yet unproven with regard to many allergens.[1] Others believe patients should be counseled about food families to avoid a cross-reactive potential.[2]

At least one *in vitro* study has demonstrated cross-reactivity among soybean, peanut, garden pea, and garbanzo bean (or chick pea).[4] Sachs and O'Connell,[3] however, suggest most legume-sensitive patients should be tested to confirm cross-reactivity to other legume types. Bernhisel-Broadbent and Sampson[5] studied 69 legume-sensitive patients and found only 2 with sensitivity to more than one legume.

Crustacea have been extensively studied in terms of their cross-reactive potential. Significant cross-reactivity has been demonstrated for crawfish, lobster, and shrimp.[3] Because of the severe nature of the allergic manifestations related to crustacean consumption, Sachs and O'Connell[3] feel open challenges to confirm cross-reactivity potential are unwarranted and cross-reactivity to various crustacea can be presumed.

Clinical manifestations of food allergy are reviewed in Chapter 1, and specific manifestations associated with major food allergens will be discussed in this chapter. It is important to remember that although seemingly rare, food-induced anaphylaxis resulting in death can occur. Yunginger et al[6] identified 7 such deaths within 16 months. (Peanut was involved in four of these deaths; the others were related to pecan, crab, or fish consumption.) Such deaths emphasize the importance of avoidance because fatal anaphylaxis in the case of true food allergy may be initiated upon consumption of very small amounts of the offending food. Patients with food allergies must also be able to self-administer epinephrine when needed.

MAJOR FOOD ALLERGENS

Cow's Milk

Cow's milk contains approximately 30-35 grams of protein per liter,[1] and over 25 protein fractions have been identified in cow's milk that have the capability to induce an allergic response.[7] Most clinical cow's milk allergy, however, is believed to be related to the allergenicity of three fractions: (1) ß-lactoglobulin (a whey protein), (2) α-lactalbumin (another whey protein), and (3) casein.[1,7,8] Bovine serum albumin and globulin may be allergenic but are considered to be less so than the above three protein types.[2,7] (The effects of processing on allergenicity of cow's milk protein are discussed in Chapter 9.)

Proteins of goat's milk, which serve as antigens, are closely related to cow's milk protein fractions. This means that persons having a cow's milk allergy will frequently be allergic to goat's milk as well.[7,9] Cow's milk protein hydrolysates commonly do not elicit an antibody response; therefore, they are used in products serving as cow's milk or cow's milk-formula substitutes. Businco et al,[10] however, have reported that Alpha-Ré®, a cow's milk whey protein hydrolysate formula product of the Nestle Corporation, did evoke anaphylactic reaction in five infants with cow's milk allergy. (Residual casein epitopes in the formula were believed to be responsible.) Chapter 2, Part II, includes a discussion of whey versus casein hydrolysate formulas.

Components in cow's milk other than its natural protein constituents may also be responsible for an allergic reaction. Examples of such substances include penicillin and proteins of ragweed, linseed, peanut, and/or wheat.[11] The US Food and Drug Administration does have regulations aimed at prevention of penicillin contamination of milk products.[7]

It has been noted that individuals with cow's milk allergy may react to other food allergens. It has been estimated that 10 to 30% of persons who are sensitive to cow's milk will also be sensitive to soy.[12]

Allergy to cow's milk is considered by some to be the most common food allergy in the United States.[9] The prevalence in infants and children is estimated to be between 1 and 3%.[2,13] Some evidence suggests that cow's milk allergy is seen in up to 30% of children with allergies.[14] Olejer in Chapter 2, Part II, provides data that suggest even higher levels of prevalence in both the total and allergic populations.

Cow's milk allergy seen in infants and children may be related not only to the allergenicity of protein fractions, but may also be related to the large amounts of cow's milk consumed relative to body weight. Also, the relative immaturity of the gastrointestinal tract may allow greater antigen uptake.[2] Roberton et al[15] found higher serum ß-lactoglobulins in preterm, as contrasted to term, neonates.

The phenomena of cow's milk allergy, although most prevalent in the pediatric age group, can occur at any age.[16] Olalde et al[17] recently presented an interesting case history of a 29-year-old patient with cow's milk allergy. The allergic manifestations in this patient were bronchospasm and urticaria.

Several immune response mechanisms may be involved in cow's milk allergy. Bahna and Heiner[13] have indicated potential involvements of type I, type III, and type IV reactions. Children who never manifest symptoms of cow's milk allergy may still demonstrate high levels of antibodies to cow's milk protein.[18]

Anderson et al[19] have identified several factors that may impact on the development of cow's milk allergy in the infant. These include diet history (ie, formula versus breastfeeding), health status (ie, the presence of gastrointestinal disease), and familial history of atopic disease. Gerrard and Shenassa[20] have postulated different types of cow's milk allergy linked to breastfeeding versus formula feeding. These researchers feel an IgE-mediated mechanism is probably associated with cow's milk allergy seen in the breastfed infant. At any rate, the prognosis for cow's milk allergy in early life is generally good with disappearance of clinical problems by age 2 years.[14]

The clinical presentation of cow's milk allergy can be extremely varied. Gastrointestinal problems are considered to be the most common clinical manifestations.[13,14] Intestinal changes may range from minor inflammation of the lamina propria to villus flattening with inflammation.[21] Specific gastrointestinal problems seen in conjunction with cow's milk allergy may include diarrhea, vomiting, steatorrhea, abdominal or stomach pain, malabsorption (particularly of zinc and calcium), colonic inflammation, protein-losing enteropathy, and bleeding (either overt or occult).[7,13,14] Occult blood loss is considered to be a common problem and an area of concern because it can be a cause of iron deficiency anemia.[14] Blood loss in the occult form may be as high as 10 ml per day and small losses (less than 5 ml/dl of stool) may go undetected using a guaiac test.[7] Wilson et al [22] report that in their pediatric practice experience, occult bleeding related to cow's milk ingestion is seen in about half the children with diagnosed iron deficiency who reportedly consume large quantities of milk per day (one quart or more).

Two forms of gastroenteropathy associated with milk ingestion have been outlined by Katz et al.[23] Milk-sensitive enteropathy, a type not associated with IgE abnormalities, is reported to appear most commonly in the first year of life. This type of enteropathy is often said to resolve with cow's milk elimination. The other outlined chronic gastroenteropathy type, labeled as eosinophilic, is associated with IgE-mediated food allergies. This latter type responds well to corticosteroid treatment.

Respiratory problems are another potential manifestation of cow's milk allergy. Respiratory symptoms may include wheezing, coughing, and nasal congestion or draining. Cow's milk has not been shown to either produce mucus or affect mucus viscosity.[14,24] Heiner's syndrome is a specifically defined respiratory disorder associated with cow's milk allergy.[7,14] Heiner's syndrome is characterized by lung infiltrates, elevated levels of eosinophils, and high levels of serum precipitins to cow's milk. Patients may have respiratory and/or gastrointestinal problems, anemia, or fail to thrive.[7,14] The development of Heiner's syndrome is believed to involve either type III or type IV immune reaction.[7]

Some patients with cow's milk allergy may have skin manifestations such as hives, angioedema, or eczema. Some patients may react to skin contact with dermatitis. Anaphylactic reaction as a clinical manifestation is rare but can occur.[14]

Sleeping problems in infants may, in some instances, be related to adverse reaction to cow's milk, and this is an area of current investigation.[25,26] Researchers in this field support the exploration of behavioral therapies for infant sleep disorders prior to experimental dietary manipulation involving cow's milk elimination. Although some have linked use of cow's milk formula to colic,[27] a definitive association has yet to be established.[26,28]

Treatment of cow's milk allergy involves elimination of the offending source from the diet.[29] This means avoidance of cow's milk, its products, and beverages and foods containing cow's milk, cow's milk products, or cow's milk protein as an ingredient. Management of cow's milk allergy in infants and toddlers is discussed in Chapters 2 and 6. General guidelines for a diet eliminating cow's milk protein are shown in Appendix A. Label reading is an important skill because milk protein content may be indicated using terms such as whey, curds, or sodium caseinate.[8] A diet that eliminates cow's milk protein sources may result in inadequate calcium, vitamin D, riboflavin, and/ or vitamin A intake.[29] Supplementation as appropriate to meet individual needs may be warranted. Consumption of alternative bioavailable calcium sources can be encouraged.

Legumes

Several legumes have been cited as food allergens. These include soybeans, peanut, green peas, taugeh (a variety of sprouted green bean used in egg rolls), garbanzo, and lima beans.[1,3,5,30] Of these, the soybean and peanut have been most extensively studied.

The allergenic protein fractions of soybeans have yet to be fully characterized. The globulin 2S component is considered by some to be the most allergenic fraction with 7S and 11S globulins and hemagglutinin (soybean trypsin inhibitor) also believed to be allergenic.[1,2] Burks et al[31] reported they could find no one soy fraction to be more allergenic than any other.

Manifestations of soybean allergy include gastroenteropathy,[32] asthma,[33] urticaria,[34] eczema, and anaphylaxis.[35] Exposure to soybeans may come from bean consumption, consumption of products containing soy (eg, tofu, miso, soy sauce, textured vegetable protein), occupational exposure to soy flour, or use of a soy-based formula.[33,36]

Because many infants with cow's milk allergy are allergic to soy, soy formulas are no longer recommended by many practitioners as a hypoallergenic alternative.[37] Some practitioners, however, continue to switch a cow's milk-sensitive infant to a soy formula and believe that such a switch is an appropriate therapy strategy. (Olejer in Chapter 2, Part II, discusses use of soy formulas for infants allergic to cow's milk.) Burks et al[38] studied the allergenicity of two types of soy-based infant formulas, liquid versus powder. *In vitro* testing in this study indicated the liquid form may be more allergenic. Donovan and Torres-Pinedo[39] report that some infants who do poorly on soy formulas seem to react adversely to the sugar components, sucrose or dextrimaltose, rather than the soy proteins. They report these infants can be helped by use of a soy-lactose formula.

The ability of soybean oils to cause allergic symptoms has been a subject of investigation. An article written by Swedish researchers indicated that soy proteins could be present in some fat products (margarines and oils).[40] After unsuccessfully challenging seven soy-allergic patients with soy oil, Bush et al[41] concluded most soybean oils were probably not likely to induce an allergic response. These researchers, however, note that certain cold-pressed soy oils may contain soy protein and therefore advise soy-sensitive patients to avoid these products.

Dietary avoidance of soy protein is central to patient management. Avoidance of soy protein means not consuming soybeans and not consuming products containing either soy or lecithin.[8] General guidelines for a diet eliminating soy protein are given in Appendix B.

The peanut is the other extensively studied allergen in the legume group. It is believed that peanuts may contain many allergenic fractions.[1] Examples of fractions studied include peanut I,[42] alpha-arachin, conarachin I, and concanavalin A-reactive glycoprotein.[43] Nordlee et al[44] studied 20 peanut products, including peanut oil. Seventeen were found to be highly allergic. The three products not found to be allergenic or of low allergenicity in this study were peanut hull flour, hydrolyzed peanut protein, and peanut oil. The authors postulated that the allergenic portion of the peanut may be destroyed during the processing of these products. Because peanut hull flour did still exhibit some allergenic potential, the authors advise avoidance by sensitive individuals. (They postulate that the allergenicity of peanut hull flour may relate to residual cotyledon.) The authors also advise further research with regard to the safety of hydrolyzed peanut protein for sensitive individuals. (Nonallergenicity of peanut oil is discussed further in Chapter 9.)

Peanut is a strong allergen. Zimmerman et al[45] report that highly allergic infants may exhibit sensitivity to peanut even when peanut does not appear to have been introduced into the diet. Bock and Atkins[46] in longitudinal studies of pediatric patients report that peanut allergy appears to persist over time.

Clinical manifestations of peanut allergy may include urticaria, angioedema, wheezing, choking, vomiting, rhinorrhea,[47] itching, dyspnea, nausea, asthma, tearing of the eyes, and anaphylaxis.[48] Development of hives from direct skin contact with peanut butter has also been reported.[49] Clinical manifestations can be so severe, patients will need to have self-injecting epinephrine available for emergency use.[48] One report indicated that aspirin use in conjunction with peanut ingestion created serious health problems for a peanut-allergic individual.[50]

Fries[48] points out that induction of allergic reaction is not the only problem with peanut ingestion. Inhalation of peanut can create serious respiratory problems and, on a worldwide basis, the peanut is cited as being the most frequently aspirated foreign object. Even peanut butter can be aspirated and cause death by strangulation.

Allergic individuals must avoid peanuts and products containing peanut proteins. To avoid inhalation problems, some recommend that persons below five years of age should not consume peanuts.[48]

Nuts and Seeds

Various nuts and seeds have been reported to contain allergens and produce clinical symptoms of allergy. Pistachio nuts and cashews have been cited as causes of urticaria, angioedema, and even anaphylaxis.[51] Macadamia nut allergy is reported to have these same manifestations.[52] Recently anaphylaxis and urticaria related to pinon (pine) nut allergy have also been reported.[53] Sesame seed ingestion has been noted to cause asthma, stinging lips, edema of the palate, and anaphylaxis in allergic individuals.[54]

Interest in cottonseed, a potent allergen, has been renewed due to its inclusion in several food products in recent years. Early reports describe the lethal potential of cottonseed protein allergy by citing deaths associated with intradermal testing.[55] Positive skin-test results to cottonseed protein have been reported to be found in 1-6% of patients treated at selected allergy clinics.[56] Clinical problems associated with cottonseed protein allergy include nausea, vomiting, angioedema, urticaria, pruritus, bronchospasm, dysphagia, and edema of the larynx.[56,57] Atkins et al[56] report that many patients first feel an abnormal burning in the mouth or describe a change in taste prior to onset of other symptoms. Label reading is important in management of cottonseed protein allergy. Cottonseed protein flour may be a component of baked goods, candy, and spices.[57] The use of cottonseed protein in cream substitutes and processed meats has been investigated.[56]

Crustacea

Several allergens have been identified in crustacea. Particularly, shrimp allergens have been studied. Types identified include Sa-I and Sa-II (both heat-stable)[58] from *Penaeus indicus* shrimp and antigen I and antigen II from an unknown shrimp variety.[1] Demonstration of allergens for specific shrimp types has been cited in Chapter 2, Part II. As mentioned previously, cross-reaction seems likely among the crustacea (shrimp, lobster, and crawfish).[3]

Shrimp allergy symptoms may become manifest as soon as 15 minutes after consumption.[59] Symptoms seen in association with shrimp allergy include pruritus, urticaria, angioedema, vomiting, nausea, diarrhea, dyspnea, tightness in the chest, hypotension associated with fainting, and anaphylaxis.[60,61]

Waring et al[60] suggest there may be two types of mechanisms by which individuals experience adverse reactions to shrimp. One mechanism would be IgE mediated, and the other would be reaction through another immune or nonimmune mechanism.

Fish

A major fish allergen that has been extensively studied and described is allergen M from codfish. Allergen M is a parvalbumin type of protein of the sarcoplasm.[1,62] Protamine sulfate may also serve as a fish allergen in some instances. Other allergens are believed to be present in fish, but to date have not been identified or described.[1] Fish allergens are considered to be heat stable.[2]

Fish may cause an allergic reaction through ingestion, inhalation, or contact.[2,34,63] Aas[63] even reported that some individuals will react to steam produced during the cooking of fish. Contact dermatitis has been reported via water in which codfish had been washed.[34] Dust from a household where fish has been cooked also may serve as another allergen exposure source. Allergy to one type of fish may or may not be associated with cross-reactivity.[62]

Clinical manifestations of fish allergy may include asthma, urticaria, nasal problems, nausea, vomiting, pruritus, angioedema, diarrhea, and headache.[2,62] Clinical manifestations may appear very quickly after ingestion.[2] Testing is recommended to correctly identify the species of fish to be avoided.[62] Once this is accomplished, dietary counseling can be initiated.

Fruits (Noncitrus) and Vegetables

Several fruits and vegetables have been cited as foods causing allergic reaction. Allergen types in most fruits and vegetables have to be identified but glycoproteins with allergenic potential have been extracted from the tomato.[1] Fruit and vegetable allergies seem to be associated with hay fever and allergies to certain pollens. Ortolani et al[64] describe associations between allergy to cherry, apple, carrot, or pear to birch and allergy to watermelon and tomato to grass. Associations were also found between birch and fennel and walnut allergies and mugwort and allergies to watermelon, celery, and apple.

Ortolani et al[64] also describe a constellation of clinical symptoms known as oral allergy syndrome, which may be seen in conjunction with fruit and vegetable allergy, particularly celery allergy. The initial symptom of oral allergy syndrome consists of swelling and irritation of the mouth and lips occurring a few minutes following consumption. This initial stage may be followed by other symptoms such as urticaria, angioedema of the pharynx, rhinoconjunctivitis, asthma, or anaphylactic shock. Pauli et al[65] also describe symptoms of urticaria, rhinitis, asthma, pruritus, conjunctivitis, and anaphylaxis with celery allergy. Of the 20 patients studied by this group, 16 of the celery-allergic subjects were also sensitive to pollen. Vallier et al[66] recently published evidence that the cross-reacting components among celery, mugwort, and birch pollen may be carbohydrates.

Egg

Hen's eggs contain many potential allergens. The allergens with primary allergenicity are contained in the egg white.[2] At least one report has cited 13 potentially allergenic components in egg white.[67] The principal allergens in the egg white are ovalbumin, ovotransferrin (conalbumin), and ovomucoid.[1,67] Egg yolk proteins may also be allergenic. Specifically cited in this regard have been the yolk proteins apovitellenin I and VI.[68] Research to date also suggests allergic cross-reactivity may exist between some egg proteins in the white and yolk.[69]

IgE antibodies to egg white have been detected in cord blood, and egg allergy is considered to be relatively common during infancy. The incidence of egg allergy appears to decline with age.[70]

Egg allergy may result not only from exposure through ingestion, but inhalation as well.[71-74] Edwards et al[71] concluded that inhalation did not significantly impact on skin-test reactivity to eggs in adults, but Kemp et al[72] reported cases of anaphylaxis in children exposed by the inhalation route to pavlova mix that was being prepared by parents (1 case) and a nurse (1 case). Hoffman and Guenther[73] describe the case of an adult patient who raised birds as a profession and subsequently developed allergy to ingested egg yolk. Allergy to egg yolk subsequent to acquisition of a parrot has also been described.[74]

Symptoms of egg allergy may include pruritus, atopic dermatitis, asthma, vomiting, hives, angioedema, diarrhea, and anaphylaxis.[70,75] Egg allergens may cause adverse reaction through both intestinal allergy and contact dermatitis.[70] Iyngkaran et al[76] present a case study of an infant in whom egg allergy appeared to elicit intestinal abnormalities. These abnormalities included villous atrophy, impaired xylose absorption, and marked decreases in lactase, maltase, and sucrase activities. Rossi et al[77] suggest that in some instances egg allergy may be linked to immune dysfunction, specifically hyperimmunoglobulinemia E in conjunction with defects in polymorphonucleocyte and T-lymphocyte function. Ford and Taylor[78] suggest that egg allergy may be more long-lived in patients who exhibit a variety of clinical symptoms.

The advisability of administering vaccines cultured in egg to egg-allergic individuals remains questionable.[79] Miller et al[80] suggest a distinction be made regarding those who most likely may safely receive egg-containing vaccines and those who may not based on intradermal skin-test results. Greenberg and Birx[81] suggest the majority of egg-sensitive children will not have a reaction to the mumps-measles-rubella vaccine because the vaccine seems to contain only very small quantities of egg. In a study of six asthmatic children with egg allergy, Murphy and Strunk[82] reported that influenza vaccine was not associated with allergic manifestations. Current advisories of the American Academy of Pediatrics and other medical/public health groups should be consulted by physicians dealing with this issue.

Egg allergy is managed by eliminating egg products (both yolk and white) from the diet. Guidelines for managing egg allergy are found in Appendix C.

Wheat and Other Grains

Wheat contains a variety of allergenic proteins and the four main fractions, gliadin, globulin, glutenin, and albumin, are all considered to have allergenic potential.[2,8] Wheat proteins that are ingested or inhaled may cause allergy.[67] Baker's asthma has been attributed to wheat allergy[83] and sometimes wheat allergy may cause gastrointestinal problems.[9] Speer[9] cites wheat allergy as being a food allergen that is likely to cause severe reaction. General patient guidelines are presented in Appendix D.

Several other grains have been associated with allergy. These include corn,[2] rice,[1] rye,[2,9] and buckwheat (buckwheat technically being classified botanically as a part of the weed group).[84] Corn allergy may prove to be an allergy that is difficult to manage if a person is sensitive not only to corn and its major products, but is sensitive to manufactured corn-product derivatives as well, eg, corn syrup or corn sugar.[36] These manufactured derivatives seem to be ubiquitous in processed foods. Guidelines to help in counseling the corn-sensitive patient are presented in Appendix E.

Rice allergens have been identified as being present in both the globulin and glutelin fractions.[1] Speer[9] points out that many people mistakingly believe that rice is a naturally totally hypoallergenic substance. Rye, although it can be allergenic, seems to cause fewer problems than other cereal grains.[9]

Buckwheat prepared as a flour is used in baking. Valdivieso et al[84] describe a case study of a woman who worked preparing crepes who developed a variety of allergic symptoms related to buckwheat exposure. Initial symptoms seemed to relate to inhalation and were respiratory in nature. Contact urticaria developed later, and finally the woman developed gastrointestinal problems (stomach pain, nausea, vomiting) and hives following buckwheat consumption.

Kola Nut Products (Chocolate and Cola)

Speer[9] lists chocolate and cola (kola nut products) as important allergen-containing food items in the American diet. Speer[9] notes both cola and chocolate can cause a variety of allergic symptoms, but the amount of cola in common beverages does not seem to induce hives.

Citrus Fruits

Allergies to citrus fruits have also been noted as common.[2,9] Symptoms of a citrus allergy may include asthma, hives, eczema, and aphthous stomatitis.[9] Avoidance of citrus fruits (and for some people other products containing citric acid) necessitates dietary instruction with regard to alternative vitamin C sources such as melon, strawberries, cabbage, broccoli, brussel sprouts, greens (mustard and collard), green pepper, and potatoes.[36] Juices other than citrus may also be vitamin C-fortified. Examples include vitamin C-fortified grape, apple, and cranberry juices.

Spices

Spices may be responsible for causing allergic reactions. Speer[9] particularly cites cinnamon, bay leaf, peppers (black and white), peppermint, oregano, sage, thyme, and cumin. Speer[9] reports cinnamon as being a common cause of hives. Dominguez et al[85] note the allergic potential of paprika, mustard, and coriander. They recently isolated a protein allergen (molecular weight of 14,000) from mustard seeds.

Exotic and Uncommon Foods

Falliers[53] has recently stressed the importance of foods being recognized as allergen-containing that once were considered rare or uncommon in the typical US diet. As Americans try more ethnic foods and grow or import new food items, different types of food allergy may become more common. Falliers[53] cites the following as foods to which allergic reactions have now been reported: kiwi fruit, papaya, mango, pomegranate, sea urchin, turtle, and sunflower seed. Fallier[53] also reports that allergic reactions to teas such as chamomile and linden have been observed.

Bee Pollen

Patients may develop allergies to products sold as nutritional supplements. Bee pollen is a classic example. The *FDA Consumer*[86] cites a case of a person with seasonal allergy who developed anaphylactic shock subsequent to bee pollen consumption.

Parenteral Nutrition

Allergic reactions to ingredients in parenteral nutrition solutions seem to be rare, but dietitians need to be aware such reactions can occur and have been reported. There was a 1987 report of a child receiving peripheral parenteral nutrition who developed anaphylaxis that appeared to be the result of an allergy to components of an amino acid solution and a multivitamin-infusion product.[87] In 1990, a case report linked another pediatric vitamin product in a parenteral solution to the development of hives.[88] Other components of parenteral nutrition that have been cited as being potentially allergenic include iron, dextran and lipid emulsions.[89,90]

PRINCIPLES OF DIETARY MANAGEMENT

Dietary management of food allergy involves avoidance of the offending allergen or allergens.[91] Dietitians can help patients with the processes of label reading, recipe modification, and special product purchase. It is also the dietitian's responsibility to ensure the diet is nutritionally adequate and provide advice on supplementation when appropriate. Dietitians need to perform nutritional assessments at appropriate intervals. Patient needs may vary in time related to allergy persistence and other concomitant medical problems. As always, dietitians also need to provide encouragement and support, especially to those who are attempting major dietary changes. Specific guidelines for counseling with regard to selected allergies are given in Appendixes A through E. Recipe sources for allergy diets are found in Appendix F.

Elemental diets may be necessary in some instances as a therapeutic modality, but are more commonly used in diagnosis.[92] Elemental diets due to flavor, social, and economic considerations are rarely accepted on a long-term basis. Every effort should be made to reserve these products for short-term therapeutic use only .

Nutritional problems have been documented in relationship to dietary manipulations used to treat food allergies. Lloyd-Still,[93] in 1979, reported on the inappropriate prescription of elimination diets for children that resulted in low calorie intakes and failure to thrive. He also speculated that the use of wheat elimination to treat chronic diarrhea may in some instances lead to a failure to correctly diagnose gluten intolerance (celiac sprue). Sinatra and Merritt[94] describe the development of kwashiorkor in four patients who were placed on a nondairy creamer low in protein. This product had been recommended for treatment of suspected milk allergy. David et al[95] compared diets of children with multiple allergy restrictions to controls and found calcium intake to be a problem for those children following the restricted diet. These researchers urge dietetic involvement in continued assessment and treatment.

Reintroduction of foods to the diet may be associated with problems. Anaphylaxis with reintroduction of corn, chicken, soy, and cow's milk has been reported.[96] Reintroduction of foods should be accomplished only under physician directive.

SUMMARY

Major and some minor food allergens have been described. Although some knowledge exists regarding specific allergen components in food, much work needs to be done in this area of identification. Avoidance of allergens while maintaining appropriate nutritional intake is the goal of dietary therapy.

REFERENCES

1. Taylor SL, Lemanske RF, Bush RK, Busse WW. Food allergens: structure and immunologic properties. *Ann Allergy.* 1987; 59:93–99.

2. Chiaramonte LT, Rao YAK. Common food allergens. In: Chiaramonte LT, Schneider AT, Lifshitz F, eds. *Food Allergy, A Practical Approach to Diagnosis and Management.* New York: Marcel Dekker, Inc; 1988: 89–106.

3. Sachs MI, O'Connell EJ. Cross-reactivity of foods—mechanisms and clinical significance. *Ann Allergy.* 1988; 61:36–40.

4. Barnett D, Bonham B, Howden MEH. Allergenic cross-reactions among legume foods—an in vitro study. *J Allergy Clin Immunol.* 1987; 79:433–438.

5. Bernhisel-Broadbent J, Sampson HA. Cross-allergenicity in the legume botanical family in children with food hypersensitivity. *J Allergy Clin Immunol.* 1989; 83:435–440.

6. Yunginger JW, Sweeney KG, Sturner WQ, et al. Fatal food-induced anaphylaxis. *JAMA*. 1988; 260(10):1450–1452.

7. Bahna SL. Milk allergy. In: Chiaramonte LT, Schneider AT, Lifshitz F, eds. *Food Allergy, A Practical Approach to Diagnosis and Management*. New York: Marcel Dekker, Inc. 1988: 107–116.

8. White JE, Owsley VB. Helping families cope with milk, wheat, and soy allergies. *MCN*. 1983; 8:423–428.

9. Speer F. Food allergy: The 10 common offenders. *Am Fam Physician*. 1976; 13(2):106–112.

10. Businco L, Cantani A, Longhi A, Giampietro PG. Anaphylactic reactions to a cow's milk whey protein hydrolysate (Alpha-Ré, Nestlé) in infants with cow's milk allergy. *Ann Allergy*. 1989; 62:333–335.

11. Collins-Williams C. Cow's milk allergy in infants and children. *Int Arch Allergy*. 1962; 20:38–59.

12. Visakorpi JK. Milk and soybean protein allergy. *J Pediatr Gastroenterol Nutr*. 1983; 2(suppl 1):S293–S297.

13. Bahna SL, Heiner DC. *Allergies to Milk*. New York: Grune & Stratton; 1980.

14. Wilson NW, Hamburger RN. Allergy to cow's milk in the first year of life and its prevention. *Ann Allergy*. 1988; 61:323–327.

15. Roberton DM, Paganelli R, Dinwiddie R, Levinsky RJ. Milk antigen absorption in the preterm and term neonate. *Arch Dis Child*. 1982; 57:369–372.

16. Rapp DJ. Milk allergy—from birth to old age. *Consultant*. 1974; 14:120–122.

17. Olalde S, Bensabat Z, Vives R, Fernandez L, Cabeza NC, Rodriguez J. Allergy to cow's milk with onset in adult life. *Ann Allergy*. 1989; 62:185a–185b.

18. Antibody formation to cow's milk protein or soya protein. *Nutri Rev*. 1983; 41(3):80–82.

19. Anderson GH, Morson-Pasut LA, Bryan H, et al. Age of introduction of cow's milk to infants. *J Pediat Gastroenterol Nutr*. 1985; 4:692–698.

20. Gerrard JW, Shenassa M. Food allergy: two common types as seen in breast and formula fed babies. *Ann Allergy*. 1983; 50:375–379.

21. Taylor GA. Cow's milk protein/soy protein allergy: gastrointestinal imaging. *Radiology*. 1988; 167:866.

22. Wilson JF, Lahey ME, Heiner DC. Studies on iron metabolism, V: further observations on cow's milk-induced gastrointestinal bleeding in infants with iron-deficiency anemia. *J Pediatrics*. 1974; 84(3):335–344.

23. Katz AJ, Twarog FJ, Zeiger RS, Falchuk ZM. Milk-sensitive and eosinophilic gastroenteropathy: similar clinical features with contrasting mechanisms and clinical courses. *J Allergy Clin Immunol*. 1984; 74:72–78.

24. Kemp A. Facts and fallacies about food allergy in children. *Austr Fam Physician*. 1984; 13(3):194–195.

25. Kahn A, Rebuffat E, Blum D, et al. Difficulty in initiating and maintaining sleep associated with cow's milk allergy in infants. *Sleep*. 1987; 10(2):116–121.

26. Kahn A, Mozin MJ, Rebuffat E, Sottiaux M, Muller MF. Milk intolerance in children with persistent sleeplessness: a double-blind crossover evaluation. *Pediatrics*. 1989; 84(4):595–603.

27. Lothe L, Lindberg T, Jakobsson K. Cow's milk formula as a cause of infantile colic: a double-blind study. *Pediatrics*. 1982; 70(1):7–10.

28. Taubman B. Parental counseling compared with elimination of cow's milk or soy milk protein for the treatment of infantile colic syndrome: a randomized trial. *Pediatrics*. 1988; 81(6):756–761.

29. Weyman-Daum M. Milk-free, lactose-free, and lactose-restricted diets. In: Chiaramonte LT, Schneider AT, Lifshitz F, eds. *Food Allergy, A Practical Approach to Diagnosis and Management*. New York: Marcel Dekker, Inc; 1988: 401–420.

30. Van Toorenenbergen AW, Dieges PH. Ig-E mediated hypersensitivity to taugeh (sprouted green beans). *Ann Allergy*. 1984; 53:239–242.

31. Burks AW, Brooks JR, Sampson HA. Allergenicity of major component proteins of soybean determined by enzyme-linked immunosorbent assay (ELISA) and immunoblotting in children with atopic dermatitis and positive soy challenges. *J Allergy Clin Immunol*. 1988; 81:1135–1142.

32. Ford RPK, Walker-Smith JA. Pediatric gastrointestinal food-allergy disease. In: Brostoff J, Challacombe SJ, eds. *Food Allergy and Intolerance*. London: Bailliere Tindall; 1987: 570–582.

33. Bush RK, Schroeckenstein D, Meier-Davis S, Balmes J, Rempel D. Soybean flour asthma: detection of allergens by immunoblotting. *J Allergy Clin Immunol*. 1988; 82:251–255.

34. Schneider AT, Silverman BA. Skin manifestations. In: Chiaramonte LT, Schneider AT, Lifshitz F, eds. *Food Allergy, A Practical Approach to Diagnosis and Management*. New York: Marcel Dekker, Inc; 1988: 193–211.

35. Mortimer EZ. Anaphylaxis following ingestion of soybean. *J Pediatr*. 1961; 58(1):90–92.

36. Dong FM. *All about Food Allergy*. Philadelphia: George F. Stickley Co; 1984.

37. Moses NS. Hypoallergenic formulas. In: Chiaramonte LT, Schneider AT, Lifshitz F, eds. *Food Allergy, A Practical Approach to Diagnosis and Management*. New York: Marcel Dekker, Inc; 1988: 453–464.

38. Burks AW, Butler HL, Brooks JR, Hardin J, Connaughton C. Identification and comparison of differences in antigens in two commercially available soybean protein isolates. *J Food Sci*. 1988; 53(5):1456–1459.

39. Donovan GK, Torres-Pinedo R. Chronic diarrhea and soy formulas-inhibition of diarrhea by lactose. *Am J Dis Child*. 1987; 141:1069–1071.

40. Porras O, Carlsson B, Fällström SP, Hanson LA. Detection of soy protein in soy lecithin, margarine and occasionally, soy oil. *Int Arch Allergy Appl Immunol*. 1985; 78:30–32.

41. Bush RK, Taylor SL, Nordlee JA, Busse WW. Soybean oil is not allergenic to soybean sensitive individuals. *J Allergy Clin Immunol*. 1985; 76:242–245.

42. Sachs MI, Jones RT, Yunginger JW. Isolation and partial characterization of a major peanut allergen. *J Allergy Clin Immunol*. 1981; 67(1):27–34.

43. Barrett D, Baldo BA, Howden MEH. Multiplicity of allergens in peanuts. *J Allergy Clin Immunol*. 1983; 72:61–68.

44. Nordlee JA, Taylor SL, Jones RT, Yunginger JW. Allergenicity of various peanut products as determined by RAST inhibition. *J Allergy Clin Immunol*. 1981; 68(5):376–382.

45. Zimmerman B, Forsyth S, Gold M. Highly atopic children: formation of IgE antibody to food protein, especially peanut. *J Allergy Clin Immunol*. 1989; 83:764–770.

46. Bock SA, Atkins FM. The natural history of peanut allergy. *J Allergy Clin Immunol*. 1989; 83:900–904.

47. Kemp AS, Mellis CM, Barnett D, Sharota E, Simpson J. Skin test, RAST and clinical reactions to peanut allergens in children. *Clin Allergy*. 1985; 15:73–78.

48. Fries JH. Peanuts: allergic and other untoward reactions. *Ann Allergy*. 1982; 48:220–226.

49. Mathias CGT. Contact urticaria from peanut butter. *Contact Dermatitis*. 1983; 9:66–68.

50. Cant AJ, Gibson P, Dancy M. Food hypersensitivity made life threatening by ingestion of aspirin. *Br Med J*. 1984; 288:755–756.

51. Food allergy—pistachios, cashews. *J Asthma*. 1985; 22:123. Letter.

52. Macadam RA. Anaphylaxis to kiwi fruit and exotic items—macadamia nuts. *J Asthma.* 1984; 21:231. Letter.

53. Falliers CJ. Pine nut allergy in perspective. *Ann Allergy.* 1989; 62:186–189.

54. Malish D, Glovsky MM, Hoffman DR, Ghekiere L, Hawkins JM. Anaphylaxis after sesame seed ingestion. *J Allergy Clin Immunol.* 1981; 67(1):35–38.

55. Harris MC, Shure N. Sudden death due to allergy tests. *J Allergy.* 1950; 21:208–216.

56. Atkins FM, Wilson M, Bock SA. Cottonseed hypersensitivity: new concerns over an old problem. *J Allergy Clin Immunol.* 1988; 82:242–250.

57. Malanin G, Kalimo K. Angioedema and urticaria caused by cottonseed protein in whole grain bread. *J Allergy Clin Immunol.* 1988; 82:261–264.

58. Nagpal S, Rajappa L, Metcalfe DD, Subba Rao PV. Isolation and characterization of heat-stable allergens from shrimp *(Penaeus indicus).* *J Allergy Clin Immunol.* 1989; 83:26–36.

59. Daul CB, Morgan JE, Hughes J, Lehrer SB. Provocation-challenge studies in shrimp-sensitive individuals. *J Allergy Clin Immunol.* 1988; 81:1180–1186.

60. Waring NP, Daul CB, De Shazo RD, McCants ML, Lehrer SB. Hypersensitivity reactions to ingested crustacea: clinical evaluation and diagnostic studies in shrimp-sensitive individuals. *J Allergy Clin Immunol.* 1985; 76:440–445.

61. Daul CB, Morgan JE, Waring N-P, McCants ML, Hughes J, Lehrer SB. Immunologic evaluation of shrimp allergic individuals. *J Allergy Clin Immunol.* 1987; 80:716–722.

62. Aas K. Fish allergy and the codfish allergen model. In: Brostoff J, Challacombe SJ, eds. *Food Allergy and Intolerance.* London: Bailliere Tindall, 1987: 356–366.

63. Aas K. Antigens and allergens of fish. *Int Arch Allergy.* 1969; 36:152–155.

64. Ortolani C, Ispano M, Pastorello E, Bigi A, Anasaloni R. The oral allergy syndrome. *Ann Allergy.* 1988; 61(2):47–52.

65. Pauli G, Bessot JC, Braun PA, et al. Celery allergy: clinical and biological study of 20 cases. *Ann Allergy.* 1988; 60:243–246.

66. Vallier P, Dechamp C, Vial O, Deviller P. A study of allergens in celery with cross-sensitivity to mugwort and birch pollens. *Clin Allergy.* 1988; 18:491–500.

67. Gjesing B, Lowenstein H. Immunochemistry of food antigens. *Ann Allergy.* 1984; 53:602–608.

68. Walsh BJ, Barnett D, Burley RW, Elliott C, Hill DJ, Howden MEH. New allergens from hen's egg white and egg yolk—in vitro study of ovomucin, apovitellenin I and VI, and phosvitin. *Int Arch Allergy Appl Immunol.* 1988; 87:81–86.

69. Walsh BJ, Elliott C, Baker RS, et al. Allergenic cross-reactivity of egg-white and egg-yolk proteins—an in vitro study. *Int Arch Allergy Appl Immunol.* 1987; 84:228–232.

70. Langeland T, Aas K. Allergy to hen's egg white: clinical and immunological aspects. In: Brostoff J, Challacombe SH, eds. *Food Allergy and Intolerance.* London: Bailliere Tindall; 1987: 367–374.

71. Edwards JH, McConnochie K, Davies BH. Skin-test reactivity to egg protein—exposure by inhalation compared to ingestion. *Clin Allergy.* 1985; 15:147–150.

72. Kemp AS, Van Asperen PP, Douglas J. Anaphylaxis caused by inhaled pavlova mix in egg-sensitive children. *Med J. Austr.* 1988; 149:712–713.

73. Hoffman DR, Guenther DM. Occupational allergy to avian proteins presenting as allergy to ingestion of egg yolk. *J Allergy Clin Immunol.* 1988; 81(2):484–488.

74. De Maat-Bleeker F, Van Dijk AG, Berrens L. Allergy to egg yolk possibly induced by sensitization to bird serum antigens. *Ann Allergy.* 1985; 54:245–248.

75. Langeland T. A clinical and immunological study of allergy to hen's egg white. *Clin Allergy.* 1983; 13:371–382.

76. Iyngkaran N, Abidin Z, Meng LL, Yadav M. Egg-protein-induced villous atrophy. *J Pediatr Gastroenterol Nutr.* 1982; 1:29–33.

77. Rossi P, Galli E, Cantani A, Perlini R, Sellitto F, Businco L. A case of hyperimmunoglobulinemia E treated with cow's milk and egg-free diet. *Ann Allergy.* 1982; 49:159–164.

78. Ford RPK, Taylor B. Natural history of egg hypersensitivity. *Arch Dis Child.* 1982; 57:649–652.

79. Greenberg LE, Moses NS. Egg-free and corn-free diets. In: Chiaramonte LT, Schneider AT, Lifshitz F, eds. *Food Allergy, A Practical Approach to Diagnosis and Management.* New York: Marcel Dekker, Inc; 1988: 441–452.

80. Miller JR, Orgel HA, Meltzer EO. The safety of egg-containing vaccines for egg-allergic patients. *J Allergy Clin Immunol.* 1983; 71(6):568–573.

81. Greenberg MA, Birx DL. Safe administration of mumps-measles-rubella vaccine in egg-allergic children. *J Pediatr.* 1988; 113(3):504–506.

82. Murphy KR, Strunk RC. Safe administration of influenza vaccine in asthmatic children hypersensitive to egg proteins. *J Pediatr.* 1985; 106(6):931–933.

83. Prichard MG, Ryan G, Walsh BJ, Musk AW. Skin test and RAST responses to wheat and common allergens and respiratory disease in bakers. *Clin Allergy.* 1985; 15:203–210.

84. Valdivieso R, Moneo I, Pola J, et al. Occupational asthma and contact urticaria caused by buckwheat flour. *Ann Allergy.* 1989; 63:149-152.

85. Dominguez J, Cuevas M, Ureña V, Muñoz T, Moneo I. Purification and characterization of an allergen of mustard seed. *Ann Allergy.* 1990; 64:352–357.

86. Larkin T. Bee pollen as a health food. *FDA Consumer.* 1984; 18(3):21–22.

87. Pomeranz S, Gimmon Z, Zvi AB, Katz S. Parenteral nutrition-induced anaphylaxis. *JPEN.* 1987; 11(3):314–315.

88. Bullock L, Etchason E, Fitzgerald JF, McGuire WA. Case report of an allergic reaction to parenteral nutrition in a pediatric patient. *JPEN.* 1990; 14(1):98–100.

89. Udall JN, Richardson DS. Allergic reactions to parenteral nutrition solutions. *Nutr Support Serv.* 1986; 6:20–22.

90. Kamath KR, Berry A, Cummins G. Acute hypersensitivity reaction to Intralipid. *N Engl J Med.* 1981; 304:360. Letter.

91. American Dietetic Association. *Food Sensitivity: A Resource Including Recipes.* Chicago: The American Dietetic Association; 1985.

92. Rao YAK, Bahna SL. Dietary management of food allergies. In: Chiaramonte LT, Schneider AT, Lifshitz F, eds. *Food Allergy, A Practical Approach to Diagnosis and Management.* New York: Marcel Dekker, Inc; 1988: 351–364.

93. Lloyd-Still JD. Chronic diarrhea of childhood and the misuse of elimination diets. *J Pediatr.* 1979; 95(1):10–13.

94. Sinatra FR, Merritt RJ. Iatrogenic kwashiorkor in infants. *Am J Dis Child.* 1981; 135:21-23.

95. David TJ, Waddington E, Stanton RHJ. Nutritional hazards of elimination diets in children with atopic eczema. *Arch Dis Child.* 1984; 59:323–325.

96. David TJ. Anaphylactic shock during elimination diets for severe atopic eczema. *Arch Dis Child.* 1984; 59:983–986.

Chapter 4

Drug Therapy of Food Allergies
Paul L. Doering

INTRODUCTION

The simplest and most logical way to prevent food allergies is to eliminate the offending agent(s) from the diet. Unfortunately, some people are unable or unwilling to completely avoid such foodstuffs. Even when a diet plan is fully implemented, a patient may inadvertently ingest a food substance to which he or she is known to be allergic. It is in these cases that medications can provide some degree of relief from the symptoms of food allergy.

In cases of anaphylactic reactions, therapy must be instituted on an emergency basis to prevent bronchospasm and shock. Other manifestations of allergy may be less dramatic and may include asthma symptoms, urticaria, rhinorrhea, and other expressions of mast cell degranulation. Food-induced migraine headache is also amenable to certain drug therapy.

Until recently, drug therapy of food allergies has focused on treating the symptoms associated with the release of histamine and other inflammatory mediators from the mast cell. In the past several years significant advances in the understanding of the mechanisms of food allergy have been made, and as a result, treatment has become more specific and more effective. This chapter highlights some of the newer forms of therapy and reviews the more traditional approaches to treating food allergies.

EPINEPHRINE AND OTHER ADRENERGICS

Epinephrine is still the drug of choice in the emergency treatment of severe anaphylactic reaction, including food-induced anaphylaxis. Symptoms such as urticaria, pruritus, angioedema, and swelling of the lips, eyelids, and tongue that may result from reactions to foods, drugs, sera, insect stings, or other allergens may be relieved by epinephrine.

Anaphylaxis is considered a medical emergency in which early recognition and treatment can be lifesaving. Often patients who might accidentally be exposed to foods to which they are known to be sensitive (eg, egg, nuts, peanuts, milk, and others) are given injectable forms of epinephrine to carry with them. Preloaded syringes designed to automatically deliver a precise dose of the drug are available on a prescription basis. One such product, the EpiPen® autoinjector system, is a prefilled syringe that delivers either 0.3 mg (adult) or 0.15 mg (children) of epinephrine. It is intended for immediate self-administration by individuals with a history of anaphylactic reactions. It is designed as emergency supportive therapy only, and patients should be advised to seek medical attention or hospital care as soon as possible after using the device.

A physician who prescribes the EpiPen® should take appropriate steps to ensure that the patient thoroughly understands the indications and use of this device. The physician should review with the patient, in detail, the instruction materials and operation of the autoinjector. Instructions call for the drug to be administered intramuscularly in the anterolateral aspect of the thigh. Because epinephrine is subject to degradation due to heat or when exposed to air, it should be periodically examined to ensure there is no discoloration, precipitation, or other indications the product is not up to its full potency. Use of the autoinjector is very simple and consists of the following steps:

1. Remove the gray safety cap.
2. Place the black tip of the syringe at a right angle to the thigh.
3. Press hard into the thigh until the autoinjector functions. Hold in place for several seconds. Then remove the autoinjector and discard.
4. Massage the injection area for 10 seconds.

In the emergency department, doses of epinephrine are administered either subcutaneously or intramuscularly. The adult dose of epinephrine for emergency treatment of sensitivity reactions is 0.1–0.5 mg (0.1–0.5 ml of a 1:1000 injection). Children should receive 0.01 mg/kg (0.01 ml/kg of a 1:1000 injection). Doses may need to be repeated at 10- to 15-minute intervals in shock and at 20-minute intervals of asthma symptoms in order to sustain the beneficial effects of the drug. Once adequate ventilation is assured, blood pressure maintenance in patients with anaphylactic shock should be achieved with other pressor agents such as norepinephrine or metaraminol. Antihistamines and corticosteroids may be useful if symptoms of allergy persist.

Other adrenergic agents, such as isoproterenol, terbutaline, albuterol, and metaproterenol, do not protect against the shock accompanying anaphylactic reactions and should not be recommended. Food-induced asthmatic attacks can be treated with adrenergic agents acting on the β-adrenergic receptors, particularly when administered by the inhalation route. Metered-dose aerosols are particularly suitable for outpatient use, while hospitalized patients may require treatment with nebulized β-adrenergic agents (Table 4-1).

Table 4-1 Metered-Dose Aerosols in the Management of Food-Induced Asthma

Brand Name	Generic Drug
Alupent®	Metaproterenol sulfate
Brethaire®	Terbutaline sulfate
Isuprel®	Isoproterenol hydrochloride
Metaprel®	Metaproterenol sulfate
Proventil®	Albuterol
Ventolin®	Albuterol

ORAL CROMOLYN

Sodium cromoglycate, or cromolyn as it is more commonly known, has been used for many years in the management of asthma. More recently, it has been given orally in the treatment of food allergy. Cromolyn can best be described as a mast cell stabilizer. It prevents the release of mediators of type I allergic reactions, including histamine and slow-reacting substances of anaphylaxis (SRS-A) from sensitized mast cells after the antigen-antibody union has taken place. Cromolyn does not alter the binding of IgE to the mast cells nor the interaction between cell-bound IgE and specific antigen. Instead, cromolyn suppresses the release of the inflammatory mediators in response to the antigen-antibody reaction.

Cromolyn is poorly absorbed from the GI tract and, until recently, was not given by the oral route. Historically, it has been used by inhalation as a prophylactic in the management of bronchial asthma. It has no role in the treatment of an acute attack of asthma, especially status asthmaticus, because it has no intrinsic bronchodilating activity. An oral version of cromolyn sodium has recently become available under the brand name, Gastrocrom.® Marketed as a capsule containing 100 mg of the drug, its contents are emptied into hot water to make a solution. Prescribers are urged to consult the labeling for this drug for specific instructions on indications, dosing, and method of administration.

In preventing asthma, cromolyn is administered as a powder that reaches the lungs after inhalation, using the special oral inhaler (Spinhaler®), and is then absorbed into the systemic circulation. Cromolyn is also used to prevent allergen-induced and exercise-induced bronchospasm.

More recently, the drug has been used in the treatment of food allergies and food-induced migraine headaches.[1-6] The exact mechanism by which some foods cause migraine attacks is unknown. However, it may be the result of a local immune complex-mediated mechanism in the gut. In food-associated migraine, there appears to be an increase in gut mucosal permeability. In healthy subjects the absorbed antigens and immune complexes are rapidly cleared from the circulation, but in susceptible individuals this process appears not to occur efficiently, leading to the development of allergic symptoms or migraine headaches.[7] Prophylactic administration of cromolyn appears to reduce antigen entry into the circulatory system and diminish immune complex formation. This reduction is a result of cromolyn's local inhibition of gut mast cell degranulation and a reduction in vascular permeability.

Monro et al[4] evaluated the efficacy of oral cromolyn pretreatment in 10 patients with food-induced migraine headaches. The dose of cromolyn used during the course of challenge testing ranged from 400 to 1600 mg/day. Each patient was given the drug for seven days prior to the challenge test. Following the course of pretreatment with cromolyn, 1 patient had complete protection with 400 mg/day, 8 experienced partial or complete protection while receiving 800 or 1600 mg/day, and 1 seemed to have no protection, but he did not adhere to his diet. Even though the cromolyn was capable of offering some forms of protection during the single-challenge test, those patients that failed to adhere to their exclusion diet while receiving cromolyn maintenance therapy all experienced a return of their migraine headaches.

In a similar study, patients were given capsules of cromolyn or placebo in a double-blind trial. Participants were pretreated with 1000 mg cromolyn (500 mg orally 2 hours and 0.5 hour before food challenge). Of the nine patients challenged, five experienced complete protection and three were partially protected, following pretreatment with cromolyn when compared to pretreatment with placebo.[6]

Mansfield et al[3] noted that of the 16 patients with positive food skin tests and 27 with negative skin tests, 11 of those with positive tests and 2 without experienced a decrease in headache frequency. Six patients were symptom free.

Freier and Berger[8] resolved whole milk intolerance in four Jewish infants with positive skin tests for lactoglobulin or milk protein. Dosage of cromolyn was 50 mg/5 ml in chloroform water every 6 hours. Kuzemko and Simpson[9] also halted a cow's milk allergy in two infants with the same treatment for at least two months. A 33-year-old female had multiple food allergies, especially fruit and fish, that were unresponsive to antihistamines. She experienced no reactions to these antigens when pretreated with 100 mg to 400 mg of oral cromolyn, but reaction followed each food challenge with placebo pretreatment.[10] Molkhou and Waguet[11] reported the use of oral cromolyn in 35 children with proven food allergy and atopic dermatitis. Oral cromolyn (200–600 mg/day) improved skin lesions and protected them from the effects of rechallenge with food allergens.

Cromolyn appears to work best in conjunction with a comprehensive dietary program to restrict or exclude those foods causing the worst problems. The dosage range of cromolyn is 50-1600 mg/day, given in 4 equally divided doses.

Intestinal mucosal biopsies of some food-sensitive patients have shown increased mucosal IgE and mast cells.[12] It seems likely that food reactions that are rapid in onset and clear within 24-48 hours after exposure are due to type I (IgE) sensitivity. The best regimen appears to be the restriction of all allergens for 2 or 3 days while taking the drug 30 minutes before meals and at bedtime. Then protection is continued if the regimen is maintained on this schedule.

The use of cromolyn by oral administration is not the usual way of administering the drug. As stated previously, the capsule is manufactured for use by asthmatics in a Spinhaler.® When used orally, the capsule cannot be swallowed whole, as would be the case with ordinary oral medications. Instead, the powder of a cromolyn capsule for use in the Spinhaler is dissolved in a small amount of hot water and administered to infants by dropper. The solution should be swished in the mouth before it is swallowed in order to coat the oral mucous membranes. Specific recommendations, including demonstration of proper administration technique, should be conveyed to the patient at the time the prescription is written. (As previously noted, an oral form of cromolyn has recently appeared on the market.)

Adverse reactions to cromolyn are minimal but have been reported. Vaz et al[13] observed adverse reactions in 7 of 24 patients in their clinical trial. These patients experienced headache, insomnia, urticaria, and rhinorrhea. It was also noted that there may be a correlation between those patients reacting adversely to food and those reacting adversely to cromolyn. One unexpected benefit noted was the reduction or complete absence of perennial allergic rhinitis in several patients while taking the drug.

ANTIHISTAMINES

Histamine$_1$ (H$_1$) antagonists are antihistamines that prevent the binding of histamine to its receptor sites. Antihistamines are more effective at preventing the actions of released histamine than in reversing symptoms once they have taken place. Reversal of symptoms, when it does occur, is most likely caused by the anticholinergic properties of these drugs and not antagonism of histamine. The anticholinergic property is responsible for the drying effect of antihistamines, which reduces the problem of nasal, salivary, and lacrimal gland hypersecretion. Antihistamines antagonize capillary permeability, wheal and flare formation, and itching.

Histamine$_2$ (H$_2$) receptor antagonists, such as cimetidine and ranitidine, may have some effect on histamine-induced nasal blockage, but not on sensory nerves. These agents currently do not have a role in treating allergic processes.

There are numerous individual antihistamines, available in a variety of dosage forms, in seemingly infinite combinations with other ingredients. Decongestants, expectorants, cough suppressants, and analgesics are often combined with antihistamines to provide multisymptom relief. Specialized dosage forms such as sustained-release tablets and capsules have been available for several years and may make taking these drugs more convenient. In general, patients should strive to take as few drugs as possible. Thus, specialized products with multiple ingredients should be avoided, unless a patient is suffering from multiple symptoms. The "shotgun" approach to symptom management invites problems with adverse reactions: single-entity antihistamine products should be used whenever possible.

Drowsiness is usually the chief complaint of patients who take antihistamines. This can interfere with a patient's ability to drive a car or operate machinery and may interfere with a patient's ability to function adequately at the workplace. The sedative effects of antihistamines vary from class to class. Table 4-2 lists common antihistamines in relation to their propensity for causing drowsiness. It should be noted that there is great patient-to-patient variability in the degree of sedation produced from the same drug and considerable variation from product to product within the same patient. Trial and error may be the best way of deciding which product is suitable for a given patient.

Some patients welcome the sedative effects of antihistamines when sleeplessness from the allergic symptoms becomes troublesome. When given at bedtime, these drugs may allow the patient to sleep restfully. The ability to produce sedation is likely related to the drug's ability to cross the blood-brain barrier.[14] Most antihistamines are lipid soluble and cross this barrier easily. Notable exceptions include terfenadine and astemizole, two of the so-called nonsedating antihistamines.

As stated above, antihistamines have prominent anticholinergic effects. These include dry mouth, blurred vision, difficult urination, constipation, and tachycardia. Some patients are predisposed to problems with antihistamines (eg, patients on concurrent medications producing CNS depressant effects or elderly males with enlarged prostate glands). Patients with glaucoma should be given antihistamines with caution, to avoid aggravating the increased intraocular pressure of this disease. Additional side effects of antihistamines are listed in Table 4-3.

Antihistamines are more effective when taken approximately one to two hours before the anticipated exposure to the offending agent. If tolerance

Table 4-2 Drowsiness from Antihistamines

High Potential

Diphenhydramine hydrochloride (Benadryl®)
Promethazine hydrochloride (Phenergan®)
Hydroxyzine hydrochloride or Pamoate (Atarax® or Vistaril®)

Moderate Potential

Azatadine maleate (Optimine®)
Tripelennamine hydrochloride (PBZ®)
Trimeprazine (Temaril®)

Low Potential

Chlorpheniramine maleate (Chlortrimeton®)
Dexchlorpheniramine maleate (Polaramine®)
Brompheniramine maleate (Dimetane®)
Triprolidine hydrochloride (Actidil®)
Cyproheptadine hydrochloride (Periactin®)

Low to None

Terfenadine (Seldane®)
Astemizole (Hisminal®)

Table 4-3 Some Side Effects of Antihistamines

Drowsiness
Dry mouth, nose, or throat
Blurred vision or other changes in vision
Confusion
Difficult urination
Dizziness
Fast heartbeat
Increased appetite (cyproheptadine hydrochloride only)
Increased sensitivity to the sun
Increased sweating
Nightmares
Unusual excitement, nervousness, restlessness, or irritability
Stomach upset

develops to the therapeutic effect, changing to an agent in a different chemical class may restore effectiveness.[15]

It is important for patients to be counseled on the safe and effective use of antihistamines. They should be advised about side effects and should be told what to do if they are experienced. They should be told in particular that driving an automobile may be hazardous, and perhaps they should let someone else drive until they see how the drug will affect them individually. They should be warned about mixing antihistamines with other drugs, including other prescription and nonprescription drugs with drowsiness as a side effect. Alcohol should be avoided when taking antihistamines.

Overall, the effectiveness of antihistamines in treatment of food allergies has been the subject of controversy. Some authorities[16] have suggested that antihistamines should be given to food-allergic children before meals to reduce the severity of the reaction, but clearly anaphylactic food allergies or severe reactions cannot be treated in this manner.

CORTICOSTEROIDS

Corticosteroids such as prednisone, dexamethasone, and methylprednisolone have been prescribed for certain types of food allergies (see Table 4-4), but side effects often limit their long-term usefulness. Patients with eosinophilic gastroenteritis and gastroenteritis due to severe milk allergy[17] are most likely to get positive results from such treatment. Whenever possible, specific food avoidance should be employed in patients with severe food allergies. In accidental exposure, such as in children who inadvertently ingest milk-containing foods in face of severe milk allergy, epinephrine is the drug of first choice, not corticosteroids.

Corticosteroid therapy is plagued by a long list of devastating side effects, overshadowing the long-term good these drugs can do. Virtually every organ

---

Table 4-4 Some Common Corticosteroid Preparations

Brand Name	Generic Name
Aristocort®	Triamcinolone
Celestone®	Betamethasone acetate
Cortef®	Hydrocortisone acetate
Decadron®	Dexamethasone
Depo-Medrol®	Methylprednisolone acetate
Various manufacturers	Prednisone
	Prednisolone

system of the body can be damaged by long-term steroid therapy. Table 4-5 lists some possible side effects of steroid therapy. It should be noted that steroid-induced side effects are a function of both dose and duration of therapy. Short-term therapy (10–14 days) is rarely associated with serious side effects, even when high doses are used. Long-term treatment, measured in months and years, is sure to produce side effects. The higher the dose, the greater the risk of more severe side effects. Steroids often produce dramatic relief of symptoms (especially in inflammatory diseases such as rheumatoid arthritis), and it is tempting for the prescriber to overlook long-term toxicity for the short-term relief steroids afford. Likewise, patients come to demand continuing treatment with these drugs, not fully understanding they are harming themselves in the process. Health care professionals must ade-

---

Table 4-5 Some Side Effects of Corticosteroids

Adrenal insufficiency
Muscle wasting
Muscle pain or weakness
Delayed wound healing
Osteoporosis
Aseptic necrosis of the femoral or humeral heads
Increased susceptibility to infections
Fluid and electrolyte disturbances
Cataract formation
Increased intraocular pressure
Cushing's syndrome
Amenorrhea
Decreased glucose tolerance
Hyperglycemia
Aggravation or precipitation of diabetes mellitus
Nausea, vomiting, anorexia, or increased appetite
Diarrhea or constipation
Abdominal distention
Pancreatitis
Gastric irritation
Ulcerative esophagitis
Peptic ulceration with possible perforation
Headache, vertigo, insomnia, and restlessness
Mental disturbances (including euphoria, mood swings, depression, anxiety, and
    personality changes)
Skin atrophy and thinning
Acne
Hirsutism
Facial erythema, striae, petechiae, ecchymoses, and easy bruising

---

quately counsel patients on the concept of benefit to risk, especially when the side effects are as numerous and severe as with corticosteroids. For food allergies, the benefits do not seem to justify routine administration of corticosteroids.

SUMMARY

Drug therapy for food allergies can be considered as an adjunct to dietary management. Theoretically, if complete avoidance of all offending foods can be accomplished, there would be no need for drug treatment. However, experience shows even the most diet-conscious patient can become accidentally exposed. Epinephrine must be used for severe reactions. Antihistamines and/or corticosteroids can help manage less severe symptoms, but neither are satisfactory for long-term administration. Oral cromolyn seems to be effective in preventing food allergies in carefully selected patients, but the patient should not interpret its availability as a green light to eat foods to which he or she knows a reaction will occur.

REFERENCES

1. Brostoff J, Carini C, Wraith DG, et al. Production of IgE complexes by allergen challenge in atopic patients and the effect of sodium cromoglycate. *Lancet.* 1979; 1:1268–1270.

2. Jones EA. Oral cromolyn sodium in milk induced anaphylaxis. *Ann Allergy.* 1984; 52:223. Abstract.

3. Mansfield LE, Vaughan TR, Waller SF, et al. Food allergy and adult migraine: double blind and mediator conformation of an allergic etiology. *Ann Allergy.* 1985; 55:126–129.

4. Monro J, Brostoff J, Carini C, et al. Food allergy in migraine. *Lancet.* 1980; 2:1–4.

5. Monro J, Carini C, Brostoff J. Migraine is a food allergic disease. *Lancet.* 1984; 2:719–721.

6. Nizami RM, Lewin PK, Baboo MT. Oral cromolyn therapy in patients with food allergy: a preliminary report. *Ann Allergy.* 1977; 39:102–105.

7. Paganelli R, Levinsky RJ, Brostoff J, et al. Immune complexes containing food proteins in normal and atopic subjects after oral challenge and effect of sodium cromoglycate on antigen absorption. *Lancet.* 1979; 1:1270–1272.

8. Freier S, Berger H. Disodium cromoglycate in gastrointestinal protein intolerance. *Lancet.* 1973; 1:913–915.

9. Kuzemko JA, Simpson KR. Treatment of allergy to cow's milk. *Lancet.* 1975; 1:337–338. Letter.

10. Kingsley PJ. Oral sodium cromoglycate in gastrointestinal allergy. *Lancet.* 1974; 2:1011. Letter.

11. Molkhou P, Waguet JC. Food allergy and atopic dermatitis in children: treatment with oral sodium cromoglycate. *Ann Allergy.* 1981; 47:173–175.

12. Shiner M, Ballard J, Smith ME. The small intestinal mucosa in cow's milk allergy. *Lancet.* 1975; 1:136–140.

13. Vaz GA, Tan LKT, and Gerrard JW. Oral cromoglycate in the treatment of adverse reactions to food. *Lancet.* 1978; 1:1066–1068.

14. Douglas WW. Histamine and 5-hydroxytryptamine (serotonin) and their antagonists. In: Gilman AG, Goodman LS, Rall TW, et al, eds. *The Pharmacologic Basis of Therapeutics.* 7th ed. New York: Macmillan; 1985: 605–638.

15. Cooper JW. Antihistamines and decongestants in the treatment of chronic rhinitis. In: Settipane GA, ed. *Rhinitis.* Providence, RI; *N Engl Reg Allergy Proc* 1982: 103–107.

16. Bahna SL, Furukawa CT. Food allergy: Diagnosis and treatment. *Ann Allergy.* 1983; 51:574–580.

17. Waldmann TA, Wochner RD, Laster L, Gordon RS. Allergic gastroenteropathy: A cause of excessive gastrointestinal protein loss. *N Engl J Med.* 1967; 276:761–769.

Chapter 5

Maternal Influences on the Development of Food Allergy in the Infant

Judy E. Perkin

A mother may influence allergic expression in her infant through a variety of mechanisms. Genetics particularly is recognized as a major contributor to allergy development[1-10] and it has been reported that allergy incidence may be as high as 68% if both parents have allergies and 55% if one parent has allergies.[3]

Heredity is believed to play a role by influencing both allergen-specific factors (such as suppressor genes and immune response) and nonspecific-allergen factors (such as general levels of responsiveness to IgE).[6] Environmental factors also influence the development of food allergy,[6] and diet is a major environmental factor of interest.

Research and clinical observations indicate in some instances diet during pregnancy and lactation may influence allergy development in an infant. It would appear that maternal diet may exert its influence either prenatally (*in utero* sensitization) or postnatally (through breastfeeding). Breastfeeding as a maternal choice may also influence allergy incidence through other components in breast milk not directly related to maternal diet.

PRENATAL SENSITIZATION

The belief that prenatal sensitization (related to maternal diet) can occur is based on knowledge that food antigens appear to cross the placenta[3,11,12] and the human fetus does have the capability to synthesize IgE.[6,13] Clinical observations of food sensitivity (such as eczema) on first known postnatal ingestion (sometimes breast milk),[11,12,14] positive testing soon after birth,[11,12,15] and high hemagglutinating antibody titers in amniotic fluid,[11] cord blood, and newborn serum also support the concept that prenatal sensitization can occur. (It should be noted that symptoms upon first postnatal exposure have also been attributed to exposure to antigens in breast milk or hidden food exposure.[14])

81

Evidence related to the ability of food antigens to cross the placenta is both direct and indirect. Matsumura et al[11] reported that food antigens have been identified by passive cutaneous anaphylaxis (PCA) reaction in amniotic fluid, cord blood, and meconium. This research team also reported the identification of hemagglutinating food antibodies in amniotic fluid and cord blood, as well as newborn sera. Michel et al[16] also provide indirect evidence for prenatal sensitization via demonstration (by RAST) of IgE antibody to cow's milk in cord samples of newborns whose mothers had no evidence of such antibodies.

IgE, as stated previously, is the major human antibody associated with allergic disease.[17] Maternal IgE does not cross the placenta.[18,19] The human fetal lungs and liver can synthesize IgE by 11 weeks, and the spleen can synthesize IgE by 21 weeks.[13] Miller et al[13] concluded from these physiological findings "that the conceptus has the potential, in terms of IgE synthesis, for developing reagin-mediated sensitivity in utero."

IgE in cord blood (or sera) is believed to be of fetal origin in most cases,[20] although there can be admixture with maternal blood in anywhere from 3% to 72% of pregnancies.[6] Cord blood has been extensively studied as a predictor of allergic disease. Most infants at birth have little or no detectable IgE in cord blood. High levels of IgE cord blood at birth have been linked to subsequent allergy development.[20] Michel et al,[16] Businco et al,[21] Hamburger,[22] and Chandra, Puri, and Cheema[23] have demonstrated that measurement of umbilical venous cord IgE can be useful in detecting allergy-prone infants.

It should be of interest to dietitians to know what foods in the mother's diet during pregnancy have been linked to allergy development in the infant. Foods implicated have been eggs,[11,15] wheat,[15] soybean,[12] milk,[12,14] and peanut.[14]

One preliminary study addressed a potential link between problems clinically associated with pregnancy and prenatal food sensitization. Baylis et al[24] conducted a retrospective study of 21 mothers of children with allergy to cow's milk matched with an equal number of controls. Nausea was found to be more persistent during the day for the allergic group mothers compared to controls; however, there was no difference found between the two groups in terms of incidence of nausea or frequency of vomiting. The researchers postulated that nausea or vomiting in response to nausea may be related to increased human chorionic gonadotropin (HCG). HCG in high levels may negatively influence the responsiveness of lymphocytes to antigens. More work is needed to substantiate any potential links such as the one just described.

It is accepted that prenatal (in utero) sensitization to food antigens can occur. However it is extremely important to note the phenomenon is believed to be very rare.[9,20] A recent study cites that no more than 2% of all newborns are believed to experience such prenatal sensitization.[20] The implications of the infrequent occurrence of this phenomenon will be explored further at the conclusion of this chapter when efforts to prevent food allergy are reviewed.

BREASTFEEDING AND ATOPIC DISEASE

Breastfeeding has been postulated to exert a protective effect with regard to infant food allergy development through a variety of mechanisms. One factor believed to be highly significant is that breastfeeding may reduce exposure to food antigens.[25] It is theorized that an exclusively breastfed infant is less subject to assault by foreign proteins than is an infant subjected to cow's milk protein formula or other antigens soon after birth.[25]

Some also believe that a breast milk component, specifically secretory IgA (SIgA), may offer protective benefits by retarding entry of antigens at mucosal surfaces.[17,25,26] SIgA is the major antibody component of human milk, and it has been demonstrated that SIgA antibodies of milk are targeted for maternal dietary proteins.[26] SIgA is believed to work by blocking contact between the intestinal mucosa and food antigens.[26,27]

The hormones associated with pregnancy and lactation, estrogen, progesterone, and prolactin, act to stimulate IgA synthesis and secretion.[28] High levels of SIgA in breast milk are believed by some to result from targeted clearance to the mammary gland (ie, by traveling lymphoid cells from Peyer's patches).[26,28] SIgA is also produced in the mammary gland itself because there are cells capable of IgA production in this location.[26]

Breast milk supplies approximately 0.5-1 g of SIgA on a daily basis.[26,28] Colostrum, secreted in the first 24 hours of life, is believed to supply up to 11g of SIgA to the newborn.[28] Cruz et al[29] among others suggest that SIgA found in breast milk relates to maternal dietary exposure. These researchers suggest allergies may be prevented if mothers consume potentially allergenic foods and subsequent production of antibodies occurs.

Although once in question, recent studies would support that intact immunoglobulins such as IgA are absorbed by the neonatal intestine.[30] Further support for the protective role of SIgA is the relatively high incidence of allergy noted in persons who are IgA deficient.[31] It has been postulated that low breast milk content of IgA relative to antigens in breast milk may play a role in allergies.[32]

Breast milk is also cited to potentially contain a factor that may allow the neonate to begin its own IgA production at an earlier point in the maturational cycle.[25] Pittard and Bill[33] demonstrated significantly increased IgA synthesis when supernates from incubated colostrum cells were put into peripheral blood leukocyte cultures.

IgG may play a role as well.[18,34] It has been postulated that maternal immunization, the active component of which is serum-specific IgG, may reduce specific IgE responses in the newborn. Breast milk may play a role in decreasing allergy incidence by supplying IgG antibodies directed against food allergens.[34]

The possibility that breast milk or colostrum may increase the rate of intestinal maturation of the neonate is another potential mechanism being investigated in regard to breast milk's role in modulating atopic manifestations. Enhancement of the maturation of intestinal epithelium is an action that has been attributed to colostrum.[35,36] Udall et al,[36] studying newborn rabbits fed bovine serum albumin, found a significant decrease in circulating concentrations of intact antigen after four hours in the breastfed compared to the bottle-fed animals at one week of age (p <.02), but not at two weeks. Udall's[36] study suggests some immediate postpartum protection associated with breastfeeding may be conferred. Although this study could not demonstrate differences in intestinal morphology between the two rabbit groups, the investigators noted changes in the glycocalyx (the glycoprotein covering of the intestinal surface) or other maturational changes might be factors in explaining the observed outcome.

This area is an important one for further study because the permeability of the infant's immature intestinal tract is believed to be a factor in allergy development.[1,37] Walker[37] cites research with fetal monkeys and human fetuses that describe morphology suggestive of structural immaturity of the cells of the intestinal epithelium. Fetal research has also demonstrated abnormally high uptake levels of large molecules by these cells. It has been suggested that this intestinal immaturity may persist into the neonatal period. Walker[37] also postulates that in the immature intestine more protein ingested by the intestinal epithelial cell may escape proteolysis and move into the circulation. It is important to note that as a result of developmentally normal increased intestinal permeability a modest and short-lived IgE response to food antigens has even been observed in healthy infants with no allergy problems.[1]

Recent studies in animals have linked changes in intestinal microvillous membrane fatty acid composition and protein composition to the maturation process.[38] Sheard and Walker[38] cite specific factors in breast milk that are believed to accelerate the process of maturation in the gastrointestinal tract. Examples of such factors are nerve and epidermal growth factors, somatomedin-C, taurine, glutamine, and amino sugars.

An additional mechanism that may be involved in the allergy-protective role of breastfeeding relates to the decreased incidence of certain types of infectious diseases (respiratory and diarrheal) that has been noted in breastfed as opposed to bottle-fed babies.[39] Infections of the gastrointestinal tract are known to increase intestinal permeability, thus potentially enabling antigens to cross the mucosal barrier with greater ease. Viral infections particularly have been associated with enhanced IgE synthesis,[39] and coincidental viral infection and manifestation of atopy have been noted in one pediatric study.[40]

A final potential protective mechanism for breastfeeding relates to anti-inflammatory properties in breast milk. Histaminase and arylsulfatase are enzyme components of breast milk that break down histamine and leukotrienes. These latter two substances are important mediators of the type I hypersensitivity reaction associated with food allergy.[41]

Does current knowledge with regard to breastfeeding practice support the protective nature of breastfeeding with regard to allergy? Although studies can be cited concluding that breastfeeding may or does help prevent or delay allergy development, other studies can be cited that fail to support this view. It is important to understand the reasons for the current unclear status of the breastfeeding-allergy connection. Underlying the confusion is incomplete knowledge about the physiological, pathophysiological, immunological, and biochemical factors involved. The processes of breastfeeding and atopy are both highly complex. The role of breastfeeding as it relates to allergic disease is particularly difficult to assess because the system involves multiple components.

One area of confusion relates to questions about human milk protein composition. Businco et al[39] state that breast milk proteins are homologous. Ponzone[42] states that while many believe human milk proteins to be homologous for the human infant, there are in fact polymorphic variants. (Voglino and Ponzone[43] have reported the existence of polymorphic variants of human casein.) Ponzone[42] has suggested human milk proteins are allologous and may have the potential to be allergenic if an infant has a different allotype than the mother.

It should also be kept in mind that over the years, as breastfeeding has been compared with formulas, formula compositions have changed. Savilahti et al[44] point out that protein concentrations of formulas have become lower over the years, perhaps making these products less allergenic. When comparisons are made with newer formulas, breastfeeding may seem less protective.

Another area of incomplete knowledge relates to the passage of food antigens (derived from the maternal diet) into the breast milk. It is recognized that food antigens can be transmitted to the infant via the mother's milk.[45,46,47] Explanation for variance in concentration of antigens in breast milk following consumption is an area of current research.[48] Antigens do not always appear in breast milk and when food antigen is transmitted in breast milk, antigen transmission does not always result in the infant's having a manifestation(s) of allergic disease.[49]

A study by Cant, Marsden, and Kilshaw[49] illustrates these points. These researchers found ovalbumin in breast milk samples from 14 out of 19 breastfeeding mothers. All 19 women were sampled after eating eggs. Concentrations of ovalbumin in breast milk were not found to be related to the allergic manifestation of eczema in infants. Prenatal sensitization has already been discussed, and this phenomenon may have played some role in explaining the divergent host responses to the presence of egg antigen in breast milk.[49] The researchers also noted that sensitization may have occurred via the environment, eg, egg antigen contaminating the hands for example. (They further suggested the importance of infant response.[49])

In other research, Kilshaw and Cant[46] have postulated that breastfed babies may be exposed to small quantities of food antigens via skin or inhalation of dust. If this environmental transmission does occur, even the most careful dietary documentation may not give the full food protein exposure picture. Kilshaw and Cant[46] documented the presence of β-lacto-globulin in nanogram amounts from finger washings of laboratory personnel who had handled milk in the home environment.

The route by which food antigens enter breast milk is postulated to proceed from the mother's gut via M cells to the mesenteric nodes and then to the thoracic duct. From the thoracic duct, the antigen is believed to be carried to the bloodstream and finally to the breast.[50] Kilshaw and Cant[46] point out that how this last step occurs—ie, food antigen transport from the bloodstream to the breast—is as yet unclear. Their research would indicate the existence of, at least in some instances, a selective protein transport system across the mammary epithelium. (The mammary epithelium has typically been characterized as being of low permeability to large protein molecules.) Kilshaw and Cant[46] have theorized food antigens either may be transported across the mammary epithelium in complex with dimeric IgA which then dissociates in the breast milk or food antigens may be carried into breast milk via macrophages.

The above discussion illustrates gaps with regard to our knowledge about antigens. The area of host response is also under investigation.

How antigens elicit host IgE changes or affect the functioning of T cells has not been fully elucidated. Plasma cell IgE production is regulated by T cells in mice, and IgE response is enhanced when there is a selective reduction in functioning of suppressor T cells.[51] It has been suggested that allergy in humans may be the result of abnormal numbers in T-cell subgroups.[51-54] Tainio,[54] in 1985, reported an altered T-cell helper-suppressor ratio was found to occur by 4 months of age in children who subsequently developed allergy. This researcher also was able to demonstrate that by 28 months of age, infants with allergy had relatively fewer T cells than their allergy-free counterparts. In atopic eczema, a deficiency of T8+-positive suppressor T cells has been found.[51,55] Juto et al[52] have put forth the idea that perhaps early introduction of cow's milk-based formula changes the reactivity and dynamics of the T-cell population, which then leads to changes in immune response.

There are diverse theories related to the effects of early antigen loading in the human infant.[56] One of the ways breastfeeding may be protective, as discussed earlier, is by lessening antigen load early in life. The theory underlying this assumption is allergic disease results from exaggerated immune response after the immature gut is exposed to antigen excess.[34,57] Some, however, theorize when large amounts of antigen are absorbed, inappropriate IgE response is actually inhibited via the activation of IgE suppressor T cells, and conversely, early exposure to only small quantities of antigen may boost IgE response.[58-62] Warner,[61(p135)] in support of the latter theory (or low-dose stimulation theory), has suggested "current recommendations for full breastfeeding and attempted reduction of exposure to foreign proteins in early infancy . . . may actually promote the development of allergy rather than protecting against it."

Gerrard and Shenassa[63,64] make the case for a distinction between cow's milk allergy in the breastfed versus the formula-fed baby based on the low-dose stimulation theory. They project that if a breastfed baby is allergic to cow's milk protein in the mother's diet, symptoms are the result of a low dose of antigen stimulating an IgE-mediated response. They postulate on the other hand that cow's milk allergy in the nonbreastfed baby is triggered by a large antigen load and is not an IgE-mediated phenomenon but rather one that is mediated instead by IgM, IgG, or other immune factors. Firer et al[65] suggest the value of breastfeeding in terms of allergy postponement or prevention may be greater if the mother does not consume cow's milk either while pregnant or breastfeeding. (She would thus avoid exposing her baby to a low cow's milk antigen dose.)

Looking at allergy in infancy is further confounded because IgE elevations in this age group do not always seem to be related to clinical presentation of allergy.[1] According to Foucard,[1(p100)] "It is quite possible that the degree of tissue sensitivity is determined by many more complex factors of which the IgE antibody response is just a part." Later in childhood, there seems to be better correlation between both total IgE and specific IgE antibodies and allergic clinical manifestations such as asthma or eczema.[62]

It should be noted that some believe serum IgE concentrations in infancy may be more definitive. Hamburger et al[3] cite data from Orgel et al,[4] who studied 34 infants with serum IgE levels ranging from <10 to >100 IU/ml. Orgel[4] found all infants with serum IgE levels of greater than 20 IU/ml measured at age 1 developed allergic symptoms by age 2 years.

Once one moves to the subject of clinical response, further problems arise. For example, how is allergy defined? Studies examining breastfeeding and allergy have documented allergy occurrence in many ways.

Clinical manifestations such as atopic dermatitis (eczema), asthma, and allergic rhinitis have all been used as allergy markers, as has subsequent development of food allergy, particularly to cow's milk.[66] The multiplicity of clinical problems used to denote allergy perhaps makes it more useful to think in terms of the specific clinical manifestation rather than using the more inclusive term of allergy.

Even if one looks at diagnosis of specific clinical manifestations (for example, eczema) the situation may be far from clear. All of the mechanisms involved in the pathogenesis of eczema (sometimes called atopic dermatitis) have yet to be fully determined.[67-70] Dietary factors are believed to play a role, but how these are related to other pathogenic mechanisms remains unclear.[69,70]

Controversy exists about the role of food allergy in the development of atopic dermatitis.[69] It has been cited that in about 43 to 83% of children with atopic dermatitis, elevated levels of serum IgE are present.[71-73] This would suggest an immediate hypersensitivity reaction in response to either dietary or environmental antigens.[68,73,74] Sampson[68] has shown that, at least in some cases, immediate food hypersensitivity (particularly in response to egg, milk, wheat, and peanut) may initiate development of eczema.

The Task Force on Pediatric Dermatology of the American Academy of Dermatology[70] suggests even when food allergy is involved in the etiology of eczema, nonimmunologic mechanisms may be involved as well. Jackson et al,[75] using a probe molecule, polyethylene glycol, documented a defect in intestinal mucosal absorption of molecules of high molecular weight. This mucosal defect was seen in eczema patients classified both with and without food allergy.

In addition to questions involved in the pathogenesis of atopic disorders potentially prevented or delayed by breastfeeding, diagnoses of allergy-related clinical conditions are not simple, clear-cut procedures. Kramer[76(p183)] has stated that the allergic clinical disorders studied in regard to breastfeeding "have no pathognomonic symptoms, signs, or laboratory tests, so their diagnosis remains somewhat subjective. . . ." For example, diagnostic criteria for eczema are not strict, and this has created confusion.[77] One researcher has suggested that in diagnosis, eczema related to use of deodorant soaps with halogenated salicylanilide ingredients may be confused with atopic eczema related to food allergy.[78] Eczema also shows spontaneous improvement that makes determination of the effects of manipulations of dietary factors (such as breastfeeding) difficult.[79]

A final questionable knowledge area relates to ascertaining the postponement or prevention of allergy. What really is an appropriate follow-up period to accurately make this determination? This is unclear. Zeiger[9(p336)] would suggest that prevention of allergy may be difficult if not almost impossible to achieve or document, because absorption of food antigens may occur to some extent throughout the lifespan and "potential sensitization of at-risk atopic

individuals may occur at any age . . . ." Businco et al[39] suggest postponement in some cases may be equivalent to prevention, especially for atopic dermatitis and cow's milk allergy, both of which commonly occur before age 2
years. Ponzone[42] also points out that certain foods (like breast milk) may
prevent symptoms as long as they are consumed, but consumption may not
correct an underlying disorder. Gruskay,[80] in reviewing studies related to
allergy prophylaxis, has stated that many studies can be criticized for conclu-
sions about prevention because follow-up periods were only 1 to 4 years.

Given the context of the above knowledge gaps and controversies, what
have major human population studies demonstrated? What have been the
methodological problems that have plagued the research in this area?

Human Studies Concluding That Breastfeeding May Prevent or Delay Allergy

The classic article relating breastfeeding to allergy prevention was that of
Grulee and Sanford,[81] published in 1936. These pediatricians examined the
relationships of three types of feeding (breastfeeding, partial breastfeeding,
and cow's milk formula feeding) to the incidence of infantile eczema in a
20,061-infant series. Of the three types of feedings, breastfeeding was associated with the lowest incidence of eczema. The infants in this series who were
fed cow's milk formula were reported to have a seven times greater incidence
of eczema compared to breastfeeders, and the incidence of eczema in those
partially breastfed was twice that of the breastfed group.

Grulee and Sanford's study[81] has been criticized on grounds that strict
diagnostic criteria were not used.[76] The diagnostic criterion for infantile
eczema cited in the study was "any lesions on the face or body at the time of
examination with 'cradle cap' excluded."[81(p223)] Other problems noted with
this study were lack of blindness about feeding regimen on the part of those
making the assessment of outcome (eczema), failure to address the issue of
outcome severity, lack of control for confounding variables (such as familial
history of atopy), and failure to sufficiently address the issue of age of eczema
onset.[76] It should also be noted that the study did not focus on the role of
breastfeeding in preventing or delaying allergy in a high-risk group, but
instead was a study of a general pediatric population.[76] From a dietary
perspective, more detail about how infant feeding information was collected
would have been helpful. Only one sentence, for example, discussed concomitant use of solids that may have been an important variable. Also the
comparison of breastfeeding with a boiled milk-cane sugar formula is not
equivalent to comparison with modern formula preparations.

On the positive side, the research is cited as important because of the large
population studied and the fact that at the time of the study the potential

relationship between feeding and eczema had not yet been publicized; therefore, women were presumably less biased with regard to choice of infant feeding mode.[82]

The 1950s and 1960s saw little breastfeeding-allergy research because formula feeding was popular during this period. Renewed interest in breastfeeding in the 1970s saw additional research in the area of potential benefits. In 1971, Murray[83] published a letter describing the results of a study regarding eosinophil numbers in nasal secretions of infants given food other than breast milk in the first month of life compared to those given only breast milk. Nasal eosinophilia was studied because the author considered this to be an indicator of allergic rhinitis. In children who had a history of allergy in the immediate family, nasal eosinophilia was present more often in the group given foods other than breast milk during month 1. Murray[83] concluded breastfeeding should be encouraged as a preventive measure against allergic rhinitis.

Studies by Blair[84] and Matthew et al[85] published in 1977 also supported the benefits of breastfeeding with regard to allergy. Blair[84] noted that breastfeeding for more than 8 weeks was significantly associated with decreased asthma incidence. Matthew et al[85] studied 49 infants of whom 23 followed an allergy prevention protocol that entailed breastfeeding for 6 months with only soy supplements (if desired). Selected weanings to certain solids occurred in this period. Examples of other environmental manipulation involved in this study were avoidance of pets and feathered bed materials. Adherence to allergy prevention protocol in the Matthew et al[85] study was found to be associated with decreased eczema incidence at 6 months and 1 year. The group following the protocol also had significantly lower mean total serum IgE levels when measured at 6 weeks of age.

In 1978, Wittig et al[5] reviewed records of 2,190 allergy patients who had a diagnosis of either asthma or allergic rhinitis. The study examined a number of risk factors including feeding modes during infancy and concluded that breastfeeding was associated with delayed onset of clinical allergy.

Chandra[86] reported in 1979 the results of a prospective study designed to assess the impact of breastfeeding on allergy incidence. Thirty-seven infants (with an allergic sibling) were reported to have been exclusively breastfed for at least 4 to 6 weeks. Allergy (eczema, recurrent wheezing) incidence in this group was compared to allergy incidence in 37 infants with comparable sibling history, but who were fed cow's milk formula. Children in both groups were followed for at least 2 years. The incidence of eczema and wheezing was found to be significantly less in the breastfed group. Also more of those formula-fed exhibited elevated levels of serum IgE.

Saarinen et al investigated incidence and severity of atopic diseases (atopic dermatitis and food allergy) in 54 infants breastfed for more than 6 months,

77 infants breastfed for 2–6 months, and 105 infants who were fed cow's milk formula beginning at less than 2 months of age. Mothers of infants in all categories were advised to introduce solid foods as follows: cooked vegetables and fruits at 3-5 months; "cereals at 5 months; meat and eggs at 6 months; dairy products at 8 months; . . . fish and citrus . . . avoided until 1 year of age."[87(p163)]

Saarinen's study found that for children both with and without familial allergy history, the incidence of atopic dermatitis (occurring up to 3 years of age) was significantly lower for those breastfed more than 6 months. For children with a family history of atopic disease, incidence of atopic dermatitis occurring by 3 years of age was also significantly lower for prolonged breastfeeders. Food allergy incidence by year 1 was significantly lower among children who were breastfed longer than 6 months.

Several studies were published in 1981 supporting that breastfeeding might be protective. Hide and Guyer[88] published a study of the incidence of allergy in Isle of Wight infants (April 1, 1977, through March 31, 1978). Types of allergy incidence for 1 year included in this study were eczema, asthma or bronchitis, and chronic rhinitis. The analysis distinguished between infants with and without a parental history of allergy. Results were analyzed with regard to both initial feeding method (breastfeeding versus formula feeding) and end of year 1 feeding method (breastfeeding only, formula feeding only, mixed formula and breastfeeding, and formula and solids feeding). It should be noted that 71% of all infants studied were in the breastfed initially category.

These researchers found the overall incidence of allergy (eczema, asthma or bronchitis, and chronic rhinitis combined) was significantly lower in infants initially breastfed. No statistically significant differences in incidence analyzed by type of allergic manifestation were found between those initially breastfed versus those initially formula fed. When data were analyzed with regard to feeding category at age 1, the breastfeeding only group had the lowest overall allergy incidence.

Kaufman and Frick[89] looked at the influence of breastfeeding versus bottle feeding on asthma incidence in infants whose mothers had allergies. It was found that infants breastfed for at least 6 weeks exclusively had a decreased incidence of asthma.

A short abstract published by Lucarelli et al[90] in 1981 reported the results of a study designed to examine the relationship of infant feeding modes to serum IgE concentrations and the development of allergic disease within the first year of life. Infants were from atopic families. The researchers reported atopic dermatitis incidence was significantly less in those infants who were breastfed. None of the feeding modes examined (breast, cow's milk formula, or soy formula), however, was found to be correlated with serum IgE levels.

In 1982, Gruskay[80] published the results of a prospective study (15 years' duration) examining the relationship of breastfeeding and formula feeding (cow's milk and soy) to allergic disease development (asthma, allergic rhinitis, and atopic dermatitis). The study involved assignment of children from allergic families ($n = 328$) to either breast, soy formula, or cow's milk formula. A control group of children ($n = 580$) without family history of allergy was also a part of this study. Breastfeeding did not appear to be exclusive in either the study breastfeeding group or the control group. Control group infants who were breastfed were supplemented with cow's milk formula and infants who breastfed from allergic families were reported to have used soy formula for supplemental feeds.

Gruskay[80] found that the incidence of overall allergy in breastfed infants with positive family histories was approximately half that of similar infants fed either cow or soy formula. Differences in these groups were not significant until beyond 3 years. Incidence of atopic dermatitis did not significantly differ in those with familial allergy history regardless of feeding mode employed.

Kajosaari and Saarinen[57] published a study addressing the respective influences of exclusive breastfeeding (no solids, no formula supplements) for 6 months versus breastfeeding with solid foods introduced by age 3 months. Diets of both of these groups were considered to be similar during the second 6 months. Incidence of allergy by age 1 was examined. Atopic eczema incidence was found to be significantly less in those solely breastfed for 6 months. Incidence of food allergy was also found to be significantly less in those exclusively breastfed. The results of this study suggest exclusivity of breastfeeding and duration may be very important and positive effects of breastfeeding may not occur if solids are given too early.

In attempting to explain potential physiological bases for results, Kajosaari and Saarinen[57] cite the work of Jackson et al[75] discussed previously. Jackson et al,[75] using polyethylene glycol, found that eczema (with or without concomitant food allergy) is associated with increased absorption of large molecules, which they believed to be suggestive of abnormalities in the distal part of the small intestine or colon. Kajosaari and Saarinen[57] postulate that even small amounts of solids given with breast milk may cause problems for some individuals. They also cite a paper by Juto and Björksten[62] that suggested in some infants feeding a combination of breast milk and solids may enhance IgE synthesis. In summary, the Kajosaari and Saarinen[57] study supports the protective value of exclusive breastfeeding with introduction of solids no earlier than age 6 months.

Businco et al[39] studied the development of atopy over a 2-year period in 101 infants with a family history of atopic disease (defined as at least one parent or sibling having atopic dermatitis, rhinitis, or asthma). Thirty-four infants were breastfed exclusively for 6 months. Mothers of these infants were advised to wean only to certain foods when the infants were between 6 and 9 months of age. Twenty-six infants received soy formula with partial breastfeeding for the first 6 months. These mothers also received instruction regarding selected 6- to 9-month weanings comparable to the breastfed group. Forty-one children were fed cow's milk formula from birth (11 partially breastfed for a short period). The lowest percentage of atopic disease diagnoses was found in the breastfed group (17.6%), and the highest for the cow's milk group (36.6%). Of those on the soy milk regimen, 24% were diagnosed with atopic conditions within the 2-year study period.

Pratt,[91] in 1984, published a study related to eczema incidence in 198 infants observed from birth through 4.5 to 5.0 years of age. When incidence of eczema was compared between all those initially breastfed (all durations) and those initially fed cow's milk, no significant difference was noted. When infants with a first-degree relative family history were exclusively breastfed for less than 12 weeks, the incidence of eczema was 24%. When exclusive breastfeeding was continued for over 12 weeks, the number with eczema decreased to 16%. Thirty-eight percent of nonbreastfed infants from allergic families developed eczema. It is presumably related to these findings that Pratt's[91] study is classified as supportive of the protective effect of breastfeeding. Pratt also found eczema incidence rose in breastfed infants (both with and without atopic history) when breastfeeding after 12 weeks was supplemented with other foods.

Pratt[91] spends time in her article discussing the issue of exclusive breastfeeding. She feels her research supports the view that breastfeeding may be beneficial when it is used to exclude other foods. She concludes that prolonged *exclusive* breastfeeding may be associated with decreased eczema incidence and suggests long-term nonexclusive breastfeeding conversely may be associated with an increased incidence of eczema. To support her view, she cites work suggesting the eczema incidence increases with increases in the number of solid foods introduced between birth and 4 months of age.[92]

Moore et al,[93] in 1985, suggest from observational data that breastfeeding may be at least one factor contributing to decreased eczema incidence in genetically prone children. These investigators analyzed data for 475 children fed in various ways, including some exclusively breastfed for at least 4 weeks. Significant less eczema was found at 3 months and at 6 months among breastfeeders but not at 12 months.

In 1988, Miskelly et al[94] published the results of a clinical trial designed to examine the exclusion effect of cow's milk from diets of infants from allergic families. The trial involved random assignment to either a control group (cow's milk formula) or intervention group (soy formula or breastfeeding). Women in the intervention group were asked to restrict daily milk intake to 1 half-pint per day during pregnancy and lactation. Intervention group mothers were also given a list of solid foods containing milk and asked not to give these to infants. Assessments were made by a physician blind to the feeding group assignments. Infants were examined 3 times at ages 3, 6, and 12 months.

Although this study was not designed to examine potential protective effects of breastfeeding, the authors did analyze the data for those choosing to breastfeed. The authors clearly state their study does not address potential benefits of exclusive breastfeeding. Breastfeeding, as practiced by mothers in this study, was not associated with decreased eczema incidence. A significantly decreased occurrence of wheezing, however, was associated with breastfeeding. The authors point out that reduction of wheezing may have been related to reduction of viral infection as opposed to allergy. Breastfeeding has been related to reduction in the incidence of infection with respiratory syncytial virus.[93-95] Children with wheeze were also given wheat or rye proteins earlier and if allergy was involved, feeding of these solids could have been responsible. The study, however, with major qualifications, does offer a suggestion that breastfeeding may be beneficial with regard to lessening the occurrence of one potential allergy symptom (wheeze).

Human Studies Concluding Breastfeeding Does Not Prevent or Delay Allergy

Halpern et al,[96] in 1973, studied 1,753 infants who were breastfed or fed soy or cow's milk formula. Some study infants were followed for as long as 7 years. The primary hypothesis being studied related to determining if deletion of cow's milk formula (substituted by either breast or soy milk) would decrease allergy incidence. The study by Halpern et al[96] found no differences related to allergy incidence among the feeding groups. It was noted, however, that allergy developed significantly later in those breastfed compared to those fed cow's milk. The researchers concluded that the type of milk fed for the first 6 months did not alter overall allergy incidence.

In 1981 Kramer and Moroz,[97] attempting to shed light on the breastfeeding and atopic eczema question, published the results of a case control study of 470 dermatology patients. Study subjects were ages 1 month to 20 years. Cases were blindly diagnosed with atopic eczema and controls were infants or children diagnosed as having a dermatologic problem unrelated to allergy. Feeding histories were ascertained by maternal recall. It was reported that the interviewer was unaware of both the study question and the case or control designations. In addition to questioning about breastfeeding practices and rationale (if practiced), information was obtained with regard to age of solids introduction, history of allergic disease in the family, and race. Infants were considered to have been breastfed if they received breast milk for 1 week after birth with no more than one formula feeding per day.

The initial analysis that compared atopic eczema incidence in breastfeeders versus controls found that breastfeeding was associated with an increased estimated relative risk for eczema development. Analysis with a stricter definition of breastfeeding (defined as at least 2 months of breastfeeding exclusively) did not alter the finding of increased estimated relative risk. When severity of eczema was examined, no significant relationship was found with regard to breastfeeding. The researchers reported no correlation between age at atopic eczema diagnosis and age of solid food introduction. In summary, this study did not support a protective role for breastfeeding.

Fergusson et al,[92] in a 2-year cohort study of over 1,000 children born in the Christchurch region of New Zealand, reported that exclusive breastfeeding for 4 months had no significant effect on eczema incidence. This study, however, found that feeding solids in the first 4 months did significantly increase eczema incidence. (Children given solids before 4 months of age were 1.5 times more likely to have eczema.)

In a 1982 study of 250 infants from families with allergy history (one or both parents or sibling), Gordon et al[98] found that breastfeeding did not decrease eczema incidence. This study, in fact, reported that 22% of infants breastfed for at least 3 months developed eczema compared with 15% of those who were formula fed. Breastfeeding was also not found to be associated with lower IgE levels. The study found that 18% of breastfed babies and 17% of formula-fed babies had high serum IgE concentrations.

Publication of the Gordon[98] study that found greater eczema incidence among breastfeeders prompted several letters to appear in *The Lancet*. Golding et al[99] reported that in an analysis of a national cohort (with 5-year follow-up), they too had seen a positive association between breastfeeding and eczema incidence. (They also noted they did not find breastfeeding to be positively associated with either asthma or wheezing.) Golding et al[99] suggested that analysis be done to determine if observed results clustered in time, and if so, these researchers postulated the potential involvement of a contaminant in breast milk as being related to eczema development. (Specifically mentioned were polychlorinated biphenyls.)

Another letter supporting Gordon's findings was that of Cogswell and Alexander.[100] These investigators commented that in a 3-year prospective study of infants from atopic families, they too found that infants breastfed for more than 3 months had a higher incidence of eczema. They also noted that some breastfed babies in their study positively skin tested to egg in the first year and such children were more prone to develop either eczema or allergy in the follow-up period. Cogswell and Alexander[100] postulated that their observation related to transfer of food antigens (specifically egg) in breast milk.

A letter from Garrow and Pratt[101] also responded to Golding's letter. These researchers felt the association reported by Golding[99] might be due to biased selection of feeding method (ie, women from atopic families choosing more frequently to breastfeed).

In 1983 Fergusson et al,[102] who had earlier studied eczema incidence, published their findings from the Christchurch, New Zealand, cohort in regard to asthma. Breastfeeding was not found to be associated with decreased asthma incidence.

The study of Taylor et al[103] is among those not supporting the protective role of breastfeeding. This study looked at allergic manifestations (eczema, hay fever, and asthma) in a national cohort of over 13,000 children and found breastfeeding to be a nonprotective factor with regard to incidence of all three manifestations. Eczema, in fact, was reported more often in the breastfed group.

Van Asperen et al[104] studied incidence of wheeze, allergic rhinitis, and atopic dermatitis in 54 infants exclusively breastfed for 2 months and 19 infants exclusively breastfed for 4 months. The influence of exclusive breastfeeding on appearance of allergic symptoms was not found to be significant.

Peters et al,[105] in 1985, reported in letter form findings from an analysis of a 1970 cohort study (Britain-national data) and spoke to the issue of increased eczema incidence in breastfed infants reported by some[99,100] previously. These researchers reported that breastfeeding was not associated with increased eczema incidence when several confounding variables were controlled. Examples of control variables used in this study were education and maternal birthplace. The researchers said that no analysis of their data could show a protective role of breastfeeding.

Hide and Guyer,[106] in 1985, published an extension of their earlier Isle of Wight study. Exclusive breastfeeding was associated with an increase in reported eczema. Asthma incidence, at 4 years of age, defined by having more than one wheezing episode, was also not found to be decreased by breastfeeding. (These researchers speculated that failure to demonstrate a breastfeeding protective effect may have been due to passage of cow's milk proteins in breast milk.)

Midwinter et al[77] studied the association between development of either asthma or eczema in 457 children with a family history of atopy. The study followed up on the children at their fifth birthday. Infant feeding method was assessed by feeding diary. Asthma and eczema were assessed on parental reports of physician diagnosis. Breastfeeding was not found to be associated with either decreased asthma or eczema incidence.

A prospective study published in 1987 by Cogswell et al[107] examined breastfeeding as one potential environmental factor influencing development of eczema and wheeze episodes in 73 children with a family history of allergic disease. Eczema was diagnosed by a physician blind to feeding method and stated criteria were used to define eczema. Wheezing was also assessed by a physician. Infants were also skin tested with several antigens, including egg and cow's milk. Feeding was assessed via review of a diary kept by parents. This study found no relationship between duration of breastfeeding (defined as ending at first formula feed) and allergy (defined as the presence of eczema or positive skin testing or asthma.)

Another prospective study published in 1987[44] followed 183 infants over a 2-year period. Infants were not chosen by family history of atopy, although it was noted that 79 infants did have a family history of atopy (one or both parents or a sibling). In children with no family history of atopy, there was a 5% incidence of atopy in those exclusively breastfed for less than 3.5 months compared with 28% atopy incidence in those breastfed exclusively for more than 9 months. In children with a history of family atopy, there was a 25% incidence of atopy in those breastfed for less than 3.5 months compared with 31% in those exclusively breastfed for more than 9 months. The authors concluded the above results did not support a protective effect of breastfeeding with regard to allergy.

Allergy and Breastfeeding: A Summary of Human Studies

The vast majority of studies to date (both pro and con with regard to breastfeeding and delay or prevention of allergy) have had a variety of methodologic problems. Some relate to biologic considerations, some relate to study design, and some relate to statistical analysis and interpretation.[76,82] A summary of major problems and comments is shown in Table 5-1. Given the state of the research, as just summarized, what have reviews in this area concluded?

Burr,[82] writing in 1983, felt most studies support delay of cow's milk introduction and delay of solids introduction. He also felt controlled random studies should be conducted and future studies should ensure that diagnosis of allergy is accomplished blindly (ie, the physician making diagnoses being unaware of feeding history).

Kovar et al,[66] in an overview examining relationships between infant feeding and health, concluded that present studies fail to prove a protective role for breast milk related to allergy development. These researchers felt if there were any protective effect, it was most probable in regard to asthma. In 1986, a Task Force on Pediatric Dermatology of the American Academy of

Table 5-1 Common Methodological Problems in Breastfeeding-Allergy Studies

Problem	Comments
Failure to assess prenatal sensitization and maternal diet during pregnancy.	Several researchers have commented that lack of a study to demonstrate a protective effect may be due to this failure. Studies in this area could be enhanced by analysis using appropriate indicators to assess prenatal sensitization and monitoring maternal diet during pregnancy.
Failure to control or monitor maternal diet during lactation and assess food antigen transmission in breast milk.	Monitoring or controlling maternal diet during lactation and measuring antigens in breast milk might clarify results. Potential reactions to food antigens transmitted in breast milk have been cited for failure to show a protective effect.
Failure to test breast milk for environmental contaminants.	It has been postulated in some studies that environmental contaminant passage may be a reason why a protective effect was unable to be demonstrated.
Failure to randomly assign to feeding method.	This has been noted as a problem with calls for future prospective studies to use random assignment. Others feel random assignment is impractical. Zeiger[9] considers failure to randomize to be the major weakness of studies to date. Failure to randomize does introduce confounding variables. It has been suggested, for example, that women with an allergic history may be more likely to breastfeed.[10] If this were true in a particular study, it could lead to conclusions of no effect or even a negative effect of breastfeeding.
Failure to use specific and appropriate diagnostic criteria.	It is possible some studies used specific appropriate criteria but failed to report this in the methodology section. It is important that specific referenced and appropriate diagnostic criteria be used. Kramer[76] also states that in cases where more than one individual is involved in diagnosis, efforts should be made to minimize interobserver error.
Failure to analyze results separately by atopic diagnosis category.	Some studies use the general categories of atopy (with several conditions listed) versus nonatopy. Failure to analyze by specific atopic categories may result in failure to show effects on one or more diagnoses.
Use of parental report or recall for diagnosis.	Reliance on parents for diagnosis is problematic. Diagnosis of an allergic condition should be made by a qualified physician.
Failure to blindly diagnose allergic condition.	This methodologic error has been cited as a major problem for studies to date, and when this error is present observer bias is an issue.

continues

Table 5-1 continued

Problem	Comments
Failure to use immunologic testing as part of the process for allergy diagnosis.	Some believe the exclusion of immunologic testing is an important omission because it can help detect the presence of antigen-specific IgE and aid in the characterization of immunologic alterations that may coexist with clinical problems.[9]
Failure to appropriately document or use dietary intake assessment methodology.	Some studies have relied on parental recall over excessively long periods. Other studies have used diet records with no explanation as to how records were kept or verified. Some studies have used past medical records that may or may not have been complete or consistent in recording feeds. Some studies seem to have assumed specific feed instructions were followed. Cross-check strategies need to be explored. Although current techniques for diet intake assessment are sorely lacking in precision, more attention needs to be paid to increasing the reliability and validity of feed information and adequately describing the methodology of dietary data collection in research papers.
Failure to control for or monitor exclusivity of breastfeeding.	A major problem is that definitions of "breastfeeding" and "breastfed" vary widely. If truly exclusive breastfeeding (ie, breast milk only) is of interest, this needs to be specified with testing for varying realistic durations. Many studies classify "breastfed" as some who received other nourishment sources (formula supplements or solids) quite early. Timing of receipt of other nourishment sources is critical and needs to be documented and categorically analyzed. Some studies really look at the effectiveness of combined regimens (breastfeeding linked with formula supplements or various patterns of solids).
Failure to examine duration of breastfeeding as a factor.	If there is a critical timing effect, it may be that duration[76] is a key issue. Future prospective studies should examine varying durations of both exclusive (breast milk only) and simultaneous breastfeeding (ie, breastfeeding with other nourishment sources, distinguishing and describing formulas and solids). In retrospective studies, the validity of duration information may be questionable.
Failure to control for or monitor solid food and formula introduction.	Failure to address the solid food and formula introduction issue in detail may bias results, if thoughts about the allergenicity of early introduction of food antigens are correct. Types and amounts of solids and formulas introduced, as well as timing of such introductions, may be important, and such information must be gathered from all available sources and be as complete and descriptive as possible. An important monitoring issue relates to incomplete data. It has been noted, for example, that infants may receive early formula feeds in the hospital (without maternal knowledge) or be given solids by other caretakers.

continues

Table 5-1 continued

Problem	Comments
Failure to designate degree of family atopy and compare similar groups.	Some studies fail to delineate subjects by family atopy, and yet most agree that if breastfeeding or other strategies can be demonstrated as preventative, they will be most effective in those considered to be high risk. Even studies that have an atopic history group seem to have broad definitions for familial atopy. Given the strong genetic component involved, it may be useful to more specifically delineate atopic family classifications, ie, bilateral (both parents), unilateral (one parent), etc.
Failure to analyze for potentially confounding variables.	Several important confounding variables have been cited that some studies failed to take into account. Examples of important variables cited by Kramer[76] are race, family history of atopy (see above), age of infants, smoking habits of parents (in evaluation of asthma), and socioeconomic status. Incidents of certain allergy-related diagnoses seem to differ among racial groups.[76] Failure to control for race, if the above holds true, would bias toward showing that breastfeeding has a protective effect.
Failure to consider or report severity of atopy.	It has been postulated that breastfeeding may be beneficial by lessening severity of atopy.[76] Most studies only focus on the measure of incidence.
Failure to have adequate follow-up time to ascertain delay or prevention or failure to frame the results clearly in these terms.	All any study may technically be able to show is delay because sensitization may potentially occur at any age[9] and follow-up through the total lifespan is impractical. Businco et al[39] have pointed out that in some instances delay may be for all practical purposes the equivalent of prevention.

Dermatology[70] concluded that most studies do not indicate breastfeeding, even when relatively long in duration, is protective with regard to atopic dermatitis.

Zeiger,[9] reviewing the subject in 1988, found weaknesses both in studies concluding breastfeeding was beneficial and those indicating it was not. He cited major weaknesses of both types of studies as failure to blindly conduct diagnosis, failure to describe or monitor dietary compliance, failure to have sample sizes of adequate number, and failure of many subjects to complete study protocols. He also criticized both study types for failure to randomize subjects, and many of the studies (both pro and con) for their failure to assess allergy presence by immunologic (IgE) testing. Zeiger[8] also observed that studies showing a protective effect were more likely to have involved both breastfeeding of longer duration and later introduction of solids. Despite the above problems with research, Zeiger[9] concluded that breastfeeding of sufficient duration (6 months) is linked to decreased eczema incidence in the first 3 years of life.

Kramer[76] cites many of the problems mentioned by Zeiger.[9] Interestingly, Kramer's review concluded that studies showing a protective effect of breastfeeding with regard to atopic eczema were more likely to have problems with methodologies related to diagnosis and blindness, but were better designed in terms of what he termed biologic standards. Kramer[76] cites the two most serious design flaws in all studies as (1) diagnosis of outcome with knowledge of feeding mode (ie, nonblind assessment) and (2) lack of control with regard to potential confounding variables. (Examples of important confounders cited by Kramer[76] included age of the infant, socioeconomic status, and history and degree of atopy in the family.) Kramer[76] states that to date "not much" can be concluded about a protective role of breastfeeding with regard to allergy.

Many problems relate to the retrospective nature of the majority of past studies. Clearly more appropriately conducted prospective research (both observational and experimental) is needed.

From the viewpoint of a dietitian, it is difficult to evaluate the majority of currently published papers because these reports provide surprisingly little information related to the methodology used to obtain a description or categorization of an infant's diet. Some articles provide no information. When dietary methodology is discussed, it is usually discussed briefly with references to use of such techniques as parental recall, diet diary, or review of medical reports. A description of how these methods were used is rarely provided. Each of these methods, even assuming they were appropriately executed, has problems that may affect reliability and validity of the data.[108,109] Researchers have generally failed to address how they have attempted to minimize these problems (for example, through appropriate cross-checks).

Some researchers have indicated diet instructions were provided and seemed to assume in data analysis these were followed. If subjects are given instructions, it is important that the study methodology monitor compliance and data be analyzed based on this knowledge of actual practices.

Not only are dietary methodology reports a problem, but so too are the terminology and detail of diet descriptions. Even the terms "exclusive breastfeeding" and "breastfeeding" seem to be used in various ways. Some use the terms to mean only breast milk as a nourishment source (no formula, no solids). Others seem to use them to mean only breast milk (as opposed to formula) with solids not of concern (eg, sometimes given and sometimes not given).

Dietitian involvement in the design and conduct of the research, as well as in reporting, could be helpful in improving future studies. Suggestions for dietitians are shown in Table 5-2. These suggestions are specific to the portions of research most closely related to the dietetic domain. Research planning decisions related to controlling or monitoring diets involve choice of research type (observational versus experimental).

In undertaking future studies, dietitians, as well as others, need to carefully frame the research questions. Kramer and Moroz[97] make an excellent point by suggesting that investigating pure or exclusive breastfeeding may not be as relevant as investigating "breastfeeding as currently practiced." One could argue that perhaps both are important and should be investigated, but the critical issue is stating both for one's self and others which concept is being studied. In many instances researchers have studied the latter and confused it with the former.

Allergies in Breastfed Infants

While it remains unclear that breastfeeding prevents or delays allergies, it is known that some exclusively breastfed infants (ie, breast milk only, no solids or formula supplements) do develop allergies. In these cases, some have postulated that allergy may develop in response to human milk proteins as antigens,[42,43] and in other cases, develop in response to food protein

---

Table 5-2   Suggestions for the Dietary Aspects of Allergy-Breastfeeding Research

- Control/monitor exclusivity of breastfeeding.
- Compare breastfeeding periods of several realistic durations.
- Control/monitor introduction of solids and formulas (both timing and types).
- Compare breastfeeders and bottle feeders with comparable solids and formula introduction regimens.
- Control/monitor maternal diet during lactation (and potentially pregnancy).
- Use appropriate dietary assessment methods and keep accurate records of infant and maternal diets. (Include a cross-check method.)
- Include a full description of dietary methodology and subject diets in research publications. Define dietary terms clearly. State methodology limitations and describe attempts made to minimize these.

Note: The decision to control or monitor will be based on research design (ie, control in experimental studies and monitor in observational studies).

antigens transmitted in the breast milk.[45-49,64] Antigen exposure through a formula or food feeding unknown to or considered unimportant by the caretaker may also be a possibility for initiating allergy in the breastfed baby.

Allergy to human milk itself is considered to be very rare. In 1948, Wergeland[110] reviewed a small number of cases attributed to this cause. Gerrard[111] reports only two families in his practice whose infants seemed to have had this problem. While clinicians should bear in mind that such allergy may infrequently occur, fear of such a highly unusual occurrence certainly should not be used as a reason to discourage breastfeeding.

Reports of allergies in solely breastfed infants more commonly involve food antigens in breast milk, and reports of this phenomenon can be traced back to 1918 (as reviewed by Gerrard).[111] In that year, Talbot reported that a 3-week old infant who was being breastfed developed eczema subsequent to maternal chocolate consumption. Another early report summarized by Gerrard[111] was that of O'Keefe who in 1920 reported eczema and positive prick tests in exclusively breastfed infants. Egg, codfish, and cow's milk were the foods implicated, and O'Keefe postulated infants were sensitized via mother's milk.

Shannon,[45] in 1921 using guinea pigs, demonstrated that food protein (in this case egg) eaten by a mother could enter breast milk. In 1930, Donnally's[112] research supporting Shannon's[45] findings demonstrated that egg white could be absorbed in an antigenically active form and be present in breast milk. In 1984, Stuart et al[47] reported the results of an analysis of milk samples from 28 women taken 7-8 days after giving birth. Using the double-antibody sandwich method, they found β-lactoglobulin in the milk of 5 women and casein in 13 of the 28 milk samples. These investigators reported the cow's milk proteins in most cases to be detectable approximately 12 hours following last maternal cow milk consumption. Their research called for follow-up studies to determine patterns of protein passage into breast milk at other time intervals after birth.

Kilshaw and Cant[46] studied samples of breast milk from 29 women who had experienced various durations of breastfeeding ranging from 1 week to 12 months after giving birth. Samples were taken before and after a specified regimen of combined egg and cow milk consumption. After consumption, samples were taken at 2, 4, and 6 hours. Ovalbumin and β-lactoglobulin were detected in the breast milk samples from over half the study subjects in concentration ranges from 100 pg/ml to 6 ng/ml. Maximum food protein levels in breast milk were observed to be measured at 4 to 6 hours after egg-milk consumption.

In 1985, Cant et al[49] reported detection of ovalbumin in breast milk in samples from 14 of 19 lactating women who were challenged with egg. Maximum concentrations were reached 2 to 4 hours after consumption and ranged from 0.2 to 4.0 ng/L. Interestingly enough, maternal milk ovalbumin concentrations did not correlate with eczematous symptoms in infants. Seventy-two percent of mothers of eczematous infants had milk that contained ovalbumin with a mean concentration of 1.6 µg/L. Seventy-five percent of mothers of noneczematous infants had milk that contained ovalbumin with a mean concentration of 2.4 µg/L. The researchers suggested infant response, rather than the amount of antigen in breast milk, may be the key factor in infant atopy development. This is in contrast to the earlier suggestion of Warner[61] that allergy in breastfed infants could be due to maternal abnormalities that result in large quantities of food antigen transmission in breast milk.

Another 1985 Cant et al[113] case report describes an exclusively breastfed infant who developed both eczema and gastrointestinal problems when the mother's diet contained cow's or goat's milk and eczema when the mother drank soy milk. Symptoms in response to diet were confirmed by double-blind challenge.

Gerrard and Perelmutter,[114] in 1986, published a study of 19 children with positive RAST and prick skin tests to peanut, egg, or cow's milk. All children reacted adversely on first known ingestion of one or more of these foods. Of these 19, 10 had been solely breastfed for at least 5 months. A retrospective look at maternal diet during pregnancy and lactation was conducted. Because the mean age of the children at time of the study was 3 years 5 months, it should be noted that maternal recall data may be of uncertain validity. Given this note of caution, what were the reported study results? The researchers reported mothers of children with milk and egg sensitivity did not consume more of these substances either prenatally or during breastfeeding than mothers of infants without these sensitivities. (Ten children studied had sensitivity to peanut only.) It was suggested that there is not a clear-cut relationship between maternal intake during pregnancy and lactation and subsequent sensitization of the child. This work supports earlier observations of Kilshaw and Cant.[46]

Clearly additional research is needed relative to this issue. Proposed mechanisms for antigen transport into breast milk have been discussed earlier in this chapter.

In 1983, Gerrard and Shenassa[63] published clinical information relative to 73 breastfed infants they ascertained were sensitive to antigens in mother's milk. The most common presenting symptoms were reported as colic, vomiting, rhinorrhea, diarrhea, bronchitis with wheeze, and eczema. Criteria used to diagnose these presenting symptoms were not reviewed. The most common food eaten by the mother that seemed to initiate infant symptoms was cow's milk. The next most common maternal dietary component that appeared to be problematic was egg, followed in descending order by citrus, wheat, and chocolate. The first line of reported treatment for these cases was suggesting the mother avoid potential offending foods or beverages (as indicated by diet-symptom history and skin testing). If that failed, the authors suggested the mother limit her diet to 3 or 4 safe foods for 12-24 hours with the hope that infant symptoms would resolve in this period and the mother could begin to reintroduce foods on a one-by-one basis with avoidance of foods that cause problems. It is noted that while daily intake of some foods may cause infants to have symptoms, less frequent intake might not. If mothers were on restricted diets for several days, the authors prescribed elemental formula to supplement the diet. In instances where the above strategies did not work, oral cromolyn was given, and if this intervention proved ineffective the infant was switched to formula.[63]

Another important but rare clinical manifestation that some suggest may be related to allergy to food proteins in breast milk is inflammatory procto-colitis. Lake et al[115] reported seeing six infants who developed this problem during the first month of life while being exclusively breastfed. In two instances, restricting maternal intake of cow's milk resolved the problem. Wilson et al[116] recently reported a case of cow's milk-induced colitis in a 4-day old solely breastfed infant presenting with severe bleeding from the rectum. The mother reported drinking four to five glasses of milk per day and passage of intact cow's milk protein through the breast milk was suspected.

Another issue regarding allergies in breastfed babies relates to breastfed infants who may be sensitized by early formula feeds or prenatally. A 1988 case report of an infant who developed anaphylactic shock 3 times illustrates this point.[117] This infant was initially given two feedings of a casein-based formula, and then exclusively breastfed for 5 days. At age 5 days the infant developed bloody stools, and medical evaluation was conducted. At that time, the infant was given nothing by mouth and intravenous fluids and antibiotics. At 8 days of age, the infant refused to nurse and was given another type of casein-based formula. The infant experienced anaphylaxis and was placed on total parenteral nutrition for 8 days. The infant began to receive ex-pressed milk with the mother eliminating cow's milk from her diet. All seemed to go well until the infant received milk that had been expressed and stored before the mother had eliminated the cow's milk. The infant again experienced anaphylaxis. At 31 days of age, the infant was not breastfed and was given a casein-hydrolysate formula. Once again, anaphylaxis occurred.

In summary, dietitians need to be aware that even while being presumably exclusively breastfed, infants may exhibit clinical problems related to allergy. Important roles for the dietitian are obtaining information about the mater-nal and infant diet to help the physician in identifying potential problem foods and providing dietary counseling once problem foods have been identified. Such help may enable breastfeeding to continue and obviate the need to switch the infant to formula. Cant et al,[79] in trials involving 37 infants, found that some breastfed infants with eczematous symptoms positively respond to maternal dietary restrictions. Unfortunately not all respond, and these researchers reported they could identify no factors that predicted responders.

DIET MODIFICATION DURING PREGNANCY AND LACTATION: STRATEGIES TO PREVENT ALLERGY

Based on the preceding review of knowledge of prenatal sensitization and the potential relationships between breastfeeding and allergy, what are current recommendations with regard to allergy prevention involving maternal diet manipulation and to what extent have they been successful?

First, who are the appropriate target groups for allergy prevention programs? Appropriate target groups identified and with whom prevention efforts have been tried are those infants who have been conceived or born to an atopic family unit (both parents, one parent and sibling, or one parent or sibling).[3,6,9,39,67,118,119,120,121] Prevention efforts may begin prenatally or postnatally. Hamburger et al[3] suggest immunologic testing to identify persons at risk for having atopic offspring. This group recommends determination of specific IgE reactivity by skin testing males and nonpregnant females and the use of serum IgE tests and RAST to determine atopic at-risk pregnant females.

Infant cord bloods are also used to target infants.[3,6,8,9,34,120] Michel et al[34] note guidelines for use of both cord blood levels of IgE and family history in decision making with regard to initiation of prevention strategies. Sampson[120] defines at-risk infants as those with both family history and levels of cord blood IgE of >2 µg/L.

The focus of early efforts at allergy prevention was changes in infant feeds or formulas. In 1953, Glaser and Johnstone[118] retrospectively looked at the effect of withholding cow's milk for various intervals with provision of either soy milk, meat-based formulas, or breast milk. These researchers did note breastfeeding mothers were advised to eliminate eggs and cheeses from the diet, as well as to limit milk intake to one pint that had been boiled for 10 minutes. Calcium and phosphorus supplements were given. Those children from whom cow's milk was withheld exhibited a significantly lower incidence of allergic diseases (atopic dermatitis and milk allergy).

In 1966, Johnstone and Dutton[121] published the results of a prospective study also designed to test the hypothesis that withholding cow's milk from infants would reduce the incidence of specific allergy diagnoses. Evaporated milk versus soy milk feedings were compared. Significantly less asthma and allergic rhinitis were reported for the soy group. Stintzing and Zetterstrom[122] published research in 1979 that supported withholding formulas with a cow's milk base for the first month (and encouraging breastfeeding) to lower the incidence of cow's milk allergy.

The debate over the allergic potential related to timing and amount of cow's milk introduction is still in progress. Readers are referred to the earlier part of this chapter that discusses the debate over antigen loading.[56-65] The idea of reducing sensitization potential by giving large doses of foreign protein foods such as cow's milk is relatively new.[1]

The year 1983 saw the publication of a landmark allergy prevention protocol by Hamburger et al.[3] The major dietary components of the Hamburger et al[3] plan were breastfeeding for at least 6 months, complete avoidance of supplemental soy or cow's milk formula (with a casein-hydrolysate formula, Nutramigen®, used if desired), addition of some solids considered relatively nonallergenic at 6 months, introduction of whole cow's milk after 12 months, and introduction of egg after 2 years. The plan permitted introduction of wheat cereal between 13 and 18 months of age. Introduction of legumes (peas and beans), corn, and citrus fruits was permitted after wheat introduction during the 13- to-18-month age period. The Hamburger et al[3] plan also contained a significant maternal dietary component and called for specific foods and beverages to be eliminated both during the last trimester of pregnancy and during breastfeeding. Foods and beverages to be eliminated from the maternal diet were eggs, peanut, and milk (and related products). Reduced consumption of wheat, soy, citrus fruit, and fish was encouraged. The protocol called for maternal calcium supplementation at the level of 500 mg twice daily. At the time of the 1983 publication, it was reported that over 300 mothers were involved in testing the protocol.

Lawrence,[119] in her 1985 classic text on breastfeeding, provides guidelines for an allergy prophylaxis regimen for the pregnant and lactating woman. She targets only women who have allergy (especially asthma or atopic dermatitis) in the immediate family unit. For these women, she suggests excluding all foods to which they are allergic and those foods to which any immediate family member is allergic. For women with cow's milk allergy or with cow's milk allergy in the family, Lawrence[119] recommends milk elimination with use of meats or soybean products to supply protein. For these women she also recommends calcium supplementation (0.4 g/day for pregnancy and 0.5 g/day for lactation). If there is no milk allergy, she still recommends that the at risk woman limit intake to 2 cups of milk prepared by boiling for 10 minutes or 2 cups of a one-half water/one-half evaporated milk mixture. (She notes potential substitutions with either soy milk or superheated commercial milk-based formulas.) Further recommendations include avoiding excessive consumption of a food or food category (especially peanut) and avoiding synthetic colorings, such as tartrazine, which may be present in vitamin supplements.

Chandra et al,[67] in 1986, published the results of a study looking at the effects of maternal avoidance of food antigens on atopic eczema incidence in infants. Study subjects were women who had given birth to an atopic child in the previous pregnancy. These 121 women were randomly allocated for either an antigen-avoidance or control group. The antigen-avoidance group was told to eliminate cow's milk, dairy products, peanut, egg, fish, and beef throughout pregnancy and during the time of lactation. (A 3g daily calcium lactate supplement was prescribed, and all women were taking multivitamin and iron preparations.) The control group received no instructions about dietary restrictions, but did receive the multivitamin and iron supplements. In the maternal antigen-avoidance group, 35 women breastfed and 20 used formulas (modified cow's milk). In the control group 36 women breastfed and 18 formula fed their infants. Breast milk samples for both groups were examined monthly for antigen presence. There were 17 cases of eczema in infants of the avoidance group, and 24 cases in controls. Statistical differences were noted, however, when breastfeeders (both categories) were compared to formula feeders (both categories). Eczema incidence was significantly less in the breastfed group. Although the authors reported that maternal dietary restriction was associated with decreased atopic eczema incidence, incidence differences between the control group and the avoidance group infants were not statistically significant. The results of this analysis were that 3 out of 20 mothers on the antigen-avoidance diet had 1 or more antigens (β-lactoglobulin, ovalbumin, or casein) present in breast milk compared to 15 of 16 controls. The authors concluded by suggesting that women at risk because of familial allergic history should be advised to follow an avoidance protocol. They support exclusive breastfeeding for at least 6 months' duration.

In 1986, Zeiger et al[6] (with Hamburger) reported on results using the Hamburger[3] protocol described earlier. The 1986 report dealt with the effectiveness of the regimen in 200 atopic mother and infant pairs who volunteered to become involved in the project. Diagnosis of atopic conditions was conducted in a blind fashion using standard criteria. After 36 months, despite a professionally intense program of prophylaxis, eczema developed in 12% of infants, infectious asthma in 24%, food allergy in 14%, and allergic rhinitis in 7%. Allergic symptoms seemed to be triggered most often by (1) egg and (2) milk. The authors cited the problems of noncompliance and hereditary predominance as potential factors that could explain their findings. (The researchers were able to monitor dietary compliance by using an enzyme-linked immunosorbent test for IgG specific to cow's milk.) This method enabled them to document a break in compliance for 30% of protocol infants at 1 year of age. The authors called for randomized prospective studies of the prevention protocol, which they now have under way.[6,9] On a pessimistic note, they concluded that because genetics is so predominant in the etiology of allergic disease, preventive efforts are often likely to fail.

A recent study by Magnusson et al (summarized by Zeiger[9] in 1988) also supports the difficulty in achieving allergic prophylaxis. This study of 212 atopic infants involved prenatal diet restriction (no cow's milk, no egg, Nutramigen®, and calcium supplements) and control of postnatal diet (breastfeeding supplemented only with Nutramigen® for three months). No significant differences were found between the group following the experimental protocol and controls in terms of incidence of positive skin tests, incidence of atopic dermatitis, or incidence of food allergy.

Lilja et al,[123] also in 1988, reported that changing maternal diet in the third trimester of pregnancy did not seem to be an effective prevention strategy. Comparing groups of atopic women who eliminated cow's milk and egg from their diet to those who did not, no significant differences in cold IgE levels were noted.

SUMMARY AND IMPLICATIONS FOR DIETETIC PRACTICE

What do we know about maternal influences on the development of food allergy in the infant? It seems from current knowledge that maternal diet can potentially influence the infant's allergic status both pre- and postnatally. Genetics, however, appears to be a dominant factor influencing allergy development.

There are identified components of breast milk that would seem to offer some protection and potentially at least delay allergy. Studies comparing incidence of allergic conditions for breastfed versus nonbreastfed infants have yielded conflicting results. Prospective studies, with better study design, are needed. An important variable is how breastfeeding is practiced. Dietitians can aid future research by fully describing how women breastfeed (indicating such factors as duration, use of supplemental formulas, and solid food introduction practices).

Practitioners can emphasize to at-risk mothers that *exclusive* breastfeeding for at least 6 months is currently recommended as an important preventive strategy and, if formula supplementation is desired, a casein hydrolysate-based formula (such as Alimentum® or Nutramigen®) might be considered.

Allergies can occur in solely breastfed infants. Physicians need to be aware of this possibility to make a timely and appropriate diagnosis. Once a diagnosis is made, the dietitian can aid the lactating woman in avoiding food offenders, and in so doing, can be supportive of continued breastfeeding. If a switch to a formula is desired by the mother or mandated by medical necessity (eg, the infant does not respond to maternal dietary manipulations), the dietitian can be involved in helping to select an appropriate formula.

To date, dietary protocols with prenatal and postnatal components aimed at prevention have not proved highly successful. Some highly motivated atopic patients, under the care of a competent allergy team, however, may benefit by following the recommendations put forward by Hamburger[3] and Zeiger.[6,8,9] It is important that dietitians work with such patients to assure nutritional adequacy of intake in the face of food and beverage restrictions.

REFERENCES

1. Foucard T. Developmental aspects of food sensitivity in childhood. *Nutr Rev.* 1984; 42(3):98–104.

2. Vandenplas Y, Sacre L. Influences of neonatal serum IgE concentration, family history and diet on the incidence of cow's milk allergy. *Eur J Pediatr.* 1986; 145:493–495.

3. Hamburger RN, Heller S, Mellon MH, O'Connor RD, Zeiger RS. Current status of the clinical and immunologic consequences of a prototype allergic disease prevention. *Ann Allergy.* 1983; 51:281–290.

4. Orgel HA, Hamburger RN, Bazaral M, et al. Development of IgE and allergy in infancy. *J Allergy Clin Immunol.* 1975; 56:296–307.

5. Wittig HJ, McLaughlin ET, Leifer KL, Belloit JD. Risk factors for the development of allergic disease: An analysis of 2,190 patient records. *Ann Allergy.* 1978; 41:84–88.

6. Zeiger RS, Heller S, Mellon M, O'Connor R, Hamburger RN. Effectiveness of dietary manipulation in the prevention of food allergy in infants. *J Allergy Clin Immunol.* 1986; 78(1):224–238.

7. Schatz M, Zeiger RS, Mellon M, Porreco R. Asthma and allergic disease: Management of the mother and prevention in the child. In: Middleton E Jr, Reed CE, Ellis EF, eds. *Allergy: Principles and Practice.* St. Louis: CV Mosby Co; 1983:935–86.

8. Zeiger RS. Offspring of high risk allergic families. In: Lifshitz F, ed. *Nutrition for Special Needs in Infancy: Protein Hydrolysates.* New York: Marcel Dekker, Inc; 1985:239–256.

9. Zeiger RS. Prevention of food allergy. In: Chiaramonte LT, Schneider AT, Lifshitz F, eds. *Food Allergy: A Practical Approach to Diagnosis and Management.* New York: Marcel Dekker, Inc; 1988:329–350.

10. Balyeat RM. The hereditary factor in allergic diseases. *Am J Med Sci.* 1928; 176:332–345.

11. Matsumura T, Kuroume T, Oguri M, et al. Egg sensitivity and eczematous manifestations in breast-fed newborns with particular reference to intrauterine sensitization. *Ann Allergy.* 1975; 35:221–229.

12. Kuroume T, Oguri M, Matsumura T, et al. Milk sensitivity and soybean sensitivity in the production of eczematous manifestations in breastfed infants with particular reference to intrauterine sensitization. *Ann Allergy.* 1976; 37:41–46.

13. Miller DL, Hirovonen T, Gitlin D. Synthesis of IgE by the human conceptus. *J Allergy Clin Immunol.* 1973; 52(3):182–188.

14. Van Asperen PP, Kemp AS, Mellis CM. Immediate food hypersensitivity reactions on the first known exposure to the food. *Arch Dis Child.* 1983; 58:253–256.

15. Kaufman HS. Allergy in the newborn: skin test reactions confirmed by the Prausnitz-Küstner test at birth. *Clin Allergy.* 1971; 1:363–367.

16. Michel FB, Bousquet J, Greillier P, Robinet-Levy M, Coulomb Y. Comparison of cord blood immunoglobulin E concentrations and maternal allergy for the prediction of atopic diseases in infancy. *J Allergy Clin Immunol.* 1980; 65(6):422–430.

17. Bellanti JA. Prevention of food allergies. *Ann Allergy.* 1984; 53:683–688.

18. Dannaeus A, Johansson SGO, Foucard T. Clinical and immunological aspects of food allergy in childhood, II: development of allergic symptoms and humoral immune response to foods in infants of atopic mothers during the first 24 months of life. *Acta Paediatr Scand.* 1978; 67:497–504.

19. Berg T. The immunoglobulin development during the first year of life. *Acta Paediatr Scand.* 1969; 58:229–236.

20. Strimas JH, Chi DS. Significance of IgE level in amniotic fluid and cord blood for the prediction of allergy. *Ann Allergy.* 1988; 61:133–136.

21. Businco L, Marchetti F, Pellegrini G, Perlini R. Predictive value of cord blood IgE levels in "at risk" newborn babies and influence of type of feeding. *Clin Allergy.* 1983; 13:503–508.

22. Hamburger RN. Diagnosis of food allergies and intolerances in the study of prophylaxis and control groups in infants. *Ann Allergy.* 1984; 53:673–677.

23. Chandra RK, Puri S, Cheema PS. Predictive value of cord blood IgE in the development of atopic disease and role of breast-feeding in its prevention. *Clin Allergy.* 1985; 15:517–522.

24. Baylis JM, Leeds AR, Challacombe DN. Persistent nausea and food aversions in pregnancy—a possible association with cow's milk allergy in infants. *Clin Allergy.* 1983; 13:263–269.

25. Atherton DJ. Breastfeeding and atopic eczema. *Br Med J.* 1983; 287(6395):775–776.

26. Hanson LÅ, Ahlstedt S, Anderson B, et al. Protective factors in milk and the development of the immune system. *Pediatrics.* 1985; 75(suppl):172–176.

27. Soothill JF. Immunological aspects of infant feeding. In: Soothill JF, Hayward AR, Wood CBS, eds. *Paediatric Immunology.* Oxford, England: Blackwell; 1983: 110–129.

28. Ogra PL, Welliver RC, Riepenhoff-Talty M, Foden HS. Interaction of mucosal immune system and infections in infancy: implications in allergy. *Ann Allergy.* 1984; 53:523–534.

29. Cruz JR, Garcia B, Urrutia JJ, Carlsson B, Hanson LA. Food antibodies in milk from Guatemalan women. *J Pediatr.* 1981; 98(4):600–602.

30. Walker WA. Allergen absorption in the intestine: implication for food allergy in infants. *J Allergy Clin Immunol.* 1986; 78(5.2):1003–1009.

31. Stokes CR, Soothill JF, Turner MW. Immune exclusion is a function of IgA. *Nature.* 1975; 255:745–746.

32. Personal Communication: Intensive Course in Pediatric Nutrition, Iowa City, Iowa, June 1989.

33. Pittard WB, Bill K. Immunoregulation by breast milk cells. *Cell Immunol.* 1979; 42:437–441.

34. Michael FB, Bousquet J, Dannaeus A, et al. Preventive measures in early childhood allergy. *J Allergy Clin Immunol.* 1986; 78(5):1022–1027.

35. Klagsbrun M. Bovine colostrum supports the serum free proliferation of epithelial cells but not of fibroblasts in long term culture. *J Cell Biol.* 1980; 84:808–814.

36. Udall JN, Colony P, Fritze L, Pang K, Trier JS, Walker WA. Development of gastrointestinal mucosal barrier, II: the effect of natural versus artificial feeding on intestinal permeability to macromolecules. *Pediatr Res.* 1981; 15:245–249.

37. Walker WA. Antigen absorption from the small intestine and gastrointestinal disease. *Pediatr Clin North Am.* 1975; 22(4):731–746.

38. Sheard NF, Walker WA. The role of breast milk in the development of the gastrointestinal tract. *Nutr Rev.* 1988; 46(1):1–8.

39. Businco L, Marchetti F, Pellegrini G, Cantani A, Perlini R. Prevention of atopic disease in "at risk newborns" by prolonged breastfeeding. *Ann Allergy.* 1983; 51:296–299.

40. Frick OL, German DF, Mills J. Development of allergy in children, I: association with virus infections. *J Allergy Clin Immunol.* 1979; 63(4):228–241.

41. Goldman AS, Thorpe LW, Goldblum RM, Hanson LA. Anti-inflammatory properties of human milk. *Acta Paediatr Scand.* 1986; 75:689–695.

42. Ponzone A. Prolonged exclusive breastfeeding and heredity as determinants in infantile atopy. *Arch Dis Child.* 1987; 62:1196.

43. Voglino GF, Ponzone A. Polymorphism in human casein. *Nature New Biol.* 1972;238:149–150.

44. Savilahti E, Tainio VM, Salmenpera L, Shimes MA, Perrheentupa J. Prolonged exclusive breast feeding and heredity as determinants in infantile atopy. *Arch Dis Child.* 1987; 62:269–273.

45. Shannon WR. Demonstration of food proteins in human breast milk by anaphylactic experiments on guinea pigs. *Am J Dis Child.* 1921; 23(3):223–224.

46. Kilshaw PJ, Cant AJ. The passage of maternal dietary proteins into human breast milk. *Int Archs Allergy Appl Immunol.* 1984; 75:8–15.

47. Stuart CA, Twiselton R, Nicholas MK, Hide DW. Passage of cow's milk protein in breast milk. *Clin Allergy.* 1984; 14:533–535.

48. Harmatz PR, Bloch KJ. Transfer of dietary protein in breast milk. *Ann Allergy.* 1988; 61(2):21–24.

49. Cant A, Marsden RA, Kilshaw PJ. Egg and cow's milk hypersensitivity in exclusively breast fed infants with eczema and detection of egg protein in breast milk. *Br Med J.* 1985; 291:932-935.

50. Gerrard JW. Cow's milk and breast milk. In: Brostoff J, Challacombe ST, eds. *Food Allergy and Intolerance.* London, England: Bailliere Tindall; 1987: 351–355.

51. Chandra RK, Baker M. Numerical and functional deficiency of suppressor T cells precedes development of atopic eczema. *Lancet.* 1983; 2:1393–1394.

52. Juto P, Möller C, Engberg S, Björksten B. Influence of type of feeding on lymphocyte function and development of infantile allergy. *Clin Allergy.* 1982; 12:409–416.

53. Strannegård Ö, Strannegård IL. T lymphocyte numbers and function in human IgE mediated allergy. *Immunol Rev.* 1978; 41:149–170.

54. Tainio VM. Lymphocyte subsets in infants: relationship to feeding, atopy, atopic heredity and infections. *Int Archs Allergy Appl Immun.* 1985; 78:305–310.

55. Butler M, Atherton D, Levinsky RJ. Quantitative and functional deficit of suppressor T-cells in children with atopic eczema. *Clin Exp Immunol.* 1982; 50:90–98.

56. Ross Laboratories. *Use of Hydrolysate Feedings in Infancy.* Columbus, OH: Ross Laboratories; 1988: 8.

57. Kajosaari M, Saarinen UM. Prophylaxis of atopic disease by six months total solid food elimination, evaluation of 135 exclusively breastfed infants of atopic families. *Acta Paediatr Scand.* 1983; 72:411–414.

58. Jarrett E. Activation of IgE regulatory mechanisms by transmucosal absorption of antigen. *Lancet.* 1977; 2:223–225.

59. Björksten F, Saarinen UM. IgE antibodies to cow's milk in infants fed breast milk and milk formulae. *Lancet.* 1978; 2:624–625. Letter.

60. Kaplan MS, Solli NJ. Immunoglobulin E to cow's milk protein in breast fed atopic children. *J Allergy Clin Immunol.* 1979; 64(2):122–126.

61. Warner JO. Food allergy in fully breast-fed infants. *Clin Allergy.* 1980; 10:133–136.

62. Juto P, Björksten B. Serum IgE in infants and influence of type of feeding. *Clin Allergy.* 1980; 10:593–600.

63. Gerrard JW, Shenassa M. Sensitization to substance in breast milk: Recognition, management, and significance. *Ann Allergy.* 1983; 51:300–302.

64. Gerrard JW, Shenassa M. Food allergy: two common types as seen in breast and formula fed babies. *Ann Allergy.* 1983; 50:375–379.

65. Firer MA, Hosking CS, Hill DJ. Effect of antigen load on development of milk antibodies in infants allergic to milk. *Br Med J.* 1981; 283:693–696.

66. Kovar MG, Serdula MK, Marks JS, Fraser DW. Review of the epidemiologic evidence for an association between infant feeding and infant health. *Pediatrics.* 1984; 74(suppl): 615–638.

67. Chandra RK, Puri S, Suraiya C, Cheema PS. Influence of maternal food antigen avoidance during pregnancy and lactation on incidence of atopic eczema in infants. *Clin Allergy.* 1986; 16:563–569.

68. Sampson HA. Role of immediate food hypersensitivity in the pathogenesis of atopic dermatitis. *J Allergy Clin Immunol.* 1983; 71(5):473–480.

69. Hanifin JM. Diet, nutrition, and allergy in atopic dermatitis. *J Am Acad Dermatol.* 1983; 8(5):729–731. Editorial.

70. American Academy of Dermatology Task Force on Pediatric Dermatology. Diet and atopic dermatitis. *J Am Acad Dermatol.* 1986; 15(3):543–545.

71. Johnson EJ, Irons JS, Patterson R, Roberts M. Serum IgE concentration in atopic dermatitis. *J Allergy Clin Immunol.* 1974; 54:94–99.

72. Church JA, Kleban DG, Bellanti JA. Serum immunoglobulin E concentrations and radioallergosorbent tests in children with atopic dermatitis. *Pediatr Res.* 1976; 10:97–99.

73. Hoffman DR, Yamamoto FY, Geller B, Haddad Z. Specific IgE antibodies in atopic eczema. *J Allergy Clin Immunol.* 1975; 55(4):256–267.

74. Hill DJ, Balloch A, Hosking CS. IgE responses to environmental antigens in atopic children. *Clin Allergy.* 1981; 11:541–547.

75. Jackson PG, Baker RWR, Lessof MH, Ferrett J, MacDonald DM. Intestinal permeability in patients with eczema and food allergy. *Lancet.* 1981; 1:1285–1286.

76. Kramer MS. Does breast feeding help protect against atopic disease? Biology, methodology, and a golden jubilee of controversy. *J Pediatr.* 1988; 112(2):181–190.

77. Midwinter RE, Morris AF, Colley JRT. Infant feeding and atopy. *Arch Dis Child.* 1987; (62):965–967.

78. Papa CM. Breast feeding and eczema/asthma. *Lancet.* 1982; 1:911. Letter.

79. Cant AJ, Bailes JA, Marsden RA, Hewitt D. Effect of maternal dietary exclusion on breast fed infants with eczema: Two controlled studies. *Br Med J.* 1986; 293:231–233.

80. Gruskay FL. Comparison of breast, cow, and soy feedings in the prevention of onset of allergic disease: A 15 year prospective study. *Clin Pediatr.* 1982; 21:486–491.

81. Grulee CG, Sanford HN. The influence of breast and artificial feeding on infantile eczema. *J Pediatr.* 1936; 9:223–225.

82. Burr ML. Does infant feeding affect the risk of allergy? *Arch Dis Child.* 1983; 58:561–565.

83. Murray AB. Infant feeding and respiratory allergy. *Lancet.* 1971; 1:497. Letter.

84. Blair H. Natural history of childhood asthma. *Arch Dis Child.* 1977; 52:613–619.

85. Matthew DJ, Norman AP, Taylor B, Turner MW, Soothill JF. Prevention of eczema. *Lancet.* 1977; 1:321–324.

86. Chandra RK. Prospective studies of the effect of breast feeding on incidence of infection and allergy. *Acta Paediatr Scand.* 1979; 68:691–694.

87. Saarinen UM, Backman A, Kajosaari M, Siimes MA. Prolonged breastfeeding as prophylaxis for atopic disease. *Lancet.* 1979; 2:163–166.

88. Hide DW, Guyer BM. Clinical manifestations of allergy related to breast and cow's milk feeding. *Arch Dis Child.* 1981; 56:172–175.

89. Kaufman HS, Frick OL. Prevention of asthma. *Clin Allergy.* 1981; 11:549–553.

90. Lucarelli S, Frediani T, Barbato MB, Marchetti F, Pellegrini G, Businco L. Serum IgE in newborns from atopic parents, development of atopy and influence of type of feeding. *Pediatr Res.* 1981; 15(8):1181.

91. Pratt HF. Breastfeeding and eczema. *Early Hum Dev.* 1984; 9:283–290.

92. Fergusson DM, Horwood LJ, Beautrais AL, Shannon FT, Taylor B. Eczema and infant diet. *Clin Allergy.* 1981; 11:325–331.

93. Moore WJ, Midwinter RE, Morris AF, Colley JRT, Soothill JF. Infant feeding and subsequent risk of atopic eczema. *Arch Dis Child.* 1985; 60:722–726.

94. Miskelly FG, Burr ML, Vaughn-Williams E, Fehily AM, Butland BK, Merrett TG. Infant feeding and allergy. *Arch Dis Child.* 1988; 63:388–393.

95. Downham MAPS, Scott R, Sims DG, Webb JKG, Gardner PS. Breastfeeding protects against respiratory syncytial virus infections. *Br Med J.* 1976; ii:274–276.

96. Halpern SR, Sellars WA, Johnson RB, Anderson DW, Saperstein S, Reisch JS. Development of childhood allergy in infants fed breast, soy, or cow milk. *J Allergy Clin Immunol.* 1973; 51(3):139–151.

97. Kramer MS, Moroz B. Do breast-feeding and delayed introduction of solid foods protect against subsequent atopic eczema? *J Pediatr.* 1981; 98(4):546–550.

98. Gordon RR, Ward AM, Noble DA, Allen R. Immunoglobulin E and the eczema-asthma syndrome in early childhood. *Lancet.* 1982; 1:72–74.

99. Golding J, Butler NR, Taylor B. Breast-feeding and eczema/asthma. *Lancet.* 1982; 1:623. Letter.

100. Cogswell JJ, Alexander J. Breastfeeding and eczema/asthma. *Lancet.* 1982; 1:910. Letter.

101. Garrow D, Pratt H. Breastfeeding and eczema/asthma. *Lancet.* 1982; 1:910. Letter.

102. Fergusson DM, Horwood LJ, Shannon FT. Asthma and infant diet. *Arch Dis Child.* 1983; 58:48–51.

103. Taylor B, Wadsworth J, Golding J, Butler N. Breastfeeding, eczema, asthma, and hayfever. *J Epidemiol Comm Health.* 1983; 37:95–99.

104. Van Asperen PP, Kemp AS, Mellis CM. Relationship of diet in the development of atopy in infancy. *Clin Allergy.* 1984; 14:525–532.

105. Peters T, Golding J, Butler NR. Breastfeeding and childhood eczema. *Lancet.* 1985; 1:49–50. Letter.

106. Hide DW, Guyer BM. Clinical manifestations of allergy related to breast and cow's milk feeding. *Pediatrics.* 1985; 76(6):973–975.

107. Cogswell JJ, Mitchell EB, Alexander J. Parental smoking, breast feeding, and respiratory infection in development of allergic diseases. *Arch Dis Child.* 1987; 62:338–344.

108. Karvetti RL, Knuts LR. Validity of the 24-hour dietary recall. *J Am Diet Assoc.* 1985; 85(11):1437–1442.

109. Krall EA, Dwyer JT. Validity of a food frequency questionnaire and a food diary in a short term recall situation. *J Am Diet Assoc.* 1987; 87(10):1374–1377.

110. Wergeland H. Three fatal cases of probable familial allergy to human milk. *Acta Paediatr Scand* 1948; 35(suppl 1):321–334.

111. Gerrard JW. Allergy in breastfed babies to ingredients in breast milk. *Ann Allergy.* 1979; 42(2):69–72.

112. Donnally HH. The question of elimination of foreign protein (egg white) in woman's milk. *J Immunol.* 1930; 19:15–40.

113. Cant AJ, Bailes JA, Marsden RA. Cow's milk, soya milk, and goat's milk in a mother's diet causing eczema and diarrhoea in her breast fed infant. *Acta Paediatr Scand.* 1985; 74:467–468.

114. Gerrard JW, Perelmutter L. IgE-mediated allergy to peanut, cow's milk, and egg in children with special reference to maternal diet. *Ann Allergy.* 1986; 56:351-354.

115. Lake AM, Whitington PF, Hamilton SR. Dietary protein-induced colitis in breast-fed infants. *J Pediatr.* 1982; 101(6):906-910.

116. Wilson NW, Self TW, Hamburger RN. Severe cow's milk induced colitis in an exclusively breastfed neonate. *Clin Pediatr.* 1990; 29:77–80.

117. Lifschitz CH, Hawkins HL, Guerra C, Byrd N. Anaphylactic shock due to cow's milk protein hypersensitivity in a breast-fed infant. *J Pediatr Gastroenterol Nutr.* 1988; 7:141–144.

118. Glaser J, Johnstone DE. Prophylaxis of allergic disease in the newborn. *JAMA.* 1953; 153(7):620–622.

119. Lawrence RA. Prenatal dietary prophylaxis of atopic disease. In: Lawrence RA, ed. *Breastfeeding: A Guide for the Medical Profession.* St. Louis: CV Mosby Co; 1985: 561–562.

120. Sampson HA. Food allergies and the infant at risk. *JAMA.* 1988; 260(23):3507.

121. Johnstone DE, Dutton AM. Dietary prophylaxis of allergic disease in children. *N Engl J Med.* 1966; 274(13):715–719.

122. Stintzing G, Zetterstrom R. Cow's milk allergy incidence and pathogenetic role of early exposure to cow's milk formula. *Acta Paediatr Scand.* 1979; 68:383–387.

123. Lilja G, Dannaeus A, Fälth-Magnusson K, et al. Immune response of the atopic woman and foetus: effects of high- and low-dose food allergen intake during late pregnancy. *Clin Allergy.* 1988; 18:131–142.

Chapter 6

Managing Food Allergies in Infants and Toddlers

Victoria Olejer

The primary objective in the treatment of individuals diagnosed with food allergies, regardless of the age of the patient, remains the complete removal of the offending food(s) from the diet. While simple in premise, this directive can be quite difficult in practice, depending on the number and identity of foods to be avoided. Dietary treatment is based on the assumption that the diagnosis was made by a qualified physician employing appropriate elimination diets followed by supervised provocation tests, ideally, double-blind, placebo-controlled food challenges (DBPCFC). A secondary objective is the appropriate medical management of symptoms resulting from poor dietary compliance, inadvertent exposures to an offending food (eg, cooking vapors, topical exposures, etc.), and possible incomplete recognition of all potentially sensitizing foods. While reputed to be of only limited benefit in preventing symptoms resulting from dietary indiscretions,[1] the judicious use of drugs and topical agents may reduce some of the discomfort and certainly much of the mortality associated with food allergies. Pharmacological adjuncts useful in treating patients are discussed in Chapter 4.

For those patients with a history of particularly severe or anaphylactic reactions, instruction directed toward key family members and caretakers (eg, teachers, sitters, day-care workers, etc.) regarding the proper procedures to be taken in an emergency is paramount.[2] Two frequently used emergency devices, available by prescription only, include the EpiPen® Jr. Autoinjector (Center Laboratories, Port Washington, NY 11050) and the Ana-Kit® Insect Sting Treatment Kit (Hollister-Stier Laboratories, Spokane, WA 99207). These devices are not designed to permit dietary infractions but, instead, when used as directed may provide valuable time for the transport of the child to where appropriate emergency care may be given. Identification bracelets, necklaces, and clothing tags listing the patient's name, address, responsible parties, and specific food allergies may also be indicated. There is no evidence at present to support either classic immunotherapy with food antigens[3] or oral desensitization or neutralization with gradually increasing amounts of food antigen[4] as valid treatment options.

The signs and symptoms of food allergy often provide the first clues to an infant's underlying atopic nature. The term, atopy, was first introduced by Coca and others in 1923 to suggest "strange disease."[5] Today, the term has been refined to indicate the existence of IgE-mediated, mast cell-dependent hypersensitivity reactions resulting from the combination of IgE antibody with specific antigen in individuals with a genetic propensity for both experiencing such reactions and producing large amounts of IgE.[6] Elevated levels of IgE alone are not automatically diagnostic of atopy, because individuals with low levels of IgE may also develop allergic symptoms.[6] The predisposition for atopy is believed to be controlled by multiple genes of unknown location, but a basic defect in T-lymphocyte function is suspected.[6,7]

Evidence of atopic diseases worldwide is estimated to occur in approximately 15% of the children in first world countries.[6,8,9] In accordance with the genetic propensity for atopy, the highest incidence is found in children with a family history of allergy. Kjellman and Johansson[10] observed a 67% incidence of atopy in 48 children of similar genetic background with a biparental history of atopy, followed prospectively from birth to 4 years of age, with the first appearance of symptoms occurring at a mean age of 9.1 months and a peak prevalence at approximately 3 years of age. If only one parent is atopic, the incidence drops to approximately 40%-50%.[11] Common clinical manifestations include atopic eczema, asthma, and rhinoconjunctivitis and may range in severity from mere annoyances to life-threatening reactions. Time and money spent in seeking treatment for these maladies can impose significant burdens on the family. It is, therefore, not surprising that research efforts have traditionally focused on identifying infants considered to be at risk of developing allergies in the hope that by eliminating or reducing an infant's exposure to allergens and certain potentiating factors, allergic sensitization may be prevented or, at least, postponed. Infants considered high allergic risk candidates include those infants born with a combination of an elevated level of cord blood (CB) IgE,[12-19] a low T-cell count,[20-22] and a positive history of allergy in two or more immediate family members (ie, mother, father, full siblings). High allergic risk infants are felt to represent an important target population toward which aggressive preventive measures should be directed.

IgE synthesis of fetal origin can occur as early as 11 weeks' gestation in the liver and lung,[23] and in amniotic fluid as early as 13 weeks' gestation.[24] Michel and coworkers reported detectable levels of CB IgE in 34% of term infants.[14] Because a placental barrier exists for both IgE and IgA, the last immunoglobulin of ontogenetic sequence, the presence of CB IgE in the absence of IgA represents fetal synthesis of IgE,[25] suggesting infants may be atopic at birth.

The accurate determination of either total or specific IgE in CB samples requires the assessment of IgA when CB IgE is elevated to rule out the possibility of a maternal-fetal blood admixture, not an uncommon occurrence.[25]

Clinical evidence for a genetic effect on IgE production in first world countries was first provided by Kjellman and Johansson,[12] who observed that neonates born with a family history of atopy tended to have higher levels of CB IgE. Differences of opinion persist concerning the level of CB IgE considered most predictive of atopy. Cutoffs of 0.75 IU/ml[13] and, particularly, 0.90 IU/ml[14,16] have emerged as the levels with the highest specificity and sensitivity for first world Caucasian infants, but these findings are still in the investigational stages. The extremely high CB IgE concentrations observed in black third world infants, independent of atopic family history and maternal parasitic infections (two potentiators of IgE synthesis), support the contention that additional research is needed to establish relevant cutoffs for different ethnic groups before broad clinical applications may be made based on CB IgE levels.[26]

In a prospective study examining the relationships between a positive family history for allergy, T-cell concentration, type of feeding, and the development of allergic symptoms, formula feeding using a cow's milk-based formula was associated with increased signs of allergic sensitization in infants with low T-cell counts.[20-22] At 1 month of age, approximately 33% of the infants with a positive family history for allergy had low numbers of T lymphocytes, while only 5% of the infants with a negative family history for allergy had similar findings. Infants with low T-cell counts also possessed higher levels of IgE than infants of similar genetic background with normal T-cell counts and infants with a negative family history for allergy. In infants with normal T-cell counts (ie, 67% of the infants with a positive family history for allergy and 95% of the infants with a negative family history for allergy), no differences in IgE level or allergy symptom scores were observed between formula-fed and exclusively breastfed infants. At 3 and 6 months of age, the exclusively breastfed infants with low T-cell counts had IgE levels and allergy symptom scores similar to the infants with normal T-cell counts. Significantly higher levels of IgE and allergy symptom scores, though, were observed in the formula-fed infants with low T-cell counts when compared to infants with similar T-cell counts who were exclusively breastfed during the same period, suggesting that breastfeeding may be protective against allergy only in infants considered at high risk for developing atopic diseases.

The immunoprotective aspects of breastfeeding over formula feeding have long been the subject of much investigation in the medical community and have been reviewed in detail in Chapter 5. It is widely accepted and promoted that breastfeeding protects against the development of atopic diseases, in general, and food allergies, in particular.[8,11,16–18,25,27–30] Despite these sentiments, considerable contradiction exists in the research literature regarding the strength of these claims. Comparisons between studies are difficult to make due to fundamental differences in experimental design, definitions of atopy and the high-risk infant, duration of breastfeeding, maternal diet permitted during breastfeeding, age of the infant when solid foods were first introduced, and the length of the follow-up period during which infants were observed for signs of atopy. Numerous studies have observed a preventive effect for breastfeeding, particularly when the diet of the breastfeeding mother has been restricted with respect to the consumption of highly sensitizing foods, while other studies that have not employed maternal dietary restrictions have failed to confirm these observations.[31,32]

It is well established that exquisitely sensitive, exclusively breastfed infants may become sensitized to foods the mother is consuming and passively transferring to the infant via her breast milk.[33–36] Low levels of breast milk IgG[37] and IgA[38] antibodies in some nursing mothers coupled with the fairly common occurrence in breast milk of at least one particularly prominent food allergen, β-lactoglobulin,[38] are suspected of playing a permissive role in these infants. Nursing mothers with low or undetectable levels of breast milk IgG and IgA antibodies may represent an additional high-risk target group for whom dietary restriction and appropriate environmental manipulation directed at reducing allergen exposure may be especially helpful in preventing or delaying the onset of allergic disease in their infants.

In summary, the exact mechanisms by which breast milk protects some infants, but not others, from allergic sensitization are not well defined, but appear to represent a complex interaction between the immune status of both the mother and the infant and numerous environmental enhancers of allergy.[39] In a comprehensive review of many of these complicating factors, Zeiger and coworkers[25] have formulated the following strategies for the prevention of allergic disease in high allergic risk infants:

- When possible, encourage exclusive breastfeeding for at least 6 months
- Encourage the complete avoidance of cow's milk, egg, fish, and peanut-containing foods from the mother's diet for the duration of the breastfeeding period
- Encourage reduced consumption of soy, wheat, citrus fruits, and cocoa in the mother's diet for the duration of the breastfeeding period
- Supplement, when necessary, the infant's diet with casein hydrolysate-based formulas, completely avoiding cow's milk- and soy-based formulas for the first year of life
- Withhold solid food introduction until the infant is 6 months of age

— Delay introduction of cow's milk, wheat, corn, and citrus fruits until 1 year of age
— Delay introduction of egg and the true nuts until 2 years of age
— Delay introduction of fish and peanut until 3 years of age.

These prophylactic measures are endorsed with only slight modifications in numerous other research camps[11,17,18,27-30,40,41] and appear to be most effective in postponing the advent of allergic diseases rather than preventing them altogether. To postpone is perceived to be near synonymous with prevention, owing to the often increased frequency and severity of allergic symptoms seen in infancy and early childhood and the difficulties in medicating this age group. Nonetheless, the hardships imposed by these dietary restrictions must be weighed against the possible prophylactic benefits on a case-by-case basis.

Maternal dietary intervention during pregnancy has not yet been demonstrated to be of significant benefit in preventing or delaying the onset of allergic diseases,[42] despite the occasional observation of intrauterine sensitization to foods.[14,17] Additional research is needed to clarify the frequency, mechanisms, and significance of intrauterine sensitization before the benefits of broad maternal dietary restrictions outweigh the risks of suboptimal nutrition accompanying such rigorous diets.

The prognosis for food hypersensitivity reactions is, fortunately, an optimistic one, particularly in the very young. Spontaneous symptom remission rates ranging from 38%-67% have been reported.[43-50] Factors thought to influence the rate of remission include the age of the patient when symptoms were first diagnosed and the identity of the sensitizing food. Tolerance to an offending food is more rapid very early in life, while symptoms that linger into childhood are less likely to resolve. Of the 20 newborn infants observed by Jakobsson and Lindberg[43] to be allergic to cow's milk, 50% achieved tolerance by 1 year of age and 60% by 2 years of age. Similarly, Ford and Taylor[44] reported a remission rate of 60% in infants diagnosed in the first year of life as compared to 33% in older children. Of the children under 3 years of age in Bock's study, an amazing 73% achieved tolerance, while only 26% of the children older than 3 years of age experienced symptom resolution.[49]

The identity of the sensitizing foods also exerts an effect on the eventual outcome. Sampson and McCaskill[46] observed a 42% remission rate in atopic dermatitis patients over a 1- to 2-year period dependent on the food antigen involved. In reviewing numerous studies examining the natural history of food allergy, Eggleston[51] calculated a 68% and 41% remission rate associated with cow's milk and egg allergy, respectively. For the majority of patients in these studies, symptoms resulting from food allergies largely resolved, only to be replaced by symptoms resulting from inhalant sensitivities,[44,48] confirming the atopic nature of these patients.

The prospect for gradual resolution of symptoms strongly points to the need for the periodic reassessment of continuing sensitization. Indeed, physicians caring for children with a history of even severe adverse food reactions are encouraged to perform periodic supervised food challenges.[47] The challenges should be conducted in a setting where emergency medical care is readily available, such as emergency rooms and outpatient clinics, with properly equipped treatment rooms staffed with personnel skilled in performing cardiopulmonary resuscitation.[47] If qualified emergency care is not available, challenges in these children are best avoided.

Some controversy exists regarding the length of time a sensitizing food should be avoided before being reintroduced into the diet in a carefully controlled systematic manner. Periods of 1 to 3 months, 6 months, and longer have been suggested depending on the allergen involved, the severity of symptoms, and the degree of difficulty associated with dietary avoidance.[52] A conservative approach employed by the author is summarized below and may serve as a general guideline.

MANAGEMENT OF FOOD ALLERGIES IN INFANTS

1. Use of alternative formulas for infants with allergies is discussed extensively in Chapter 2, Part II.
2. Avoid, at all costs, any food that results in anaphylaxis. These foods should not be rechallenged.
3. It may be necessary for mothers of exquisitely sensitive, breastfed infants to adhere to individualized elimination diets before maximum symptom relief can be achieved in the infant.
4. Infants in whom food sensitivities were diagnosed prior to 6 months of age should not be rechallenged with an offending food until they are at least 12 months old.
5. Wait at least 6 months before rechallenging an offending food in infants older than 6 months of age diagnosed with food sensitivities.
6. Always use single-ingredient foods when introducing a new food into the diet or when challenging with a previously unsafe food.
   - Allow one to two small feedings per day for 7 consecutive days when introducing a new food into the diet, allowing no more than one new food per week.
   - When challenging with a previously unsafe food, begin the challenge sequence with a very small sample size (eg, 1/2 teaspoon), gradually increasing the serving size over several hours to equal the amount of food that is customarily consumed or history suggests results in symp-

toms. If no symptoms occur, continue one to two feedings per day for a period of 7 consecutive days.

- If a reaction occurs anytime during the introduction or challenge of a food, discontinue any further feeding of that food.
- Wait for all symptoms resulting from a previous positive food challenge to completely go away before proceeding to the next food in the introduction or challenge sequence.

MANAGEMENT OF FOOD ALLERGIES IN TODDLERS AND OLDER CHILDREN

1. Because optimal nutrition is based on maximum variety in the diet, no food should be eliminated from the diet unless it is absolutely necessary. With the exception of any food that results in anaphylaxis, offending foods should be rechallenged at 6- to 12-month intervals.

2. Each challenge food is returned to the diet for a period of 3 consecutive days in the following manner:

Day 1:

Breakfast:	1/16 of a portion
10:00 A.M.:	1/8 of a portion
Noon:	1/4 of a portion
2:00 P.M..:	1/2 of a portion
4:00 P.M.:	1 whole portion
Dinner:	1 whole portion
HS:	2 whole portions

Days 2 and 3: Consume at least 3 portions of challenge food per day.

3. Portions represent serving sizes considered to be meal-sized portions and have largely been taken from diabetic exchange lists, so the amount of protein, carbohydrate, and fat contributed by various members of individual food groupings would be approximately the same.

4. Challenges resulting in a positive reaction at any time during the 3-day period are to be discontinued immediately. Symptom resolution should be complete before proceeding to the next food in the challenge sequence.

5. Open oral challenges resulting in a positive reaction should be repeated to confirm the reaction. Double-blind, placebo-controlled food challenges represent the gold standard and should be employed in equivocal challenges or when bias is suspected.

Elimination diets used in managing patients with food allergy generally mirror diets employed in the diagnosis phase with the exception that, in the management phase, only those foods documented to result in symptoms are eliminated from the diet. Parents of children with mild-to-moderate food sensitivities may be encouraged to experiment with various forms of an offending food (eg, cooked vs raw; refined vs unrefined; individual fractions of a food) to determine if certain forms are more tolerable than others. For example, both peanut oil and sunflower oil have been reported to be tolerated by individuals who anaphylax to whole peanut[53] and sunflower,[54] respectively, presumably due to the degree of refinement of the oils. Because the purity of an oil is difficult for the consumer to predict, caution is still the best advice. Additionally, parents should be counseled that periods of heightened sensitivity to a food may occur during times of illness, excessive fatigue, increased antigen load related to inhalant sensitivities, emotional stress, etc. Reassessment of continuing sensitization is best avoided during these times.

For many families, the prospect of long-term elimination of what may be favored foods is viewed with great apprehension, particularly if milk, egg, or wheat are among the foods to be avoided. Inclusion of a registered dietitian on the treatment team not only improves compliance by ensuring strict dietary avoidance through education and substitution, but is essential for assuring the nutritional adequacy of the diet. Implementation of the following suggestions in a patient's treatment plan should facilitate compliance.

RECOMMENDATIONS FOR ENHANCING PATIENT COMPLIANCE

1. Provision of individualized patient education materials regarding:
   - Derivatives of foods whose names bear little or no resemblance to the name of the parent food from which they were derived
   - Frequently encountered hidden sources of foods the patient must avoid
   - Alternative food sources, product suggestions, recipes, sample menus, etc.
   - Proper measures to be taken in an emergency
2. Encourage:
   - Thorough label reading at all times
   - An adventurous approach in experimenting with alternative foods
   - Appropriate coping behaviors
   - Participation in a support group
   - Semiannual nutrition assessment visits for individuals eliminating three or more major foods from the diet

In summary, as evidence accumulates regarding the benefits of early antigen avoidance, particularly in high allergic risk populations, future management approaches may have their greatest impact in preventing or delaying the appearance of food allergy rather than simply treating existing food sensitivities.

REFERENCES

1. Sogn DS. Medications and their use in the treatment of adverse reactions to foods. *J Allergy Clin Immunol.* 1986; 78(1):238–243.

2. Yunginger JW, Sweeney KG, Sturner WQ, et al. Fatal food-induced anaphylaxis. *JAMA.* 1988; 260(10):1450–1452.

3. Johnstone DE. Uses and abuses of hyposensitization in children. *Am J Dis Child.* 1972; 123:78–83.

4. Golbert TM. A review of controversial diagnostic and therapeutic techniques employed in allergy. *J Allergy Clin Immunol.* 1975; 56:170–190.

5. Coca AF, Cooke RA. On the classification of the phenomena of hypersensitiveness. *J Immunol.* 1923; 8:163–178.

6. Frick OL. Predisposing factors in the development of allergy. In: Lessof MH, Lee TH, Kmeny DM, eds. *Allergy: An International Textbook.* Sussex, UK: John Wiley & Sons, Ltd.; 1987: 347–358.

7. Strannegård Ö, Strannegård IL. T lymphocyte number and function in human IgE mediated allergy. *Immunol Rev.* 1978; 41:149–170.

8. Kjellman N-IM. Atopic disease in seven-year-old children: Incidence in relation to family history. *Acta Paediatr Scand.* 1977; 66:465–471.

9. Slavin RG, Smith LJ. Epidemiologic considerations in atopic disease. In: Bierman CW, Pearlman DS, eds. *Allergic Diseases of Infancy, Childhood and Adolescence.* Philadelphia: WB Saunders Co; 1980:165–172.

10. Kjellman N-IM, Johansson SGO. Soy versus cow's milk in infants with a biparental history of atopic disease: Development of atopic disease and immunoglobulins from birth to four years of age. *Clin Allergy.* 1979; 9:347–358.

11. Businco L, Cantani A. Prevention of atopy—Current concepts and personal experience. *Clin Rev Allergy.* 1984; 2:107–123.

12. Kjellman N-IM, Johansson SGO. IgE and atopic allergy in newborns and infants with a family history of atopic disease. *Acta Paediatr Scand.* 1976; 65:601–607.

13. Dannaeus A, Johansson SGO, Foucard T. Clinical and immunological aspects of food allergy in childhood. II. *Acta Paediatr Scand.* 1978; 67:497–504.

14. Michel FB, Bousquet J, Greillier P, Robinet-Levy M, Coulomb Y. Comparison of cord blood IgE concentrations and maternal allergy for the prediction of atopic disease in infancy. *J Allergy Clin Immunol.* 1980; 65(6):422–430.

15. Croner S, Kjellman N-IM, Eriksson B, Roth A. IgE screening in 1701 newborn infants and the development of atopic disease during infancy. *Arch Dis Child.* 1982; 57:364–368.

16. Kjellman N-IM, Croner S. Cord blood IgE determination for allergy prediction—a follow-up to seven years of age in 1651 children. *Ann Allergy.* 1984; 53:167–171.

17. Businco L, Marchetti F, Pellegrini G, Perlini R. Predictive value of cord serum IgE levels in "at risk" newborn babies and influence on type of feeding. *Clin Allergy.* 1983; 13:503–508.

18. Chandra RK, Puri S, Cheema PS. Predictive value of cord blood IgE in the development of atopic disease and role of breast-feeding in its prevention. *Clin Allergy.* 1985; 15:517–522.

19. Strimas JH, Chi DS. Significance of IgE level in amniotic fluid and cord blood for the prediction of allergy. *Ann Allergy.* 1988; 61:133–136.

20. Juto P, Moller C, Engerg S, Björksten B. Influence of type of feeding on lymphocyte function and development of infantile atopy. *Clin Allergy.* 1982; 12:409–416.

21. Björksten B, Juto P. Immunoglobulin E and T cells in infants. In: Kern JW, Ganderson MA, eds. *Proceedings of the XI International Congress of Allergy and Immunology.* London: McMillan Press; 1983:144–148.

22. Björksten B. Immune responses to ingested antigens in relation to feeding pattern in childhood. *Ann Allergy.* 1986; 57:143–146.

23. Miller DL, Hirvonen T, Gitlin D. Synthesis of IgE by the human conceptus. *J Allergy Clin Immunol.* 1973; 52(3):182–188.

24. Singer AD, Hobel CJ, Heiner DC. Evidence for secretory IgE in utero. *J Allergy Clin Immunol.* 1974; 53:94.

25. Zeiger RS, Heller S, Mellon M, O'Connor R, Hamburger RN. Effectiveness of dietary manipulation in the prevention of food allergy in infants. *J Allergy Clin Immunol.* 1986; 78(1):224–238.

26. Haus M, Heese HDV, Weinberg EG, Potter PC, Hall JM, Malherb D. The influence of ethnicity, an atopic family history, and maternal ascariasis on cord blood serum IgE concentrations. *J Allergy Clin Immunol.* 1988; 82(2):179–189.

27. Businco L, Marchetti F, Pellegrini G, Cantani A, Perlini R. Prevention of atopic disease in "at-risk newborns" by prolonged breastfeeding. *Ann Allergy.* 1983; 51:296–299.

28. Saarinen U. Prophylaxis for atopic disease: Role of infant feeding. *Clin Rev Allergy.* 1984; 2:151–167.

29. Miskelly FG, Burr ML, Vaughan-Williams E, Fehily AM, Butland BK, Merrett TG. Infant feeding and allergy. *Arch Dis Child.* 1988; 63:388–393.

30. Hattevig G, Kjellman B, Sigurs N, Björksten B, Kjellman N-IM. Effect of maternal avoidance of eggs, cow's milk and fish during lactation upon allergic manifestations in infants. *Clin Exp Allergy.* 1989; 19:27–32.

31. Van Asperen PP, Kemp AS, Mellis CM. Relationship of diet in development of atopy in infancy. *Clin Allergy.* 1984; 14:525–532.

32. Savilahti E, Tainio VM, Salmenperä L, Siimes MA, Perheentupa J. Prolonged exclusive breast feeding and heredity as determinants in infantile atopy. *Arch Dis Child.* 1987; 62:269–273.

33. Matsumura T, Kuroume T, Oguri M, et al. Egg sensitivity and eczematous manifestations in breast-fed newborns with particular reference to intrauterine sensitization. *Ann Allergy.* 1975; 35:221–229.

34. Kilshaw PJ, Cant AJ. Passage of maternal dietary proteins into human breast milk. *Int Arch Allergy Appl Immunol.* 1984; 75:8–15.

35. Cant AJ, Marsden RA, Kilshaw PJ. Egg and cow's milk hypersensitivity in exclusively breast fed infants with eczema and detection of egg protein in breast milk. *Br Med J.* 1985; 291–937.

36. Cavagni G, Paganelli R, Caffarelli C, et al. Passage of food antigens into circulation of breast-fed infants with atopic dermatitis. *Ann Allergy.* 1988; 61:361–365.

37. Casimir G, Gossart B, Vis HL, et al. Antibody against beta lactoglobulin (IgG) and cow's milk allergy. *J Allergy Clin Immunol.* 1985; 75(1):206. Abstract.

38. Machtinger S, Moss R. Cow's milk allergy in breast-fed infants: the role of allergen and maternal secretory IgA antibody. *J Allergy Clin Immunol.* 1986; 77(2):341–347.

39. Björksten B, Kjellman N-IM. Perinatal factors influencing the development of allergy. *Clin Rev Allergy.* 1987; 5:339–347.

40. Kajosaari M, Saarinen UM. Prophylaxis of atopic disease by six months total solid food elimination-evaluation of 135 exclusively breastfed infants of atopic families. *Acta Paediatr Scand* 1983; 72:411–414.

41. Kjellman N-IM. Food allergy—Treatment and prevention. *Ann Allergy.* 1987; 59(Part II):168–174.

42. Falth-Magnusson K, Kjellman N-IM. Development of atopic disease in babies whose mothers were receiving exclusion diet during pregnancy—A randomized study. *J Allergy Clin Immunol.* 1987; 80(6):868–875.

43. Jakobsson I, Lindberg T. A prospective study of cow's milk protein intolerance in Swedish infants. *Acta Paediatr Scand.* 1979; 68:853–859.

44. Ford RPK, Taylor B. Natural history of egg hypersensitivity. *Arch Dis Child.* 1982; 57:649–652.

45. Bock SA. The natural history of food sensitivity. *J Allergy Clin Immunol.* 1982; 69:173–177.

46. Sampson HA, McCaskill CC. Food hypersensitivity and atopic dermatitis: evaluation of 113 patients. *J Pediatr.* 1985; 107:669–675.

47. Bock SA. Natural history of severe reactions to foods in young children. *J Pediatr.* 1985; 107:676–680.

48. Businco L, Benincori N, Cantani A, Tacconi L, Picarazzi A. Chronic diarrhea due to cow's milk allergy. A 4- to 10-year follow-up study. *Ann Allergy.* 1985; 55:844–847.

49. Bock SA. Prospective appraisal of complaints of adverse reactions to foods in children during the first three years of life. *Pediatrics.* 1987; 79:683–688.

50. Kjellman N-IM, Björksten B, Hattevig G, Falth-Magnusson K. Natural history of food allergy. *Ann Allergy.* 1988; 61(Part II):83–87.

51. Eggleston PA. Prospective studies in the natural history of food allergy. *Ann Allergy.* 1987; 59(Part II):179–182.

52. Bock SA, Sampson HA, Atkins FM, et al. Double-blind, placebo-controlled food challenge (DBPCFC) as an office procedure: A manual. *J Allergy Clin Immunol.* 1988; 82(6):986–997.

53. Taylor SL, Busse WW, Sachs MI, Parker JL, Yunginger JW. Peanut oil is not allergenic to peanut-sensitive individuals. *J Allergy Clin Immunol.* 1981; 68(5):372–375.

54. Halsey AB, Martin ME, Ruff ME, Jacobs FO, Jacobs RL. Sunflower oil is not allergenic to sunflower seed-sensitive patients. *J Allergy Clin Immunol.* 1986; 78(3):408–410.

Chapter 7

Adverse Reactions to Food Additives and Other Food Constituents

Judy E. Perkin

INTRODUCTION

In some instances individuals appear to be sensitive to food or beverage additives through mechanisms not, for the most part, classified as immuno-logically mediated.[1] This chapter includes a review of substances most commonly associated with these adverse reactions. This chapter also reviews selected natural food constituents for which adverse reactions have been described. The majority of the adverse reactions discussed in this chapter seem to be food intolerances. (See Chapter 1.)

ASPARTAME

In 1985, the Food and Drug Administration (FDA) established the Adverse Reaction Monitoring System (ARMS). Aspartame has headed the list in terms of the ingredient most complained about (80% of ARMS complaints as of November 1988).[2] Soft drinks have been cited most as the aspartame-containing food culprit, and headaches are the most common adverse reaction reported.[2]

Aspartame is a nutritive artificial sweetener. Although it is caloric (4 Kcal/g), its sweetness relative to sucrose (180-200 times sweeter) makes it an attractive very low calorie sweetener.[3-5]

Aspartame chemically is L-aspartyl–L-phenylalanine methyl ester. The components of aspartame are two amino acids, phenylalanine and aspartic acid and an alcohol methanol.[6] When consumed by humans, aspartame may be absorbed and metabolized via two different pathways.[7] Both pathways ultimately result in the appearance of aspartate, phenylalanine, and methanol in the portal blood. Pathway number one involves hydrolysis to the three major component parts by enzymes in the intestinal lumen. Pathway number two involves demethylation of aspartame within the intestinal lumen to form methanol and aspartyl-phenylalanine. The dipeptide, aspartyl-phenylalanine in pathway two is absorbed and subsequently (within the enterocyte) hydrolyzed to the components phenylalanine and aspartate.[7] Tobey and Heizer[8] report that intact transport of the dipeptide (pathway two) may occur commonly. Their experiments further suggest that an enzyme in the cortisol of the enterocytes may be involved in aspartyl-phenylalanine hydrolysis. Tobey and Heizer[8] suggest, at least in some instances, that adverse reactions to aspartame may be the result of deficiency in cytosol hydrolase activity.

The question of aspartame safety or adverse reaction needs to be viewed in two ways. One is safety from a public health (or population-based) perspective, and one is safety from an individual perspective. From current evidence, it seems that aspartame can be safely consumed in reasonable quantities by the majority of the population. Case reports and metabolic studies indicate that for some individuals, who may be seen in a clinical setting, adverse reactions can occur. (It should be noted from the outset that individuals who are homozygous for phenylketonuria because they have to limit their phenylalanine intake are warned not to consume aspartame.[3])

Population-focused recommendations for consumption limits have been established by both the World Health Organization (WHO) and the FDA. The WHO maximum level of acceptable intake is 40 mg/kg of body weight.[9] The FDA maximum acceptable daily intake level is 50 mg/kg of body weight.[4,10] The FDA's acceptable daily intake factor was calculated to include a safety factor of 100-fold.[10] A can of soft drink contains approximately 200 mg of aspartame.[10] Using this figure and assuming no other aspartame dietary sources a 50 kg (110 lb) adult would have to consume 12.5 soft drinks per day to achieve this maximum acceptable daily intake level.

The American Dietetic Association position paper related to sweeteners states that if aspartame is used to replace dietary sucrose taken in average amounts, aspartame intake would be in the range of 3 to 11 mg/kg/day.[5] A position statement of the American Diabetes Association cites statistics that indicate that most adults consume less than 3.5 mg of aspartame per kilogram of body weight per day.[11]

Two population groups for whom potential adverse effects related to aspartame consumption have been of particular concern are pregnant women and children.[7,10,12–18] The aspartate component of aspartame appears to be of no concern during pregnancy because this component does not cross the placenta readily.[12] In monkeys, even when aspartate was given in levels of 100 mg/kg/hr, little crossed the placenta.[19] Methanol would also not appear to be a problem because the amount generated from the consumption of one aspartame-containing soft drink is similar to the methanol content of one banana.[12] Theoretically methanol might be a problem if very large quantities of aspartame were consumed and if methanol concentrated on the fetal side of the placenta. Information to date does not suggest a problem with this component. (The mechanics of placental methanol transfer are not currently known.[12])

Safety related to the phenylalanine component for pregnant women is more controversial, and fetal exposure is a concern because the fetal side of the placenta concentrates phenylalanine in a ratio of 2:1.[4] Pardridge[13,16] has voiced concern about potential effects of elevated maternal plasma phenylalanine concentration on the brains and subsequent mental development of offspring. Others[4,12,14,15] feel maternal plasma phenylalanine levels, even presuming high aspartame intakes, are within a safe range of <600 µmol/dl. It is further cited by those who see no danger of aspartame consumption in pregnancy that no epidemiologic studies have indicated adverse effects of aspartame consumption to date.[12]

One study has cited that by 1 year of age, infants can absorb and metabolize aspartame at adult levels of proficiency.[20] Stegink,[7] based on survey patterns of children's beverage consumption, analyzed the effects of a 4-year-old child drinking three successive 12-oz aspartame-containing beverages. Stegink[7] projected no significant increases in plasma levels of phenylalanine with this intake pattern.

Kruesi and Rapoport[17] reviewing the literature up to 1986 found no significant behavioral effects linked to aspartame consumption. Kruesi et al,[18] in a study of 30 preschool males, concluded that aspartame ingestion (30 mg/kg) was not related to disruptive behavior. Interestingly, in this study motor activity, as assessed by an acetometer device, was decreased following aspartame ingestion. Observers could not detect this decreased activity, however, and the investigators considered it to be of minimal importance. A study by Ferguson et al[21] using a lower dose of aspartame also failed to find behavioral problems in children.

The issue of aspartame's safety for children remains alive. In March 1989, *American Health*[22] reported children may be at risk of exceeding the FDA's advisable daily intake. The article quotes Dr. William Pardridge of UCLA as suggesting that many children probably consume more than 23 mg/lb/day.

Individual adverse-reaction reports related to aspartame have encompassed a large variety of complaints. The most commonly reported adverse reaction appears to be headache.[2] Bradstock et al[23] (in 1986) published an article analyzing 231 consumer complaints received about aspartame. In this analysis, 91 complaints were classified as neurological or behavioral, and headaches were cited in 45 cases.

The postulated mechanism for aspartame's potential influence on headache is via norepinephrine and similar amine compounds. Aspartame consumption may be linked to increases in serum tyrosine that is a norepinephrine precursor.[24] (It should be noted, however, that some researchers link phenylalanine to decreased rather than potentially increased catecholamine synthesis. These individuals say phenylalanine in aspartame does not have the same effects on brain as phenylalanine consumed in a protein source and in humans aspartame consumption most likely reduces tyrosine uptake by the brain.[25,26])

Schiffman et al,[24] in 1987, published the results of a double-blind crossover trial in 40 subjects who had attributed headaches to aspartame. Aspartame challenges in this study were given at the level of 30 mg/kg of body weight over a 4-hour period. The headache incidence after aspartame was not significantly different from placebo and was in actual numbers less, 35% incidence after aspartame compared to 45% incidence after placebo. This study also failed to support a potential norepinephrine-headache link. Despite preceding treatment (aspartame or placebo), subjects who developed headaches exhibited lowered plasma concentrations of both epinephrine and norepinephrine preceding headaches. Steinmetzer and Kunkel[27] have questioned the Schiffman study findings for a variety of reasons. Most importantly was the evaluation time used. Steinmetzer and Kunkel[27] suggest reactions may occur up to 72 hours after intake, and the Schiffman study allowed only 48 hours between challenges. They also question the value of a single challenge and the composition of the diet during trials (eg, was intake of other potentially vasoactive substances controlled?).

In 1988, Koehler and Glaros[28] published the results of a community-based double-blind crossover trial comparing headache incidence after consumption of 300 mg of aspartame and placebo. (Dosage was not given on a kilogram of body weight basis.) In this study, five subjects experienced no increase in headache following aspartame ingestion and six did. These researchers postulate individual threshold differences may be involved.

Other clinical reports[29-31] support the view that aspartame may trigger headache in susceptible individuals. Ferguson,[29] in 1985, described an eating disorder in which aspartame consumption (10 packets of sweetener per day), spitting up of carbohydrate, and concomitant tranylcypromine use were associated with headache. The patient's headaches ceased when saccharin, as opposed to aspartame, was used as the artificial sweetener. Johns,[30] in 1986, described a patient in whom migraines were associated with aspartame consumption of approximately 1,000 to 1,500 mg/day. [The patient reported consuming on some days 6 to 8 cans (12 oz each) of diet soda and 15 aspartame tablets.] Challenge with a 500-mg aspartame solution in a clinical setting also provoked headaches in this patient. Finally, Lipton et al[31] report aspartame as a dietary factor potentially involved in headaches of 8.2% of 171 patients evaluated at the Montefiore Headache Unit.

Another concern with regard to adverse reaction to aspartame relates to increases in seizure susceptibility for certain individuals. Maher[9] states that the phenylalanine component of aspartame may lower thresholds for seizure occurrence. He bases this statement on what he cites as phenylalanine's ability to inhibit catecholamine synthesis and a demonstration of lowering of seizure thresholds in mice.[26]

Wurtman,[32] in 1985, reported cases of three individuals experiencing grand mal seizures at times of varying levels of aspartame consumption. One individual was cited as consuming four quarts of diet soda containing aspartame and also about four quarts of aspartame-sweetened lemonade daily. One individual reportedly drank four to five glasses of aspartame-sweetened lemonade, and the third individual was cited as consuming at least 900 ml of iced tea containing aspartame as a sweetener. Wurtman's letter postulates, but does not prove, a role for aspartame. Walton,[33] in 1986, also published an individual case report of grand mal seizure, which he postulated could be associated with consumption of aspartame-sweetened ice tea (about 1 gal/day). The Epilepsy Institute, however, has stated the position that it does not believe aspartame is unsafe for persons with epilepsy.[34]

Aspartame may also affect appetite. A 1986 letter[35] reporting on the effects of appetite control in 95 subjects stated that in some subjects aspartame may stimulate appetite. Ryan-Harshman et al,[36] however, failed to demonstrate such effects in two subsequent studies with male volunteers. Because aspartame is used as a part of diets aimed at weight control, further research in this area should prove interesting.

Allergy-like symptoms reportedly associated with aspartame consumption are probably of most interest to dietitians and other health professionals reading this volume. Bradstock et al[23] (in their 1986 Centers for Disease Control-based analysis) reported receipt of 23 such complaints from consumers (with rash being the most common symptom). In 1985, there was a report of a confirmed case (by challenge) of a patient with granulomatous panniculitis manifested by leg nodules associated with aspartame ingestion.[37] (This patient was consuming 36 to 44 oz/day of aspartame-sweetened soft drink.) Kulczycki,[38] in 1986, reported a case of urticaria confirmed by double-blind challenge to be induced by aspartame. Symptoms in this patient occurred 1 to 2 hours after ingestion of relatively small quantities of aspartame-containing substances (for example, diet soda). Kulczycki[38] postulates that formation of amide bonds between endogenous proteins and aspartame or the aspartame decomposition product, diketopiperazine, might be responsible for the allergic reaction. Studies to date do not indicate that aspartame degranulates either mast cells or basophils.[34]

The clinician concerned with adverse reaction to aspartame may be dealing with individuals sensitive to smaller amounts than defined standards for acceptable levels of intake established for the general population or alternatively may be dealing with persons who are consuming aspartame in excessively large quantities. It would be advisable, if a person is determined to be aspartame sensitive, for that person to restrict or completely avoid aspartame, depending on the level of sensitivity. Some individuals may simply be consuming too much aspartame, and counseling may involve suggesting safe levels based on population standards. A list of representative products containing aspartame is shown in Appendix G.

Dietitians should be alert to additional products with aspartame appearing on the market. Usage in the following product categories is being proposed: baked goods and mixes, instant cereals, malt beverages with fruit juice and alcohol, and candies.[39] A new development that allows aspartame to be released in a controlled manner during the baking process via a coated or encapsulated form should hasten the potential for baking use.[40]

SULFITES

Sulfites are number two in the count of food additives responsible for the most complaints to the FDA (as of November 1988).[2] Although aspartame has been the additive about which the most complaints have been received, FDA considers reactions attributed to sulfites to be of greater severity.[2]

Estimates on the magnitude of the population who should be classified as sulfite sensitive vary. The FDA considers about 1% of the US population may be sulfite sensitive.[2] Studies of asthmatic patient populations reviewed in the *Annals of Allergy* (1987) cite sulfite sensitivity prevalence figures ranging from 2 to 5%.[41] Bush et al,[42] in 1986, cite a prevalence of less than 3.9% sulfite sensitivity in asthmatics and stated that steroid-dependent asthmatics were the subgroup of asthmatics most at risk. The FDA has estimated that 5% of asthmatics are sulfite sensitive. Persons who are not asthmatic can be sulfite sensitive as well.[43] Bush et al[44] state, however, that such adverse reactions to sulfite in the nonasthmatic are rare.

Although most reports[45-47] cite the 1976 report of Prenner and Stevens[48] as being the initial report of reaction to ingested sulfites, Simon[49] credits Kochen[50] with the earliest sulfite ingestion adverse-reaction report. The Prenner and Stevens[48] note involved an individual consuming a restaurant meal (containing metabisulfite) who reacted adversely with symptoms of urticaria, pruritus, and anaphylaxis. The Kochen[50] report involved a child who developed asthmatic attacks after eating foods with sulfur dioxide. The first death attributed to inhaled sulfur dioxide (SO_2) was that of Pliny the Elder (an asthmatic) in 79 AD. In this case, inhalation of volcanic gas containing sulfur dioxide, as opposed to ingestion of sulfites, was responsible.[46]

The ubiquitous distribution of sulfites in the food supply creates a problem for the sulfite-sensitive individual. Sulfites (which include sulfur dioxide, potassium sulfite, sodium sulfite, potassium metabisulfite, potassium bisulfite, sodium metabisulfite, and sodium bisulfite) are approved by the FDA as food additives with a variety of purposes. Additive purposes include control of browning (both enzymatic and nonenzymatic),[41,44] modification of dough texture,[51] sanitation and exertion of an antimicrobial effect,[41,44] and bleaching.[44] Sulfites are also used as preservatives in a variety of both inhalable and injectable drugs and, in some instances, in parenteral solutions.[45]

Food sulfites are not completely denatured by cooking.[52] At least one source does say, however, that sulfite residues can be reduced by high heat cooking.[53] Sulfites can also bind to food constituents, and thus may not be removed by washing.[53]

Form of sulfite, as well as quantity, may be important in terms of causing a clinical reaction. Taylor et al[51] have noted that the presence and quantity of free, or unbound, sulfite may be especially important. These investigators found that reactions to foods containing sulfites could not be correlated with levels of total SO_2 equivalents. Taylor et al[51] noted several substances in food to which sulfite may bind. These include protein, starch, and sugars. Protein or starch bound sulfites seem to cause fewer clinical problems than sulfites bound to sugars.

Many food types contain sulfites. Current FDA regulations state that sulfite presence in excess of 10 ppm expressed as total SO_2 must be stated on the product label.[51] Appendix H contains an example list of products currently listing sulfites on the label.

Several food and beverage products have been particularly highlighted because of their sulfite content. Dried apricots have been cited as having the highest residual sulfite content of any currently marketed food product.[51] Wines are another food product class widely known to contain sulfites. Sulfur dioxide gas is used to sterilize wine barrels, and sulfites in wine also react to slow oxidation.[54] Most wines contain about 10 mg of sulfite per ounce.[49] An analysis of wines from various countries revealed that US wines contained an average of 145 mg/L of sulfur dioxide. Rumanian wines were at the high end with an average of 159 mg/L, and the Spanish wine samples assayed for this study had the lowest average sulfite content at 60 mg/L.[54] Tsevat et al[55] have reported a fatal anaphylactic reaction to white wine (few sips) in a 33-year-old asthmatic.

Sulfites are not authorized for use in thiamin-containing foods because sulfite presence in a food destroys thiamin.[48,49] Sulfites break the thiamin molecule into two fragments that have no vitamin activity.[56] Fresh red meats, for example, should not contain sulfites. Simon[49] points out that foods such as meats, however, may have sulfite added.

A test strip (Sulfitest®) is available for use by consumers to test foods and beverages. Color changes in the plastic strip indicate the presence of sulfites. The test as currently available is not reported to be either highly sensitive or specific.[53] A false-negative reading would be of particular concern for a sulfite-sensitive individual. The FDA does not currently recommend use of the strips due to the above problem.[57]

Because of their antioxidant properties, sulfites may be used in drugs, as well as foods.[41,45] There has been a particular concern about sulfite exposure via parenteral solutions or peritoneal dialysis. Gunnison and Jacobsen[45] have noted that a patient infused with certain types of amino acids or electrolyte solutions might receive 500 mg of sodium bisulfite within a few hours and 500 mg of sulfite per day could also be absorbed following infusion of 10 L of dialysate. Cole[58] has noted that when sulfites are introduced parenterally, tissues are exposed to high levels of free sulfite because the enterohepatic detoxification mechanism is bypassed. There is loss of sulfite in drug preparations over time due to autoxidation. This is particularly true of preparations packaged in plastic bags.[45]

Other classes of pharmaceutical products about which specific and frequent concerns regarding sulfite content have been expressed include bronchodilators,[41,46,49,59-61] ophthalmic solutions,[62] epinephrine products,[59] and local dental anesthetics.[63,64] It should be noted that there may be sulfite-free products in these categories and pharmaceutical firms in recent years have removed sulfites from many products. Current information about sulfite content of pharmaceuticals should be reviewed by health professionals treating sulfite-sensitive individuals.

Ingestion is a mode of entry for food, beverage, and pharmaceutical sulfites. Sulfites in pharmaceuticals may also be administered subcutaneously, intravenously, ophthalmically, or be available in inhalable form.[45] Skin contact may be another route of entry, leading to development of an adverse reaction, and food and pharmaceutical industry workers are at a particular risk. Reports of sulfite-associated contact dermatitis in individuals representing both of these groups have been published.[65,66]

It should also be borne in mind that while the sulfite-sensitivity problems discussed in this chapter relate to exogenous sulfite exposure, endogenous sulfite production does occur. Endogenous sulfite is produced via the catabolism of the sulfur-containing amino acids and other sulfur-containing compounds. The major precursor for endogenous sulfite is cysteine.[45] Approximately 1,000 mg of endogenous sulfite are produced on a daily basis.[49] Gunnison and Jacobsen[45] warn that in some individuals excess production of sulfites via endogenous pathways after eating high-sulfur foods may occur.

A variety of reactions to sulfites have been reported in both asthmatics and nonasthmatics. These are summarized in Table 7-1. It should be remembered that present knowledge indicates sulfite sensitivity is more common among asthmatics.[67] Almost all asthmatics seem to be sensitive to inhaled sulfites, so some restrict the term sulfite sensitive to those asthmatics who react to ingested sulfites in capsule form.[45] It should be kept in mind, however, that reactions to sulfites in foods and beverages may be via inhalation. Sulfites placed in solution such as saliva form sulfur dioxide gas. The higher the temperature and the lower the pH, the more sulfur dioxide gas will be produced.[41,44,49] Simon[49] has also indicated some adverse reactions to sulfites may be explained by inhalation of sulfur dioxide gas formed in the stomach, which is later brought up through burping and inhaled. Freedman[68] has reported inhalation reactions related to consumption of orange drink solutions. (Note: Orange drinks in the U.S. generally do not contain sulfites.[44])

Bronchospasm in asthmatics has been one of the most extensively studied clinical reactions. Bronchospasm is believed to be due to physiological actions of one or more of the following constituents: bisulfite or sulfite ions, the hydrogen ion, dissolved sulfur dioxide, or sulfurous acid.[45] Stimulation of the parasympathetic nervous system is believed to play a role in bronchospasm induction.[45,46,69] Settipane[46] also believes parasympathetic stimulation could induce other symptoms as well such as urticaria or angioedema.

Schwartz[70] made an important contribution to extend knowledge of potential clinical manifestations in 1983. He presented two case studies illustrating

Table 7-1   Examples of Clinical Responses to Sulfites

Asthmatics	*Nonasthmatics*
Bronchospasm/bronchoconstriction	Contact dermatitis
Respiratory function decline	Decreased blood pressure
Flushing	Neurological problems
Dizziness	Urticaria
Loss of consciousness	Angioedema
Anaphylaxis	Feeling of chest tightness
Wheezing	Abdominal cramps
	Diarrhea
	Dizziness
	Nausea
	Dyspnea
	Diminished liver function
	Anaphylactoid reaction (rare)

that hypotension and gastrointestinal complaints may be the initially observed problems in a patient adversely reacting to sulfites.

Sulfite sensitivity has been linked to both anaphylaxis and death.[48,56,61,71–73] The link of sulfites to anaphylaxis has prompted investigation to see if sulfites could potentially be related to a syndrome known as idiopathic anaphylaxis (IA). (IA is diagnosed if known causes such as bee stings, food, exercise, and others have been excluded.) Sonin and Patterson[74] studied 12 patients with IA, and sulfites were not implicated. Meggs et al[75] studied 8 patients with systemic mastocytosis and 25 patients with unexplained IA and found sulfite sensitivity to be rare.

Sulfite reactions appear rapidly. Reactions after ingestion usually occur in about 30 to 60 minutes.[52] The inhalation route may provoke reaction in 2 minutes,[46] and reactions with intravenous injection have also been noted within minutes.[56]

Sulfite sensitivity may be demonstrated by spirometry following an oral challenge.[45] Simon[49] outlines a suggested challenge procedure. Challenges should be performed in a hospital or medical setting, and the patient should be in a fasted state. Morning is the recommended time for challenge. A double-blinded capsule and/or beverage challenge is another recommendation.[51]

The mechanisms for sulfite sensitivity are not clearly understood, and it would seem that clinical responses may be induced in one of several ways. The majority of reactions in asthmatics are believed to be attributable to inhaled sulfur dioxide.[41]

Another mechanism suggested to explain some reactions is partial sulfite oxidase deficiency.[41,42,44,47,49,52,56] Sulfite oxidase is an enzyme found between the inner and outer mitochondrial layers for which molybdenum serves as a cofactor.[49] Simon[49] assayed sulfite oxidase levels in skin fibroblasts of sulfite-sensitive asthmatics and found activity to be low.

A small number of reactions are believed to be IgE mediated.[41,42,48,52,56,76] Because sulfites are too small to be antigenic, it is thought these molecules must become haptens for an IgE-mediated reaction to occur.[41] Most asthmatics with demonstrated sulfite sensitivity during an acute reaction will have normal levels of IgE, eosinophils, and histamine.[46] Sher and Schwartz[61] have suggested that in some cases a nonreaginic anaphylactoid reaction (involving direct complement or immune complex release) may be involved.

Persons who are sulfite sensitive need to avoid sulfite-containing foods and beverages. Taylor et al[51] have suggested that diets for some sulfite-sensitive asthmatics may contain some items with low residual sulfite levels. Because patient sensitivity thresholds to sulfites may vary, some individuals need to be more cautious than others. Simon[49] suggests that foods containing less than 10 ppm should not be a problem, even for highly sensitive individuals.

In addition to dietary strategies, a number of agents have been used in preventive efforts. Vitamin B_{12} administered orally in doses of 1,000 to 5,000 μg is one agent that has proved useful in some instances.[77] Vitamin B_{12} is believed to be protective because it catalyzes the nonenzymatic oxidation of sulfite to sulfate.[44] Other preventive treatments used include oral sodium cromoglycate, doxepin, and atropine.[76]

The preceding discussion has focused on adverse reactions to small amounts of sulfites. If high enough levels of sulfites are consumed, even individuals not clinically classified as sulfite sensitive will show adverse symptoms. Bush et al[44] have noted that inhalation of 6 to 12 ppm will cause nose, throat, and bronchial irritation. Ingestion of 400 to 600 mg in one day in nonsensitive individuals may be associated with gastrointestinal hemorrhaging or nausea and vomiting.

The FDA has made several moves to protect the health and safety of sulfite-sensitive individuals. In 1986, the FDA prohibited the use of sulfites on fresh fruits and vegetables, and in 1987, all canned, frozen, or prepared foods had to list sulfites as an ingredient when the product contained in excess of 10 ppm.[73] In June 1987, pharmaceutical firms were required to produce warning statements for sulfite-containing prescription drugs.[67] In December 1988, the FDA promulgated proposals concerning limits of sulfites in certain foods. Proposed limits and bans on potato products are an area of particular concern. The March 1988 *FDA Consumer*[67] reported potato products were associated with 12% of complaints.

One asthmatic died after eating sulfite-containing cottage fries and the FDA has wanted to ban use of sulfites on fresh potatoes.[67] Representatives of the fresh potato industry have sought to use some level of sulfites on their products[78] and several companies requested that residual levels for dehydrated potatoes be raised from 500 ppm to 600 ppm.[79] In March 1990, however, the FDA announced that fresh potatoes would be included in the list of foods from which sulfites are banned.[80]

In response to FDA proposals, other food manufacturers are making requests. The Association for Dressings and Sauces and other food organizations have requested clarification with regard to direct addition of sulfites versus carryover in ingredients used in a product.[81] The American Frozen Food Institute is seeking FDA approval for a residual level of 250 ppm in frozen mushrooms.[82] The American Bakeries Association is requesting clarification with regard to combining sulfite-containing products.[83] The National Restaurant Association is asking the FDA to clarify that labeling requirements do not extend to restaurant premises.[84] Other products being discussed in the rule promulgation process include canned quahog clams and cod cakes,[85] gelatin,[86] dried fruits,[87,88] and maraschino cherries.[89] Generally recognized as safe (GRAS) levels are being considered.[90]

Endorsements for FDA actions have come from the American Dietetic Association, the Joint Council of Allergy and Immunology, and the American Academy of Allergy and Immunology's Broncho-Provocation Committee. The American Dietetic Association has noted the benefits of more comprehensive labeling to both dietitians and consumers.[89] FDA is also proposing that information on sulfite content be available for bulk items as well as for traditionally labeled.[90]

Substitutes for sulfites are being explored. Honey has been reported to be an alternative antibrowning agent in fruit juices and wines.[91] The use of proteolytic enzymes is also being explored as a replacement for sulfite use in shrimp, vegetables, and fruit products.[92] Some sulfite-free wine products are now available.

Dietitians play an important role in helping sulfite-sensitive individuals avoid foods and beverages that may contain harmful sulfite levels. Dietitians should carefully monitor progress in FDA labeling regulations and should encourage reporting of adverse sulfite reactions to the FDA.

OTHER FOOD ADDITIVES

Food additives, other than aspartame and sulfites, have accounted for 5% of adverse reactions reported to the FDA Adverse Reaction Monitoring System since 1985.[2] Common food additives falling under this category include food colorings, monosodium glutamate (MSG), and nutrient supplements.

Tartrazine (FD&C Yellow No. 5) and Other Food Colorings

Tartrazine, more commonly known as FD&C yellow no. 5, is an artificial coloring agent used in a wide variety of foods and drugs.[1] Chemically, tartrazine is a pyrazole derivative and a coal tar aniline dye.[93,94] Appendix I provides examples of food sources of tartrazine. Use of tartrazine produces a bright yellow color, and tartrazine is also used to produce other food colors such as green, turquoise, maroon, and rust.[1,95] Lack of yellow color, therefore, is not a guarantee of tartrazine's absence. The FDA does require that FD&C yellow no. 5 be specifically stated by name on food ingredient labels.[96] Tartrazine may be used as a coloring agent in drugs, as well as food.[97,98]

Clinical manifestations are varied and may include urticaria,[94,99,100] allergic vascular purpura (or Schönlein-Henoch purpura),[93,101–103] angioedema,[1,99] photosensitivity,[104] and anaphylaxis.[98,99] The reader should be aware that some reported manifestations may be indicative of reactions in a small number of patients. Respiratory problems subsequent to tartrazine ingestion have been reported by several authors. Cited problems include mild bronchospasm[99] and asthma.[105,106] Research subsequent to initial reports[107–110] would indicate the adverse effect on respiration in asthmatics may not be as much of a problem as once thought.[110,112] The area does remain controversial, and Stevenson et al[110] present an excellent overview of the current two schools of thought. Hariparsad et al[113] suggest there may be some low level of bronchial reactivity in some asthmatics that they could assess via histamine-inhalation challenge, but not by the commonly used forced expiratory parameters. This research tested 10 asthmatic children who reported wheeze or coughing subsequent to orange drink consumption. Oral tartrazine and placebo were used.

Another focus of investigation has been the role of tartrazine in the etiology of chronic idiopathic urticaria (CIU).[114–120] Deoglas[115] states that doses of tartrazine of 1 to 10 mg have been associated with urticaria. Genton et al,[116] in studying patients with CIU, reported 10 positive oral provocation tests with tartrazine. These same researchers reported that 14 patients with urticaria responded positively to a combination of nonsteroidal anti-inflammatory drugs and a food additive-free diet. Gibson and Clancy[117] found that 26% of 66 patients reacted positively to a test challenge of 10 mg of tartrazine. There may be a subset of patients for whom tartrazine causes or exacerbates CIU. Dietary histories are not usually useful in helping to identify these patients.[118] Podell[118] recommends use of either a simple elimination diet (pear-rice-lamb) or a six to eight food diet with no manufactured foods for two weeks to aid in diagnosis. If there is no reaction (eg, the urticaria does not resolve) after two weeks, tartrazine as a cause or contributor can be ruled out. A reaction will necessitate a testing reintroduction schedule.

Tartrazine, among other food additives, has been linked to behavior problems in children. David,[121,122] testing behaviors using a double-blind challenge, found tartrazine had no effect on problems such as temper tantrums, poor sleeping, and constant running and climbing. Proposed diet and hyperactivity relationships are discussed in Chapter 11.

Tartrazine adverse reaction is believed by some in selected cases to be cross-reactive with aspirin or other nonsteroidal anti-inflammatory drugs.[99,105,106,123–125] The majority of reports supporting cross-reactivity cite that cross-reaction with tartrazine occurs in about 5% to 25% of aspirin-sensitive patients. Reports by other investigators[109–111,126] support a very low percentage or zero cross-reactivity between aspirin and tartrazine. Gerber et al,[127] as well as Stevenson et al,[110] indicate tartrazine's major metabolite sulfanilic acid does not inhibit cycloxygenase (an enzyme involved in arachidonic acid metabolism) as does aspirin. A metabolic similarity in this regard might be expected if cross-reactivity did occur.[127] Rosenhall[128] reports that persons reacting adversely to tartrazine may react adversely to other azo dyes.

The mechanism(s) underlying adverse reactions to tartrazine are unknown. Some suggest there is scant evidence to suggest an immunologic basis at present.[1] Gibson and Clancy,[117] however, suggest that although most tartrazine reactors are nonatopic, an IgE-mediated mechanism may be involved. These researchers, as well as Criep,[93] suggest that tartrazine may act as a hapten covalently bonded to a host protein carrier. Weliky and Heiner,[129] using tartrazine, provoked a short antibody response in rats and demonstrated binding to IgE by tartrazine conjugates. Kreindler et al[130] were not able to demonstrate that tartrazine was related to histamine release in the mast cells of Sprague-Dawley rats. Murdoch et al[131] demonstrated *in vivo* release of histamine after ingestion of 200 mg of tartrazine in 10 adults with no history of adverse reaction and postulated a pharmacologic rather than immunologic mechanism. In studying tartrazine-associated histamine release in subjects with and without urticaria, histamine release from leukocytes, however, could not be associated with symptoms. Murdoch[132] concludes that a factor other than histamine must be related to the appearance of clinical symptoms. Neuman et al[97] have suggested that symptoms of adverse tartrazine reaction may relate to excessive bradykinin production.

Food colorings other than tartrazine have also been implicated as causing adverse reactions in some individuals.[1,133] These are summarized in Table 7-2.

Table 7-2 Food Colorings (Other Than FD&C Yellow No. 5) Implicated in Adverse Reactions

Amaranth	(FD&C Red #2)*
Brilliant blue	(FD&C Blue #1)
Bonceau	(FD&C Red #4)
Erythrosin	(FD&C Red #3)†
Indigotine	(FD&C Blue #2)
Sunset yellow	(FD&C Yellow #6)

*As of February 1986, the FDA halted usage of FD&C Red #2.
†A proposed partial ban of FD&C Red No. 3 was announced in Spring 1990.[133]

Monosodium Glutamate (MSG)

Monosodium glutamate is the sodium salt form of glutamic acid.[134] Monosodium glutamate is used as a food additive because of its flavor-enhancing properties.[1,134] Average daily per capita consumption is estimated to be 0.3 to 1 g. Higher levels (4-6 g) may be consumed if foods highly flavored with MSG are chosen.[134]

The most commonly reported adverse reaction associated with MSG consumption is Chinese restaurant syndrome.[1,135-139] (A Chinese food meal may contain from 5 to 10 g of MSG.[1]) Symptoms of Chinese restaurant syndrome may include nausea, headache, sweating, thirst, facial flushing, tightness and burning in the face and chest, abdominal pain, sensation of crawling in the skin, or development of tears in the eyes.[138] In 1977, Gann[140] reported ventricular tachycardia in a patient as part of the Chinese restaurant syndrome complex, and Goldberg[141] also reported cardiovascular anomalies such as atrial fibrillation, sinus tachycardia, and supraventricular tachyarrhythmia occurring with Chinese restaurant syndrome. Kerr et al[139] estimate approximately 1.8% of the adult population may have the Chinese restaurant syndrome reaction.

Symptoms of Chinese restaurant syndrome are typically said to occur 15 to 30 minutes after consuming a food or meal containing large amounts of MSG.[1,135,136] Symptoms more frequently develop when ingestion occurs on an empty stomach, and Zautcke et al[136] feel this may explain why many reports cite soup frequently as an involved food. (Won ton soup may contain as much as 3 g of MSG.[1])

The symptom complex of Chinese restaurant syndrome and its etiology have been subjects of research and debate. Wilkin,[142] after studying 24 subjects (18 with a history of Chinese restaurant syndrome), found facial flushing to be a rare phenomenon. Wilkin[142] highlighted the potential role of L-pyroglutamate (an MSG conversion product) in MSG adverse reactions. In Wilkin's study, L-pyroglutamate at one-fourth the concentration of MSG, provoked the symptoms of tightness, swelling, and burning. (Boiling, such as in soup preparation, can result in L-pyroglutamate formation.) Kenny[143] indicated that MSG adverse reaction may be more likely to occur in individuals with impaired salivary flow or gastrointestinal reflux (heartburn). Other substances, besides MSG, speculated (but not proven) to be involved in the Chinese restaurant syndrome include aspartame, alcohol, and excessive sodium.[136] Other theories of Chinese restaurant syndrome causation relate to a potential inborn metabolic error or vitamin B_6 deficiency.[136] Chin et al[144] have reported that high levels of histamine (as opposed to MSG) in Chinese food may be responsible for Chinese restaurant syndrome symptoms. The condiments of tamari and soy sauce may contain particularly high levels of histamine. The European Glutamate Manufacturers' Association was recently cited for its belief that present evidence does not support a link between Chinese restaurant syndrome and MSG consumption.[145]

Other adverse reactions in selected individuals have been reported to be linked with MSG ingestion. These include angioedema,[146] headache,[147] orofacial granulomatosis,[148] and asthma.[1,143,144] Asthma as a reaction to MSG may appear 1 to 2 hours after ingestion or may appear as long as 12 hours after ingestion.[149,150]

The mechanism related to adverse reactions is unclear. Ghadimi and Kumar[138] have suggested a transitory excess of acetylcholine may be responsible because MSG is an acetylcholine precursor. Allen et al[150] suggest MSG-induced asthma may occur secondary to the peripheral excitation of irritant receptors in the lung.

Concern has recently been expressed regarding potential effects of ingestion of large doses of MSG during pregnancy.[151] Giving MSG subcutaneously to pregnant rats, Toth et al[151] produced neuronal necrosis in both mothers and fetuses. The significance of these results for human pregnancy deserves further study.

Monosodium glutamate is currently on the FDA's Generally Recognized As Safe (GRAS) list; therefore it may or may not be listed on food labels, which makes avoidance difficult.[1] Products such as Accent® definitely contain MSG and should be avoided by the MSG-sensitive individuals. Consumer concern about MSG has sparked the recent development of a flavor enhancer that can be substituted for MSG in a wide variety of products (including Oriental foods).[152]

Benzoates

The term benzoates refers to the following substances: sodium benzoate, benzoic acid, and 4-hydroxybenzoic acid.[1] Benzoates are believed to cause adverse reactions in some individuals.

Reactions reportedly associated with benzoate ingestion include purpura[101,102] and urticaria.[100,115,117,120] Rosenhall,[128] in reporting results of 637 food preservative challenge tests (in 504 subjects with rhinitis or asthma), found 12 (2%) definitely positive responses to benzoates (sodium benzoate and 4-hydroxybenzoic acid).

Benzoates are used as preservatives and antimicrobial agents for food products and pharmaceuticals.[1,153] Sodium benzoate may be used as a component of therapy for children with an enzyme defect in the urea cycle.[154] Benzoates also occur naturally in certain foods such as cranberries, prunes, raspberries, and cinnamon.[1]

In 1981, Lahti and Hannuksela[153] reported results of oral double-blind challenges with placebo (lactose) and benzoic acid in patients with atopic urticaria and other dermatologic problems. No significant differences were observed between the two substances. In 1986, another study[155] by these researchers (using wheat starch as a placebo) found a positive reaction to benzoates in only one urticaria patient. Current data indicate adverse reaction to benzoates occurs infrequently. Examples of products containing benzoates are shown in Appendix J.

BHT, BHA, and Thickeners

The antioxidants BHT and BHA may be linked to adverse reactions in a small number of individuals.[1] Some patients with chronic urticaria react positively to these substances.[156] Dong[95] has cited that thickeners such as vegetable gums may also elicit adverse reactions in some individuals.

The first part of this chapter discusses adverse reactions to food additives. Food contaminants and naturally occurring food constituents have also been linked to adverse reactions.

FOOD CONTAMINANTS

Food contaminants related to adverse reactions may include pharmaceuticals (eg, penicillin in a soft drink[157] and streptomycin in beef[158]), animal hairs, insect parts, and molds.[95] Molds are generally classified as aeroallergens, but some believe adverse reactions can also occur with ingestion.[159] Guidelines for avoiding mold ingestion are given in Table 7-3. Dietitians should realize that not all physicians feel that patients sensitive to molds in the air and environment may also be sensitive to ingested molds. This area is controversial and, some feel, not well documented. Therefore, dietary mold avoidance is not always used as part of current conventional therapy for mold allergy.[160,161]

NATURALLY OCCURRING FOOD OR BEVERAGE CONSTITUENTS

Naturally occurring food or beverage constituents may cause adverse reactions or allergy-like symptoms. Avoidance of selected foods and beverages containing these constituents may be helpful for selected individuals.

Table 7-3 Guidelines for Dietary Mold Avoidance

1. Eat canned foods immediately
2. Eat fresh fruits soon after preparation
3. Do not eat leftover foods
4. Do not consume meats or fish that have been stored for over 24 hours
5. Exclude the following foods:
   —Beer
   —Breads, soured or made with large quantities of yeast
   —Buttermilk
   —Cider
   —Cheeses (all types)
   —Dried fruit
   —Mushrooms
   —Sauerkraut
   —Sour cream
   —Soured milk
   —Vinegar and foods that contain vinegar
   —Wine and other alcoholic beverages

Histamine

Histamine occurs in some foods naturally[162-164] and may be present in wines, particularly red wines.[165,166] Examples of foods with a high histamine content include Parmesan, blue, Roquefort, and Monterey Jack cheeses; spinach; eggplant; tomatoes; and chicken livers. Examples of wines which may have high levels of histamine are Chianti and burgundy.[164] Most individuals do not have adverse reactions to dietary components that contain histamine because the histamine is metabolized through methylation by n-methyltransferase or oxidized by histaminase.[167] The drug isoniazid, however, is a strong histaminase inhibitor, and Uragoda[167] reports histamine poisoning in two tuberculosis patients associated with food consumption. The patients had consumed tuna fish that contained histamine. Symptoms included headache and reddening of the eyes, face, and palms. Enzyme insufficiency (histaminase) may therefore relate to symptoms. Other problems that may predispose to problems with ingested histamine or other biogenic amines may include abnormal intestinal permeability and portacaval shunt.[163] Malone and Metcalfe[164] have reported that clinical signs of histamine toxicity may occur in some individuals when 32 to 250 mg of histamine are consumed. Certain foods are also known as histamine releasers. These include alcohol, chocolate, egg whites, fish and shellfish, pineapple, strawberries, and tomatoes.[162] Intake of high amounts of starch has also been related to histamine production by gut bacteria.[162,163]

Scombroid fish poisoning is a type of foodborne illness that involves conversion of histidine to histamine and is characterized as histamine poisoning. Fishes involved commonly include mackerel, bonito, and tuna but sardines, bluefish, and mahimahi have been implicated as well.[168] The histidine to histamine conversion occurs when the fish are not properly cooled and are kept at high temperatures. Symptoms of scombroid poisoning include headache, flushing, and throbbing pain in the neck. Symptoms generally appear within minutes or up to 3 hours after ingestion.[162,168,169] Chin[144] has postulated a link between high histamine consumption and Chinese restaurant syndrome symptoms. (See previous discussion under monosodium glutamate.)

Certain factors may favor nonspecific histamine release. These include (1) lectins (discussed later in this chapter), (2) bacterial endotoxins, and (3) enzyme and mineral deficiencies.[163] Japanese individuals may experience facial flushing, tachycardia, and muscle weakness after alcohol ingestion. These symptoms have been linked to a deficiency of alcohol dehydrogenase and histamine liberation.[163,170] Magnesium deficiency in rats has been associated with increased histamine release and sensitivity.[171] Humans who exhibit allergic symptoms, but fail to be diagnosed as truly allergic, have also been noted by some to have decreased levels of cellular magnesium.[163]

Tyramine and Phenylethylamine

Tyramine is a vasoactive biogenic amine found in foods such as cheeses (cheddar, Gruyere, Brie, Camembert, Roquefort), wine (especially red wines), herring, and baker's yeast.[163] Tyramine has been implicated in the etiology of migraines and urticaria.[163] Patients taking monoamine oxidase inhibitors are advised to avoid foods or beverages that are high in tyramine as intake by such patients is associated with adverse reactions such as headache, hypertension, flushing, and death.[163]

Phenylethylamine is a vasoactive amine found in chocolate and some fermented cheeses.[163] Phenylethylamine ingestion has been implicated in dietary-related migraine.[172]

Octopamine and Phenylephrine

Octopamine and phenylephrine are vasoactive amines present in citrus fruits. They may be associated with adverse reactions particularly headache.[162]

Alcohol

Alcohol adverse reactions that may be associated with alcohol dehydrogenase deficiency[170] have been discussed previously. Some individuals can also suffer from bronchoconstriction after alcohol ingestion. Observed bronchoconstriction, however, seems unrelated to excess histamine release, and the exact mechanism for this type of reaction has not been elucidated.[173]

A 1980 report outlines a serious anaphylactic episode in a 31-year-old female 15 minutes after wine consumption.[174] This report suggested allergic sensitivity, but was unable to demonstrate IgE specific to wine. There are also small amounts of proteins found in wine that may be associated with potential allergic (IgE-mediated) reactions. These protein materials include pectin enzymes, isinglass (gelatin produced from the swim bladder of the sturgeon), egg white, and potassium or sodium caseinate.[175]

Caffeine

Caffeine, taken in excess, can be associated with adverse reactions. Problems seen include anxiety, heart palpitations, headache, and insomnia.[162] Excess caffeine intake may also be associated with Ebkom's syndrome, which is characterized by uncomfortable creeping sensations in the legs, arms, or shoulders.[162] There has also been a case report of generalized urticaria appearing 15 minutes after caffeine consumption. Caffeine as a causative agent was confirmed by a double-blind challenge.[176]

Lectins

A lectin is defined as a protein with the capacity to bind to the terminal carbohydrate portion of a glycoprotein. Lectins can be of either plant or animal origin.[177] Names of common lectins and their food sources are *Pisum sativum* agglutinin (green peas), phytohaemagglutinin (kidney beans), *Lens culinaris* agglutinin (lentils), and wheat germ agglutinin (wheat). Tomato is also a common source of dietary lectin.[178]

Some lectins can trigger mast cell degranulation and histamine release, and conversely, sometimes lectins act to desensitize mast cells and block their response to antigens.[178] Pokeweed mitogen, a lectin found in the poke plant used as a salad green, has been found to stimulate IgE antibody synthesis *in vitro*.[179]

Notable adverse reactions are associated with the ability of lectins to reduce the absorptive capacity of the intestine. The lectin hemagglutinin in raw or poorly cooked red kidney beans has been implicated in the etiology of gastroenteritis.[180] Such reports should encourage dietitians to aid patients or clients who need help identifying proper cooking techniques for legumes. [A personal experience of the author related to a university student who was advised to increase intake of dried beans and peas. In a subsequent dietetic counseling session, the student said the beans were tried but were "hard." Fortunately, this patient did not develop gastrointestinal symptoms from eating the raw beans. Cooking procedures were explained and the student was able to successfully (and enjoyably) increase dietary intake of dried (properly cooked) beans.] Soaking beans is also important in reducing lectin content.[178,180] Lectin-containing foods are frequently consumed raw (tomato), or the lectins are heat resistant (wheat germ agglutinin).[178]

The role of lectins in regard to human physiology and pathophysiology has yet to be fully elucidated. Lectins may have beneficial effects, but also have the ability to induce adverse reactions. Lectins have also been postulated to be an etiologic factor for celiac sprue.[178] (Celiac sprue is discussed later in this chapter.)

Psoralens

Psoralens, or linear furocoumarins, are found in several vegetables. Examples are celery, parsnip, and parsley.[181] Psoralens are believed to have toxic properties, but the only adverse reaction reported to date in humans is dermatitis in persons handling vegetables.[181,182] Although very rare, the potential dangers associated with psoralens are relevant to the dietitian in food service management concerned with the health of employees handling vegetables. Adverse reactions from oral ingestion would seem to be rare or nonexistent.

Salicylates

Salicylates have been implicated in several adverse reactions. Research related to hyperactivity is reviewed in Chapter 11. Other problems potentially linked to salicylates include urticaria, wheeze, and angioedema.[183,184] Salicylate adverse reactions have largely been studied in regard to aspirin (acetylsalicylic acid).[184] Aspirin intolerance involves the enzyme cycloxygenase pathway. Salicylate in foods does not appear to affect this pathway; therefore, aspirin-intolerant individuals are not routinely placed on a low salicylate diet.[163] Food salicylate consumption is generally estimated to be 10 to 200 mg/day, and aspirin dosage is generally 600 to 625 mg at one time, with potential for multiple daily intake.[184] This fact, coupled with the different forms of salicylate in aspirin and food, leaves it unclear if food salicylates are involved in adverse reactions.

Exorphins (Opioid Peptides)

Opioid peptides are food peptides that have actions similar to morphine.[185,186] The major sources of exorphins are wheat (glutenin and gliadin), milk (for example, cow's milk and human milk), and meat. Table 7-4 summarizes major exorphin types identified to date.

The most discussed, potentially adverse reaction to exorphins involves schizophrenia. In 1966, Dohan[187] proposed that cereals (such as wheat) with what he termed as a "pathogenicity factor" could interact with a genotype for schizophrenia to produce clinical mental disease. Zioudrou et al[185] in 1978 reported finding opioid peptides in wheat gluten and α-casein and indicated this finding provided potential biochemical evidence for Dohan's hypothesis.

Studies subsequent to Dohan's hypothesis have not provided definitive support for Dohan's views.[188] Dohan and associates[189,190] did publish two dietary trial studies supporting their view, and Singh and Kay[191] also published data in 1976 that supported Dohan. The Singh and Kay[191] study, however, has been questioned. Levy and Weinreb[192] state that the Singh and Kay data show decreasing, rather than increasing, mental pathology with gluten challenge, and Smith[193] has criticized the statistical methodology of the Singh and Kay study. Studies that have found no support for Dohan's hypothesis are those of Potkin et al[194] and Osborne et al.[195] Potkin et al[194] tested eight chronic schizophrenic patients on a milk-, cereal grain-, and gluten-free diet with gluten and placebo challenges. These researchers could find no deterioration of clinical mental status with gluten challenge. They also could detect no intestinal inflammatory responses. The Osborne[195] study

---

Table 7-4 Major Exorphin Types

Milk	α-casein exorphin
	ß-casomorphin
Beef	Cytochrophin
	Hemorphin
Wheat	Gluten exorphin

tested the effect of a gluten-free diet in five patients with diagnosis of schizophrenia. (The theory being tested by the Osborne group was that gluten absence might enhance absorption of the neuroleptic drug butaperazine.) The Osborne group could not demonstrate the efficacy of eliminating gluten in schizophrenia.

More research on this topic is needed related to Dohan's hypothesis. Future studies need to be double-blind and use objective criteria for improvement. Length of diet may be an important factor. Dohan and Grasberger[189] have suggested a gluten-free, cereal-free, and milk-free diet may need to be followed for 6 to 12 months before improvement can be noted. Potkin et al[194] have suggested if patients are going to do so, they will in one month. It may be, also, that only a subpopulation of schizophrenics experiences adverse reactions to the opiate peptides.[195] Singh[196] has put forth the hypothesis that paranoid schizophrenics and those with schizoaffective disorders are more likely to benefit from dietary restrictions involving the opioid peptides.

Opioid peptides (exorphins) may elicit allergy-like adverse reactions. This is postulated because some opioids stimulate degranulation of mastocytes and produce cutaneous wheal and flare.[186] Paroli[186] has suggested that the β-casomorphins particularly may induce an adverse reaction of this type.

Gliadin and Other Prolamins

Prolamins are alcohol-soluble fractions of gluten. Some prolamins have been associated with adverse reactions (specifically celiac sprue and dermatitis herpetiformis). Prolamins in cereal grains that have been associated with adverse reactions include gliadin (wheat), secalin (rye), and hordein (barley).[197]

Gliadin is one of the most extensively studied prolamins, and it is currently believed that four gliadin fractions have the potential to be toxic to intestinal mucosa.[197,198] Secalin (rye) and hordein (barley) are closely related to wheat gliadin. The prolamins in oats (avenin) and corn (zein) do not appear to be closely related, and thus seem to have less potential for adverse reaction.[197] More details on food products and potential problems are discussed in the latter part of this section dealing with current dietary guidance principles.

Celiac sprue (or celiac disease) is a prolamin-associated adverse reaction characterized by atrophy of the gut villi.[199] Genetic factors appear to be associated with celiac disease. A high level (70%) concordance has been found in monozygotic twins, and association of certain genetic markers with celiac disease has also been demonstrated.[200] Theories related to timing of wheat introduction in population groups are discussed in Chapter 10. Environmental factors have also been studied in regard to celiac sprue expression.

One hypothesis is that infection may initiate disease expression in the genetically susceptible individual.[200] One study has demonstrated homology for a 12-amino acid sequence in gliadin and human adenovirus type 12,[201] and serologic markers of adenovirus infection in patients with celiac disease have been found.[202]

Greco et al[203] have identified bottle feeding as an environmental risk factor for those genetically susceptible for celiac disease. These same researchers did not find early gluten introduction to be a risk factor. Gluten passage in human milk has been documented, and some believe this may facilitate appropriate immune responsiveness in the postweaning period.[203]

How does a prolamin (most commonly gliadin) initiate an adverse reaction in a person genetically and presumably environmentally primed? Although the biochemical bases for adverse reaction have not been elucidated with certainty, several mechanisms have been proposed.

One proposed mechanism is that celiac disease results from a lack of a small intestinal enzyme[204] or some type of abnormal intestinal metabolism of gliadin.[200] Problems that may occur include (1) incomplete digestion of toxic peptide fractions, (2) increased transglutaminase activity and subsequent cross-linking of gliadin peptides to intestinal cell membranes, or (3) abnormal cellular uptake or transport of gliadin within the intestinal cell.[200] Bailey et al,[204] studying mucosal biopsies from five adult celiac patients, found reduction in polypeptide synthesis by small intestinal mucosa $2^{1}/_{2}$ hours after gluten challenge, but not before challenge. These researchers concluded that abnormalities in metabolism of small intestinal mucosa were secondary effects rather than initiators of pathogenesis.

Another proposed mechanism for celiac sprue causation speculates that gliadin may behave in a lectin-like manner and bind to carbohydrate portions of glycoproteins or glycolipids on the intestinal cell surface.[200,204] Auricchio et al,[200] however, speculate that this mechanism is unlikely because lectin proteins generally have two carbohydrate-specific binding sites and L-gliadin peptides only have 25 amino acids making folding for two binding sites difficult. Biochemical research into this hypothesis continues, and Barresi et al[205] published data describing labeled lectin distribution in intestinal cells of children with celiac sprue.

Altered immune response may be involved in the pathogenesis of celiac sprue. Patients with untreated disease have large amounts of IgA, IgG, and IgM in the mucosal cells of the jejunum.[200] (Chapter 1 discusses the potential involvement of a type IV cell-mediated immune reaction.) These patients also have elevated serum levels of gliadin antibodies. Raised antibody levels may be due to increased uptake by damaged mucosa or some have suggested suppressor T-cell dysfunction. Whether antibody abnormalities are involved in pathogenesis of celiac disease or are involved in a secondary effect is not clear. Characteristic mucosal damage could be initiated via antibody-related cytotoxicity or formation of immune complexes. Cell-mediated immunity also may play a role, and cell-mediated immunity to gliadin has been demonstrated. Some have speculated that gut changes may be related to increased intraepithelial lymphocyte numbers.[200] The ability of corticosteroids to inhibit the damaging effects of gliadin *in vitro,* demonstrated in 1976, suggests an immunologic basis.[206]

Celiac disease has been described as a disease of both children and adults.[197,200,207-209] Clinical presentation varies at different ages. The disease in childhood is characterized by diarrhea, vomiting, distention of the abdomen, anorexia, and growth failure. Frequency of various symptom categories changes with age. Prior to age 6 months, chronic diarrhea is the most frequently reported symptom. Between ages 10 and 18 years, growth failure is the symptom most often reported. DeLuca et al[208] report that growth failure may be the sole clinical symptom. These researchers recommend a small bowel biopsy as part of the workup for children presenting with retarded growth. Severe hypoplasia of tooth enamel is another problem seen more frequently in children with celiac disease. Because the enamel defect is correctable with gluten withdrawal, this symptom seems to be part of the adverse reaction picture.[200]

Paré et al[209] have reported on clinical signs and symptoms associated with adult celiac sprue. Major symptoms at presentation (in order of reported percentage of patients with the symptom) were weakness and feeling tired, abdominal distention and gas, weight loss, diarrhea, abdominal pain, and borborygmus. Other less common symptoms were constipation, bone pain, and diarrhea.

The other prolamin-associated adverse reaction is dermatitis herpetiformis. Dermatitis herpetiformis is defined as an itchy blister-type rash in which IgA is demonstrable at the junction of the dermis and epidermis.[197,210] The rash usually occurs over the buttocks, knees, and elbows.[197] Dermatitis herpetiformis patients who have intestinal abnormalities are considered to have asymptomatic celiac disease (or gluten-sensitive enteropathy). The diagnosis of dermatitis herpetiformis is generally reserved for those patients with granular IgA deposits. Patients with linear IgA deposits (about 10% to 15% of those with the characteristic skin symptoms) generally do not have intestinal abnormalities and are given the diagnosis of linear IgA dermatosis.[210] In addition to diet therapy, dapsone (a sulfa drug) is used in the treatment of dermatitis herpetiformis.

The lifelong gluten-free diet is considered the mainstay of treatment for celiac disease. The gluten-free diet is also recommended for treatment of dermatitis herpetiformis. The diet for dermatitis herpetiformis is usually followed for 8 months to 5 years.[197,210,211] The diet that can be followed to achieve best results depends on prolamin content of foods and beverages and individual differences in levels of tolerance.[197]

It is generally recognized that wheat flours (whole wheat, white, and graham) and products containing wheat flours (breads, cakes, and cookies) should be avoided. Wheat flours contain the starch endosperm portion of the wheat grain where gliadin is present.[197] Wheat bran theoretically should not contain gliadin, but because it may be contaminated with gliadin, many times it is placed on the list of foods that celiac disease and dermatitis herpetiformis patients are advised to avoid.[197] Rye and barley, as mentioned previously, contain prolamins that are similar to gliadin. Triticale is a cross between wheat and rye and is recommended to be excluded. The evidence linking the prolamin-hordein in barley to celiac disease is not clear; however, due to the antigenic similarities between hordein and gliadin, most authorities do recommend elimination. Malt (made from sprouted barley) is to be excluded. Malt extract, a different product, does not need to be excluded.[197]

Oats, which contain the prolamin avenin, remain controversial in terms of avoidance or nonavoidance in the gluten-free diet.[197] It may be that a subgroup of individuals experiences problems with oats and should avoid them. Prolamins of millet, corn, and rice do not appear to cause adverse reaction and can be used by individuals with celiac sprue or dermatitis herpetiformis.[197]

A low-gluten diet (as opposed to a gluten-free diet) has been suggested by some as a viable alternative for celiac disease treatment. In 1985, Kumar et al[212] assessed 85 patients and concluded that many were tolerating small amounts of gluten. These same researchers also formally placed 8 patients on a 2.5-g gluten diet and indicated that 6 patients did well. Montgomery et al[213] compared 12 patients on a low-gluten diet (2.5-5 g/day) with 13 patients on the more conventional gluten-free diet. No significant differences were found in terms of antigluten antibody titers (IgG, IgM, and IgA) or villous height or depth of intestinal crypts. These researchers did report that the low-gluten diet was associated with some infiltration of jejunal mucosa by lymphocytes.

More research is needed to clarify the efficacy of the low-gluten diet. The use of such a diet could aid in achieving patient compliance. Additional research is also needed with regard to nutritional adequacy of gluten-avoidance diets as practiced.[197]

Lactose

Lactose is a water-soluble disaccharide composed of glucose and galactose.[214,215] It is found primarily in the whey portion of dairy foods.[215] Appendix K provides an overview of the lactose contents of some commonly consumed foods and beverages.

Adverse reaction to lactose is primarily related to absence or loss of intestinal lactase activity. Lactase enzyme in the intestinal brush border breaks down lactose into its monosaccharide components in order for absorption to occur.[216] When lactase is absent or deficient, lactose cannot be fully digested or absorbed. Undigested lactose reaching the colon is acted on by colonic bacteria to form short-chain fatty acids, hydrogen gas, and lactic acid. It is believed that if the capacity of colonic bacteria to achieve the above breakdown is exceeded, diarrhea, and pain and abdominal bloating may become manifest due to the presence of a carbohydrate (lactose) osmotic load.[215,217,218] Individual reaction to the point of clinical manifestation of symptoms is variable and depends on many factors such as degree of lactase deficiency, lactose dosage, and concomitant foods or ingredients consumed.[215,218]

Because lactose is found in milk or dairy products, adverse reaction to lactose may be confused with cow's milk allergy. Table 7-5 contrasts causes, clinical manifestation, and treatment of these two problems.[218] Cow's milk allergy is discussed extensively in Chapter 2, 3, and 6.

Table 7-5 Comparison of Milk Allergy and Primary Lactose Intolerance

	Milk Allergy	*Lactose Intolerance*
Age	Early infancy	After age 2 y
Cause	Milk protein (lactalbumin)	Milk sugar (lactose)
Inherited		
Symptoms	Variable	Yes
Diarrhea	Yes	Yes
Vomiting	Yes	Uncommon
Abdominal pain	Yes	Yes
Abdominal bloating	Yes	Yes
Dermatitis	Yes	No
Rhinitis	Yes	No
Asthma	Yes	No
Urticaria	Yes	No
Anaphylaxis	Yes	No
Duration	Usually declines rapidly after first year	Indefinite after onset
Milk protein contraindicated	Yes	No
Milk consumption contraindicated	Yes	Not if amount is moderate

Source: Reprinted from "The Acceptability of Milk and Milk Products in Populations with a High Prevalence of Lactose Intolerance" by N. Scrimshaw and E. Murray, 1988, *American Journal of Clinical Nutrition,* Suppl. 48 (4), p. 1084, © *Am J Clin Nutr,* American Society for Clinical Nutrition.

Lactase deficiency can be characterized as congenital, primary, or secondary (sometimes termed acquired).[217] Primary lactase deficiency that manifests after the weaning period is considered the most common type and may affect as much as 70% of the world's population.[215]

Congenital lactase deficiency is a rare defect characterized by persistence of lactase deficiency (very low levels of lactase) throughout the lifespan and occurs in the presence of normal small intestine morphology.[217] Intestinal symptoms, notably diarrhea, occur as soon as milk is given. Congenital lactase deficiency is believed to be transmitted as a recessive gene with more males than females reportedly affected.[217]

The existence of primary lactase deficiency (the most common type of lactose intolerance) in various ethnic groups has been extensively studied. Chapter 10 discusses primary lactase deficiency from an anthropological perspective. Readers are also referred to the excellent review on this topic by Scrimshaw and Murray.[218]

Clinical manifestations related to the degree of primary deficiency appear to be subject to modulation. Modulation in regard to types of dairy products or other foods are discussed later in this chapter.

Worthy of mention at this point are the phenomena of colonic adaption and proposed pregnancy-associated physiologic adaption. Scrimshaw and Murray[218] document that persons who are lactose intolerant when fed lactose-containing foods may adapt to increased dosages. Postulated mechanisms for adaptation include (1) increased production of bacteria that favor lactic acid production or (2) increased acidity of the colon. Villar et al[219] described adaptation to higher lactose loads (18 g) in pregnancy among women who were classified as having problems with lactose digestion (by breath H_2 test). These researchers postulate that progesterone may be involved and may favor adaptation through decreasing intestinal transit time and changing in intestinal morpholology (increased villus height in the duodenum) and function (lactase activity).

Secondary (or acquired) lactase deficiency may occur in a variety of clinical states or with consumption of certain pharmaceuticals. Table 7-6 summarizes some of these conditions. Alcoholism particularly has been cited.[220,221] Most cases of secondary lactase deficiency are associated with morphological changes in the small intestine.

Another adverse reaction to lactose that is not associated with lactase deficiency is known as severe lactose intolerance with lactosuria.[217] The basic pathological defect in this disorder appears to be abnormal gastric permeability to lactose. The disorder is a rare one with a genetic basis.[217]

Speculation also exists with regard to cataracts being an adverse reaction to lactose intake in persons with an abnormality or abnormalities in galactose utilization.[218] The theory was first proposed by Skala and Prchal.[222] Studies to date have not clearly resolved that such a connection does exist.[218]

Table 7-6 Conditions and Factors Associated with Secondary Lactase Deficiency

---

- Alcoholism[217,220,221]
- *Ascaris lumbricoides* infection[218]
- Celiac sprue[217]
- Cow's milk protein allergy[217]
- Drugs
  —colchicine[217]
  —aminosalicylic acid[218]
  —antibiotics (neomycin, kanamycin)[218]
- Gastrointestinal surgery[217]
- Hypoxia[217]
- Ionizing radiation (cancer therapy)[218]
- Iron deficiency[217]
- Protein calorie malnutrition (kwashiorkor)[217]
- Rotavirus diarrhea and other infectious diarrheas[218]
- Tropical sprue[218]

The lactose tolerance test for adults involves giving a 50-g lactose load and measuring influence on blood sugar.[218] (The lactose load for children is 2 g/kg body weight.) The lactose level (equivalent to the amount of lactose in approximately one liter of milk) has been criticized as being unphysiologic. Other tests used to assess lactase activity are the breath hydrogen test, intestinal biopsy, perfusion of the intestine, small bowel x-ray (after ingestion of lactose with barium), [^{14}C] lactose absorption, and urinary galactose.[218]

The influence of lactase deficiency on absorption of other nutrients has been the subject of concern. It has been postulated that the problem of diarrhea and decreased transit time may lead to malabsorption. Research to date, however, does not suggest lactase deficiency negatively influences absorption of protein, vitamins, and fat.[218] Ziegler and Fomon[223] did find that when lactose-free formulas were tested (compared to lactose-containing ones), fecal excretion of magnesium was significantly higher on lactose-free formula. Absorption of zinc, manganese, and copper also seemed to be better from the lactose-containing formula, but absorption differences were not significant.

Calcium absorption and intake related to lactase deficiency has been a special area of concern. In 1968, Birge et al[224] studied 19 patients with osteoporosis compared to 13 normal controls. Nine of the 19 patients with osteoporosis were found to be lactose intolerant. Birge et al[224] postulated that long-term avoidance of calcium products may play a role in osteoporosis development in at least a subset of individuals. Newcomer et al[225] studied lactase activity in 30 women with osteoporosis and 31 control subjects. Incidence of lactase deficiency was significantly higher in the group of women with osteoporosis. Again these researchers postulated that lowered intake of calcium-containing dairy products secondary to lactose intolerance may have played a role in the etiology of osteoporosis.

The role of lactose in calcium absorption has yet to be fully elucidated, but in 1988 Scrimshaw and Murray[218] concluded that the majority of evidence indicated lactose either favorably affected calcium absorption or had no effect in both those with and without lactase deficiency. Heightened passive diffusion is the proposed mechanism by which lactose may enhance calcium absorption.[218,226] Griessen et al[227] studied calcium absorption from milk containing lactose and milk containing glucose in seven lactase-deficient subjects, compared to eight lactase-sufficient controls. This work does not support the notion that calcium absorption is impaired by lactose even in those lactase deficient. The authors suggest further that their findings with regard to glucose support the use of hydrolyzed dairy products by individuals unable to tolerate higher levels of lactose. Savaiano and Kotz[215] have pointed out that many lactase-deficient individuals can tolerate 1 glass (8 oz) of milk. If such tolerance is noted, milk consumption should be encouraged to promote adequate calcium intake.

As indicated throughout this discussion, lactase deficiency represents a wide spectrum, and many lactase-deficient individuals can tolerate some degree of lactose. A totally lactose-free diet may be indicated in some cases.[214] Individualized assessment is critical in determining appropriate dietary recommendations. Dietary strategies for use with lactase-deficient individuals need to consider effects of processing, enzyme additions, and total dietary nutrient content, as well as amounts of lactose in food and beverages and individual abilities related to tolerance.

Fermentation of dairy products is an example of a processing mode that may have (in some instances) beneficial effects. Yogurt, particularly, has been studied in this regard, and yogurt is tolerated by many lactase-deficient individuals.[215,228,229] Bourlioux and Pouchart[230] report that in the case where yogurt is produced using whole milk that has skim milk powder added, lactose content in the original milk-fortified mixture is 6.5% in contrast with the lactose content of the final yogurt product, which is 5.2%. The ß-galactosidase activity of microbes in yogurt is believed to be helpful in enhancing lactose tolerance because this substance promotes digestion of the lactose within the intestinal lumen.[228] It should be noted that yogurts vary in their ß-galactosidase activity. Martini et al,[231] for example, found ß-galactosidase activity to be higher in unflavored yogurt when compared to strawberry flavor. Frozen yogurt does not have ß-galactosidase activity. It has been suggested that mucosal cell lactase may be stimulated by a component of yogurt or a lactase of a microbial origin in yogurt may adhere to intestinal mucous cells.[232]

Buttermilks are also cultured (or fermented) dairy products, but current evidence suggests these products are not better tolerated by lactase-deficient individuals. Most lactic streptococci strains used in making buttermilk (*Streptococcus cremoris* and *Streptococcus lactis*) contain phospho-ß-galactosidase. This enzyme form does not appear to operate effectively *in vivo* to break down lactose for the human host.[215,233] Gendrel et al[234] reported that a dried low-fat milk product fermented with *Lactobacillus bulgaricus* and *Streptococcus thermophilus,* however, may be a new alternative for some lactose-intolerant individuals.

Sweet acidophilus milk is a nonfermented modified milk product that has also been studied. Use of this product appears to confer no advantage over that of regular milk for the lactose-intolerant individual.[215] Use of frozen concentrate starters in processing (with subsequent ß-galactosidase activity loss) has been stated as a potential factor in failure to convey positive benefit.[215] McDonough et al,[235] however, demonstrated that if sweet acidophilus milk was prepared with sonicated *Lactobacillus acidophilus* cells, lactase activity could be increased dramatically. Measurements of breath hydrogen in lactose-intolerant subjects also indicated improved tolerance for the sweet acidophilus milk made with sonicated cells.

Dairy products can also be altered through use of enzymes that digest lactose.[215] Such alteration usually increases the potential for tolerance in lactase-deficient individuals. Hydrolysis of milk (using ß-galactosidase and refrigeration of the product for 12 to 24 hours) is one strategy that has been used.[226] A yeast (*Candida pseudotropicalis*) is the source of enzyme that can also work to hydrolyze lactose. This product is being used by the food industry during processing to reduce the lactose content of milk, whey, and milk powder.[236] Use of ß-galactosidases given orally at time of milk consumption also seems to be a viable method of improving tolerance.[237]

Lactose tolerance also seems to be affected by the presence of other foods. Martini and Savaiano,[238] feeding 5 test solutions or meals with 12 lactase-deficient subjects, found that the number of subjects with symptoms was greatly reduced when 19 g of lactose in a food supplement was given with a meal. Lee and Hardy[239] report that cocoa in milk improves lactose tolerance. Proposed mechanisms include delayed gastric emptying (due to solids in cocoa or gum in chocolate milk), potential ability of cocoa to increase lactase activity *in vivo,* and alteration of colonic bacteria, producing less hydrogen gas.

As mentioned previously dietitians need to individualize diets for lactose-intolerant individuals. Dairy products (containing lactose) are important sources of calcium, riboflavin, protein, phosphorus, and other nutrients.[237] Strategies that ensure adequacy of these nutrients should be employed.

Trehalose

Trehalose is a disaccharide known as 1-α-glucosido-1-α-glucoside.[240] Humans are known to ingest trehalose only in young mushrooms, although this disaccharide is present in other plants and in some insects. (As mushrooms age, trehalose is converted to glucose.[240,241]) Trehalase deficiency has been documented and the suggestion has been made that such deficiency is inherited as an autosomal trait.[241] Symptoms of trehalase deficiency include diarrhea, vomiting, and abdominal pain. One patient report describes diarrhea beginning during the meal that contained young mushrooms.[240] Trehalase deficiency seems to be rare and occurrence of symptoms easily preventable by elimination of young mushrooms from the diet.

CONCLUSION

Individuals can experience adverse food reactions to food additives, food contaminants, and natural food constituents. The mechanisms underlying these reactions are for the most part unknown. Dietitians can aid individuals in developing nutritionally adequate, appropriate plans for avoidance.

REFERENCES

1. Schneider AT, Codispoti AJ. Allergic reactions to food additives. In: Chiaramonte LT, Schneider AT, Lifshitz F, eds. *Food Allergy, A Practical Approach to Diagnosis and Management.* New York: Marcel Dekker, Inc; 1988: 117–151.

2. Folkenberg J. Reporting reactions to additives. In: *An FDA Consumer Special Report—Safety First: Protecting America's Food Supply.* Rockville, MD: Department of Health and Human Services, November 1988, HHS Publication No. (FDA) 88–2224.

3. AMA Council on Scientific Affairs: Aspartame—review of safety issue. *JAMA.* 1985; 254(3):400–402.

4. Alfin-Slater RB, Xavier Pi-Sunyer F. Sugar and sugar substitutes—comparisons and indications. *Postgrad Med.* 1987; 82(2):46–56.

5. American Dietetic Association. Appropriate use of nutritive and non-nutritive sweeteners. *J Am Diet Assoc.* 1987; 87(12):1689–1690.

6. Janssen PJCM, van der Heijden CA. Aspartame: Review of recent experimental and observational data. *Toxicology.* 1988; 50:1–26.

7. Stegink LD. The aspartame story: A model for the clinical testing of a food additive. *Am J Clin Nutr.* 1987; 46:204–215.

8. Tobey NA, Heizer WD. Intestinal hydrolysis of aspartylphenylalanine—the metabolic product of aspartame. *Gastroenterology.* 1986; 91:931–937.

9. Maher TJ. Natural food constituents and food additives: the pharmacologic connection. *J Allergy Clin Immunol.* 1987; 79(3):413–422.

10. Franz, M. Is it safe to consume aspartame during pregnancy? A review. *Diabetes Ed.* 1986; 12(2):145–147.

11. American Diabetes Association. Position Statement—Use of noncaloric sweeteners. *Diabetes Care.* 1987; 10(4):526.

12. London RS. Saccharin and aspartame—Are they safe to consume during pregnancy? *J Reprod Med.* 1988; 33(1):17–21.

13. Pardridge WM. The safety of aspartame. *JAMA.* 1986; 256:2678. Letter.

14. Levy HL, Waisbren SE. The safety of aspartame. *JAMA.* 1987; 258(2):205. Letter.

15. Stegink LD, Krause WL. The safety of aspartame. *JAMA.* 1987; 258(2):205–206. Letter.

16. Pardridge WM. The safety of aspartame. *JAMA.* 1987; 258(2):206. Reply.

17. Kruesi MJP, Rapoport, JL. Diet and human behavior: how much do they affect each other? *Ann Rev Nutr.* 1986; 6:113–130.

18. Kruesi MJP, Rapoport JL, Cummings, EM, et al. Effects of sugar and aspartame on aggression and activity in children. *Am J Psychiatry.* 1987; 144(11):1487–1490.

19. Stegink LD, Pitkin RM, Reynolds WA, Brummel MC, Filer LJ. Placental transfer of aspartate and its metabolites in the primate. *Metabolism.* 1979; 28:669–676.

20. Filer LJ, Baker GL, Stegink LD. Effect of aspartame loading upon plasma and erythrocyte free amino acid concentrations in one-year-old infants. *J Nutr.* 1983; 113:1591–1599.

21. Ferguson HB, Stoddart C, Simeon JG. Double blind challenge studies of behavioral and cognitive effects of sucrose-aspartame ingestion in normal children. *Nutr Rev.* 1986; 44 (suppl):144–150.

22. Gautier R. Do too many new NutraSweet products appeal to kids? *Am Health.* 1989; 8(2):154–155.

23. Bradstock MK, Serdula MK, Marks JS, et al. Evaluation of reactions to food additives: The aspartame experience. *Am J Clin Nutr.* 1986; 43:464–469.

24. Schiffman SS, Buckley CE, Sampson HA, et al. Aspartame and susceptibility to headache. *N Engl J Med.* 1987; 317(19):1181–1185.

25. McKean CM. The effects of high phenylalanine concentrations on serotonin and catecholamine metabolism in the human brain. *Brain Res.* 1972; 47:469–476.

26. Maher TJ, Wurtman RJ. Possible neurologic effects of aspartame: A widely used food additive. *Environ Health Perspect.* 1987; 75:53–57.

27. Steinmetzer RV, Kunkel RS. Aspartame and headache. *N Engl J Med.* 1988; 318(8):1201. Letter.

28. Koehler SM, Glaros A. The effect of aspartame on migraine headache. *Headache.* 1988; 28:10–13.

29. Ferguson JM. Interaction of aspartame and carbohydrates in an eating disordered patient. *Am J Psychiatry.* 1985; 142(2):271. Letter.

30. Johns JR. Migraine provoked by aspartame. *N Engl J Med.* 1986; 315:456. Letter.

31. Lipton RB, Newman LC, Solomon S. Aspartame and headache. *N Engl J Med.* 1988; 318(18):1200–1201. Letter.

32. Wurtman RJ. Aspartame: Possible effect on seizure susceptibility. *Lancet.* 1985; 2:1060. Letter.

33. Walton RG. Seizure and mania after high intake on aspartame. *Psychosomatics.* 1986; 27:218–220.

34. Garriga MM, Metcalfe, DD. Aspartame intolerance. *Ann Allergy.* 1988; 61(Part II):63–69.

35. Blundell JE, Hill AJ. Paradoxical effects of an intense sweetener (aspartame) on appetite. *Lancet.* 1986; 1:1092–1093. Letter.

36. Ryan-Harshman M, Leiter LA, Anderson GH. Phenylalanine and aspartame fail to alter feeding behavior, mood, and arousal in men. *Physiol Behav.* 1987; 39:247–253.

37. Novick NL. Aspartame-induced granulomatous panniculitis. *Ann Intern Med.* 1985; 102(2):206–207.

38. Kulczycki A. Jr. Aspartame-induced urticaria. *Ann Intern Med.* 1986; 104(2):207–208.

39. Stamp JA. Sorting out the alternative sweeteners. *Cereal Foods World.* 1990; 35(4):395–400.

40. Duxbury DD. Encapsulated aspartame for bakery applications. *Food Processing.* 1990; 51(2):58.

41. Simon RA. Sulfite sensitivity. *Ann Allergy.* 1987; 59:100–105.

42. Bush RK, Taylor SL, Holden K, Nordlee JA, Busse WW. Prevalence of sensitivity to sulfiting agents in asthmatic patients. *Am J Med.* 1986; 81:816–820.

43. FDA Drug Bulletin. 1984; 14:24.

44. Bush RK, Taylor SL, Busse W. A critical evaluation of clinical trials in reactions to sulfites. *J Allergy Clin Immunol.* 1986; 78(1):191–202.

45. Gunnison AF, Jacobsen DW. Sulfite hypersensitivity. A critical review. *CRC Crit Rev Toxicol.* 1987; 17(3):185–214.

46. Settipane GA. Adverse reactions to sulfites in drugs and foods. *J Am Acad Dermatol.* 1984; 10(6):1077–1080.

47. Wolf SI, Nicklas RA. Sulfite sensitivity in a seven-year-old child. *Ann Allergy.* 1985; 54:420–423.

48. Prenner BM, Stevens JJ. Anaphylaxis after ingestion of sodium bisulfite. *Ann Allergy.* 1976; 37:180–182.

49. Simon RA. Sulfite sensitivity. *Ann Allergy.* 1986; 56:281–288.

50. Kochen J. Sulfur dioxide, a respiratory tract irritant, even if ingested. *Pediatrics.* 1973; 52:145–146.

51. Taylor SL, Bush RK, Selner JC, et al. Sensitivity to sulfited foods among sulfite-sensitive subjects with asthma. *J Allergy Clin Immunol.* 1988; 81(6):1159–1167.

52. Bahna SL. Food sensitivity—handling reactions to foods and food additives. *Postgrad Med J.* 1987; 82(5):195–205.

53. Parathyras AJ. Diet for sulfite sensitivity. In: Chiaramonte LT, Schneider AT, Lifshitz F, eds. *Food Allergy: A Practical Approach to Diagnosis and Treatment.* New York: Marcel Dekker, Inc; 1988:435–440.

54. Gershwin ME, Ough C, Bock A, Fletcher MP, Nagy SM, Tuft DS. Grand Rounds: Adverse reactions to wine. *J Allergy Clin Immunol.* 1985; 75(3):411–420.

55. Tsevat J, Gross GN, Dowling GP. Fatal asthma after ingestion of sulfite-containing wine. *Ann Intern Med.* 1987; 107(2):263. Letter.

56. Dalton-Bunnow MF. Review of sulfite sensitivity. *Am J Hosp Pharm.* 1985; 42:2220–2225.

57. Personal Communication, Dr. Linda Tollefson, Food and Drug Administration, August 1989.

58. Cole DEC. Sulfites and parenteral nutrition. *Can Med Assoc J.* 1986; 134:17–18.

59. Jamieson DM, Guill MF, Wray BB, May JR. Metabisulfite sensitivity: case report and literature review. *Ann Allergy.* 1985; 54:115–121.

60. Koepke JW, Staudenmayer H, Selner JC. Inhaled metabisulfite sensitivity. *Ann Allergy.* 1985; 54:213–215.

61. Sher TH, Schwartz HJ. Bisulfite sensitivity manifesting as an allergic reaction to aerosol therapy. *Ann Allergy.* 1985; 54:224–226.

62. Onorato DJ. Ophthalmic medications that contain sulfites. *Arch Ophthalmol.* 1985; 103:1274–1276.

63. Schwartz HJ, Sher TH. Bisulfite sensitivity manifesting as allergy to local dental anesthesia. *J Allergy Clin Immunol.* 1985; 75:525–527.

64. Seng GF, Gay BJ. Dangers of sulfites in dental local anesthetic solutions: warning and recommendations. *J Am Dent Assoc.* 1986; 113:769–770.

65. Apetato M, Marques MSJ. Contact dermatitis caused by sodium metabisulphite. *Contact Dermatitis.* 1986; 14(3):194.

66. Nater JP. Allergic contact dermatitis caused by potassium metabisulfite. *Dermatologica.* 1968; 136:477–478.

67. Lecos CW. An order of fries—hold the sulfites. *FDA Consumer.* 1988; 22:9–11.

68. Freedman BJ. Asthma induced by sulphur dioxide, benzoate and tartrazine contained in orange drinks. *Clin Allergy.* 1977; 7:407–415.

69. Nadel JA, Salem H, Tamplin B, Tokiwa Y. Mechanism of bronchoconstriction during inhalation of sulfur dioxide. *J Appl Physiol.* 1965; 20(1):164–167.

70. Schwartz HJ. Sensitivity to ingested metabisulfite: variations in clinical presentation. *J Allergy Clin Immunol.* 1983; 71(5):487–489.

71. Gilbert RP, Hegman G, Forsyth CE. Greater awareness of sulfite allergy needed. *West J Med.* 1987; 146(2):236.

72. Tichenor WS. Sulfite sensitivity—'minor problem' proves major hazard for some. *Postgrad Med J.* 1985; 78(5):320–325.

73. Shultz CM. Sulfite sensitivity. *Am J Nurs.* 1986; 86(8):914.

74. Sonin L, Patterson R. Metabisulfite challenge in patients with idiopathic anaphylaxis. *J Allergy Clin Immunol.* 1985; 75(1):67–69.

75. Meggs WJ, Atkins FM, Wright R, Fishman M, Kaliner MA, Metcalfe DD. Failure of sulfites to produce clinical responses in patients with systemic mastocytosis or recurrent anaphylaxis: Results of a single-blind study. *J Allergy Clin Immunol.* 1985; 76(6):840–846.

77. Simon R, Goldfarb G, Jacobsen D. Blocking studies in sulfite sensitive asthmatics. *J Allergy Clin Immunol.* 1984; 73(1):136. Abstract.

76. Schwartz HJ. Observations on the use of oral sodium cromoglycate in a sulfite-sensitive asthmatic patient. *Ann Allergy.* 1986; 57:36–37.

78. Potato processors urge sulfite level relief. *Food Chem News.* 1989; 31(7):21–22.

79. Analysis-based sulfite increase asked for dehydrated potatoes. *Food Chem News.* 1989; 31(2):32.

80. Potatoes included in sulfite ban. *Comm Nutr Inst Nutr Week.* 1990; 20(11):2.

81. Sulfite comments note concern about "carryover." *Food Chem News.* 1989; 31(1):51–53.

82. AFFI seeks inclusion of frozen, unblanched mushrooms in sulfite rule. *Food Chem News.* 1989; 31(1):53.

83. ABA asks clarification on combining of sulfite GRAS foods. *Food Chem News.* 1989; 31(2):33.

84. NFPA objectives to proposed 6-month effective date following final rule. *Food Chem News.* 1989; 31(2):34–35.

85. Canned quahog clams, cod cakes sulfite rule inclusion urged. *Food Chem News.* 1989; 31(3):39.

86. Gelatin sulfite level seen inconsistent with other countries' limits. *Food Chem News.* 1989; 31(3):40.

87. Dried fruit groups urge raising proposed 2,000 ppm sulfite limit. *Food Chem News.* 1989; 31(4):33–34.

88. Separate sulfite limit asked for dried apricots. *Food Chem News.* 1989; 31(4):34–35.

89. FDA urged to codify sulfite maraschino cherry prior to sanction. *Food Chem News.* 1989; 31(6):47–48.

90. Sulfites proposed as safe. *FDA Consumer.* 1989; 23(2):3.

91. Honey halts browning in juice, wine. *Food Proc.* 1989; 50(3):42.

92. Duxbury DD. Protease enzymes offer fruit, vegetable, shrimp preservative alternative. *Food Processing.* 1990; 51(4):44.

93. Criep LH. Allergic vascular purpura. *J Allergy Clin Immunol.* 1971; 48(1):7–12.

94. Lockey SD. Allergic reactions due to FD&C yellow no. 5 tartrazine, an aniline dye used as a coloring and identifying agent in various steroids. *Ann Allergy.* 1959; 17:719–721.

95. Dong FM. *All about Food Allergy.* Philadelphia: George F Stickley Co; 1984.

96. US Department of Health and Human Services, Public Health Service, Food and Drug Administration, Center for Food Safety and Applied Nutrition. *A Food Labeling Guide.* Washington, DC: 1988; HHS Publication No. (FDA) 88-2222.

97. Neuman I, Elian R, Nahum H, Shaked P, Creter D. The danger of "yellow dyes" (tartrazine) to allergic subjects. *Clin Allergy.* 1978; 8:65–68.

98. Pohl R, Balon R, Berchou R, Yeragani VK. Allergy to tartrazine in antidepressants. *Am J Psychiatry.* 1987; 142(2):237–238.

99. Desmond RE, Trautlein JJ. Tartrazine (FD&C yellow #5) anaphylaxis: A case report. *Ann Allergy.* 1981; 46:81–82.

100. Michaëlsson G, Juhlin L. Urticaria induced by preservatives and dye additives in food and drugs. *Br J Dermatol.* 1973; 88:525–532.

101. Michaëlsson G, Pettersson L, Juhlin L. Purpura caused by food and drug additives. *Arch Dermatol.* 1974; 109:49–52.

102. Kubba R, Champion RH. Anaphylactoid purpura caused by tartrazine and benzoates. *Br J Dermatol.* 1975; 93(suppl 11):61–62.

103. Parodi G, Parodi A, Rebora A. Purpuric vasculitis due to tartrazine. *Dermatologica.* 1985; 171:62–63.

104. Pereyo N. Tartrazine, the complement system and photosensitivity. *J Am Acad Dermatol.* 1987; 17(1):143.

105. Chafee FH, Settipane GA. Asthma caused by FD&C approved dyes. *J Allergy.* 1967; 40:65–72.

106. Stenius BSM, Lemola M. Hypersensitivity to acetylsalicylic acid (ASA) and tartrazine in patients with asthma. *Clin Allergy.* 1976; 6:119–129.

107. Spector SL, Wangaard CH, Farr RS. Aspirin and concomitant idiosyncrasies in adult asthmatic patients. *J Allergy Clin Immunol.* 1979; 64:500–506.

108. Weber RW, Hoffman M, Raine DA, Nelson HS. Incidence of bronchoconstriction due to aspirin, azo dyes, non-azo dyes, and preservatives in a population of perennial asthmatics. *J Allergy Clin Immunol.* 1979; 64:32–37.

109. Morales MC, Basomba A, Pelaez A, Garcia-Villalmanzo I, Campos A. Challenge tests with tartrazine in patients with asthma associated with intolerance to analgesics (ASA-Triad). *Clin Allergy.* 1985; 15:55–59.

110. Stevenson DD, Simon RA, Lumry WR, Mathison DA. Adverse reactions to tartrazine. *J Allergy Clin Immunol.* 1986; 78(1):182–191.

111. Virchow C, Szczeklik A, Bianco S, et al. Intolerance to tartrazine in aspirin-induced asthma: results of a multicenter study. *Respiration.* 1988; 53:20–23.

112. Parker SL, Sussman GL, Krondl M. Dietary aspects of adverse reactions to foods in adults. *Can Med Assoc J.* 1988; 139:711–718.

113. Hariparsad D, Wilson N, Dixon C, Silverman M. Oral tartrazine challenge in childhood asthma: Effect on bronchial reactivity. *Clin Allergy.* 1984; 14:81–85.

114. Baumgardner DJ. Persistent urticaria caused by a common coloring agent. *Postgrad Med.* 1989; 85(6):265–266.

115. Deoglas, HMG. Dietary treatment of patients with chronic urticaria and intolerance to aspirin and food additives. *Dermatologica.* 1977; 154:308–310.

116. Genton C, Frei PC, Pecoud A. Value of oral provocation tests to aspirin and food additives in the routine investigation of asthma and chronic urticaria. *J Allergy Clin Immunol.* 1985; 76(1):40–45.

117. Gibson A, Clancy R. Management of chronic idiopathic urticaria by the identification and exclusion of dietary factors. *Clin Allergy.* 1980; 10:699–704.

118. Podell RN. Unwrapping urticaria—the role of food additives. *Postgrad Med.* 1985; 78(8):83–97.

119. Verschave A, Stevens E, Degreef H. Pseudo-allergen-free diet in chronic urticaria. *Dermatologica.* 1983; 167:256–259.

120. Ros AM, Juhlin L, Michaëlsson G. A follow-up study of patients with recurrent urticaria and hypersensitivity to aspirin, benzoates, and azo dyes. *Br J Dermatol.* 1976; 95:19–24.

121. David TJ. Reactions to dietary tartrazine. *Arch Dis Child.* 1987; 62:119–122.

122. David TJ. Food additives. *Arch Dis Child.* 1988; 63:582–583.

123. Settipane GA, Pudupakkam RK. Aspirin intolerance, III: subtypes, familial occurrence and cross-reactivity with tartrazine. *J Allergy Clin Immunol.* 1975; 56(3):215–221.

124. Condemi JJ. Aspirin and food dye reactions. *Bull NY Acad Med.* 1981; 57(7):600–607.

125. Oskas RM. Possible reaction with NSAIDs and tartrazine. *Drug Intell Clin Pharm.* 1985; 19:478–479. Letter.

126. Mathison DA, Stevenson DD, Simon RA. Precipitating factors in asthma-aspirin, sulfites, and other drugs and chemicals. *Chest.* 1985; 87(1)(suppl):50S–54S.

127. Gerber JG, Payne NA, Oelz O, Nies AS, Oates JA. Tartrazine and the prostaglandin system. *J Allergy Clin Immunol.* 1979; 63(4):289–294.

128. Rosenhall L. Evaluation of intolerance to analgesics, preservatives and food colorants with challenge test. *Eur J Respir Dis.* 1982; 63:410–419.

129. Weliky N, Heiner DC. Hypersensitivity to chemicals. Correlation of tartrazine hypersensitivity with characteristic serum IgD & IgE immune response patterns. *Clin Allergy.* 1980; 10:375–394.

130. Kreindler JJ, Slutsky J, Haddad ZH. The effect of food colors and sodium benzoate on rat peritoneal mast cells. *Ann Allergy.* 1980; 44:76–81.

131. Murdoch RD, Pollock I, Naeem S. Tartrazine induced histamine release in vivo in normal subjects. *J Royal Coll Phys London.* 1987; 21(4):257–260.

132. Murdoch RD, Lessof MH, Pollock I, Young E. Effects of food additives on leukocyte histamine release in normal and urticaria subjects. *J Royal Coll Phys London.* 1987;21(4):251–256.

133. Partial ban of red no. 3 proposed. *FDA Consumer.* 1990; 24(3):3.

134. Allen DH, Delohery J, Baker G. Monosodium L-glutamate-induced asthma. *J Allergy Clin Immunol.* 1987; 80(4):530–537.

135. Kwok RHM. Chinese restaurant syndrome. *N Engl J Med.* 1968; 278:796. Letter.

136. Zautcke JL, Schwartz JA, Mueller E. Chinese restaurant syndrome: A review. *Ann Emerg Med.* 1986; 15:1210–1213.

137. Schaumburg H, Byck R, Gerstl R, Mashman JH. Monosodium L-glutamate: Its pharmacology and role in Chinese restaurant syndrome. *Science.* 1969; 163:826–828.

138. Ghadimi H, Kumar S. Current status of monosodium glutamate. *Am J Clin Nutr.* 1972; 25:643–646.

139. Kerr G, Wu-Lee M, El-Lozy M. Prevalence of the "Chinese restaurant syndrome." *J Am Diet Assoc.* 1979; 75:29–33.

140. Gann D. Ventricular tachycardia in a patient with the "Chinese restaurant syndrome." *South Med J.* 1977; 70:879–881.

141. Goldberg L. Supraventricular tachyarrhythmia in association with the Chinese restaurant syndrome. *Ann Emerg Med.* 1982; 11:333.

142. Wilkin JK. Does monosodium glutamate cause flushing (or merely "glutamania")? *J Am Acad Dermatol.* 1986; 15:225–230.

143. Kenney RA. Placebo-controlled studies of human reaction to oral monosodium L-glutamate. In: Filer LJ, Garattini S, Kare MR, Reynolds WA, Wurtman RJ, eds. *Glutamic Acid: Advances in Biochemistry and Physiology.* New York: Raven Press; 1979: 363–373.

144. Chin KW, Garriga MM, Metcalfe DD. The histamine content of oriental foods. *Food Chem Toxicol.* 1989; 27(5):283–287.

145. Tuley L. The ABC of MSG. *Food Manufacture.* 1990; 65(3):23–25.

146. Squire EN. Angio-oedema and monosodium glutamate. *Lancet.* 1987; 1:988. Letter.

147. Diamond S, Prager J, Freitag FG. Diet and headache—is there a link? *Postgrad Med.* 1986; 79(4):279–286.

148. Sweatman MC, Tasker R, Warner JO, et al. Oral-facial granulomatosis. Response to elemental diet and provocation by food additives. *Clin Allergy.* 1986; 16:331–338.

149. Allen DH, Baker GJ. Chinese restaurant asthma. *N Engl J Med.* 1981; 305:1154–1155. Letter.

150. Allen DH, Delohery J, Baker G. Monosodium L-glutamate-induced asthma. *J Allergy Clin Immunol.* 1987; 80(4):530–537.

151. Toth L, Karcsu S, Feledi J, Kreutzberg GW. Neurotoxicity of monosodium-L-glutamate in pregnant and fetal rats. *Acta Neuropathol.* 1987; 75:16–22.

152. Duxbury DD. Stable flavor enhancer has wide application as MSG replacer. *Food Processing.* 1989; 50(4):78–80.

153. Lahti A, Hannuksela M. Is benzoic acid really harmful in cases of atopy and urticaria? *Lancet.* 1981; 2:1055. Letter.

154. Elsas LJ, Acosta PB. Nutrition support of inherited metabolic diseases. In: Shils ME, Young VR, eds. *Modern Nutrition in Health and Disease.* Philadelphia: Lea & Febiger; 1988: 1337–1379.

155. Hannuksela M, Lahti A. Peroral challenge tests with food additives in urticaria and atopic dermatitis. *Int J Dermatol.* 1986; 25:178–180.

156. Thune P, Granholt A. Provocation tests with antiphlogistica and food additives in recurrent urticaria. *Dermatologica.* 1975; 151:360–367.

157. Wicher K, Reisman RE. Anaphylactic reaction to penicillin (or penicillin-like substance) in a soft drink. *J Allergy Clin Immunol.* 1980; 66(2):155–157.

158. Tinkelman DG, Bock SA. Anaphylaxis presumed to be caused by beef containing streptomycin. *Ann Allergy.* 1984; 53:243–244.

159. Rockwell WJ. Reactions to molds in foods. In: Chiaramonte LT, Schneider AT, Lifshitz F, eds. *Food Allergy, A Practical Approach to Diagnosis and Management.* New York: Marcel Dekker Inc; 1988:153–168.

160. Damson JF. Review of therapeutic procedure for mould allergy. In: Al-Doory Y, Domson JF, eds. *Mold Allergy.* Philadelphia: Lea & Febiger; 1984:187–201.

161. Mygind N. *Essential Allergy—An Illustrated Text for Students and Specialists.* Oxford: Blackwell Scientific Publications; 1986.

162. Finn R. Pharmacologic actions of foods. In: Brostoff J, Challacombe SJ, eds. *Food Allergy and Intolerance.* London: Bailliere-Tindall/WB Saunders; 1987:425–430.

163. Moneret-Vautrin DA. Food intolerance masquerading as food allergy: False food allergy. In: Brostoff J, Challacombe SJ, eds. *Food Allergy and Intolerance.* London: Bailliere-Tindall/WB Saunders; 1987:836–849.

164. Malone MH, Metcalfe DD. Histamine in foods: Its possible role in nonallergic adverse reactions to ingestants. *N Engl Reg Allergy Proc.* 1986; 7(3):241–245.

165. Zee JA, Simard RE, L'Heureux L, Tremblay J. Biogenic amines in wines. *Am J Enol Vitic.* 1983; 34(1):6–9.

166. Ough CS, Crowell EA, Kunkee RE, Vilas MR, Lagier S. A study of histamine production by various wine bacteria in model solutions and in wine. *J Food Processing Preservation.* 1987; 12:63–70.

167. Uragoda CG. Histamine poisoning in tuberculosis patients after ingestion of tuna fish. *Am Rev Respir Dis.* 1980; 121:157–159.

168. Taylor SL, Stratton JE, Nordlee JA. Histamine poisoning (scombroid fish poisoning): An allergy-like intoxication. *J Toxicol Clin Toxicol.* 1989; 27(4–5):225–240.

169. Dysnsza H, Shimizu Y, Russell FE, Graham HD. Poisonous marine animals. In: Graham HD, ed. *The Safety of Foods.* Westport, CT: AVI Publishing Co, Inc; 1980: 625–651.

170. Harada S, Agarwal DP, Goedde HW. Alcohol deydrogenase deficiency as cause of facial flushing reaction to alcohol in Japanese. *Lancet.* 1981; 2:982. Letter.

171. Bois P. Effect of magnesium deficiency on mast cells and urinary histamine in rats. *Br J Exp Pathol.* 1963; 44:151–155.

172. Perkin JE, Hartje J. Diet and migraine: a review of the literature. *J Am Diet Assoc.* 1983; 83:459–463.

173. Geppert EF, Boushey HA. An investigation of the mechanism of ethanol-induced bronchoconstriction. *Am Rev Respir Dis.* 1978; 118:135–139.

174. Clayton DE, Busse W. Anaphylaxis to wine. *Clin Allergy.* 1980; 10:341–343.

175. Watts DA, Ough CS, Brown WD. Residual amounts of proteinaceous additives in table wine. *J Food Sci.* 1981; 46:681–687.

176. Pola J, Subiza J, Armentia A, et al. Urticaria caused by caffeine. *Ann Allergy.* 1988; 60:207–208.

177. Gjesing B, Løwenstein H. Immunochemistry of food antigen. *Ann Allergy.* 1984; 53:602–608.

178. Freed DLJ. Dietary lectins and disease. In: Brostoff J, Challacombe SJ, eds. *Food Allergy and Intolerance.* London: Bailliere-Tindall/WB Saunders; 1987:375–400.

179. Zuraw BL, Nonaka M, O'Hair C, Katz DH. Human IgE antibody synthesis *in vitro:* stimulation of IgE responses by pokeweed mitogen and selective inhibition of such responses by human suppressive factor of allergy (SFA). *J Immunol.* 1981; 127(3):1169–1177.

180. Noah ND, Bender AE, Reaidi GB, Gilbert RJ. Food poisoning from raw red kidney beans. *Br Med J.* 1980; 2:236–237.

181. Ivie GW, Holt DL, Ivey MC. Natural intoxicants in human foods: psoralens in raw and cooked parsnip root. *Science.* 1981; 213:909–910.

182. Pathak MA, Daniels F, Fitzpatrick TB. The presently known distribution of furocoumarins (psoralens) in plants. *J Invest Dermatol.* 1962; 39:225–239.

183. Wright R, Robertson D. Non-immune damage to the gut. In: Brostoff J, Challacombe SJ, eds. *Food Allergy and Intolerance.* London: Bailliere-Tindall/WB Saunders; 1987:248–254.

184. Swain AR, Dutton SP, Truswell AS. Salicylates in foods. *J Am Diet Assoc.* 1985; 85:950–959.

185. Zioudrou C, Streaty RA, Klee WA. Opioid peptides derived from food proteins—The exorphins. *J Biol Chem.* 1979; 254(7):2446–2449.

186. Paroli E. Opiod peptides from food (the exorphins). *Wld Rev Nutr Diet.* 1988; 55:58–97.

187. Dohan FC. Cereals and schizophrenia: Data and hypothesis. *Acta Psychiatr Scand.* 1966; 42:125–152.

188. Pearson DJ, Rix KJP. Psychological effects of food allergy. In: Brostoff J, Challacombe SJ, eds. *Food Allergy and Intolerance.* London: Bailliere-Tindall/WB Saunders; 1987:688–708.

189. Dohan FC, Grasberger JC. Relapsed schizophrenics: earlier discharge from the hospital after cereal-free, milk-free diet. *Am J Psychiatry.* 1973; 130:685–688.

190. Dohan FC, Grasberger JC, Lowell FM, Johnson HT, Arbegast AW. Relapsed schizophrenics: More rapid improvements on a milk and cereal-free diet. *Br J Psychiatry.* 1969; 115:595–596.

191. Singh MM, Kay SR. Wheat gluten as a pathogenic factor in schizophrenia. *Science.* 1976; 191:401–402.

192. Levy DL, Weinreb HJ. Wheat gluten-schizophrenia findings. *Science.* 1976; 194:448. Letter.

193. Smith JM. Wheat gluten-schizophrenia findings. *Science.* 1976; 194:448. Letter.

194. Potkin SG, Weinberger D, Kleinman J, et al. Wheat gluten challenge in schizophrenic patients. *Am J Psychiatry.* 1981; 138(9):1208–1211.

195. Osborne M, Crayton JW, Javaid J, Davis JM. Lack of effect of a gluten-free diet on neuroleptic blood levels in schizophrenic patients. *Biol Psychiatry.* 1982; 17(5):627–629.

196. Singh MM. Celiac-type diets in schizophrenia. *Am J Psychiatry.* 1979; 136:733. Letter.

197. Campbell JA. Diet therapy of celiac disease and dermatitis herpetiformis. *Wld Rev Nutr Diet.* 1987; 51:189–233.

198. Ciclitira PJ, Evans DJ, Fagg NLK, Lennox ES, Dowling RH. Clinical testing of gliadin fractions in coeliac patients. *Clin Sci.* 1984; 66:357–364.

199. Husby S. Dietary antigens: uptake and humoral immunity in man. *APMIS.* 1988; 96(suppl 1):5–40.

200. Auricchio S, Greco L, Troncone R. Gluten-sensitive enteropathy in childhood. *Pediatr Clin North Am.* 1988; 35(1):157–187.

201. Kagnoff MF, Austin RK, Hubert JJ, Bernardin JE, Kasarda DD. Possible role for a human adenovirus in the pathogenesis of celiac disease. *J Exp Med.* 1984; 160:1544–1557.

202. Kagnoff MF, Paterson YJ, Kumar RJ, Unsworth DJ. Role of an intestinal adenovirus in the pathogenesis of celiac disease. *Clin Res.* 1987; 35:590A.

203. Greco L, Auricchio S, Mayer M, Grimaldi M. Case control study on nutritional risk factors in celiac disease. *J Pediatr Gastroenterol Nutr.* 1988; 7:395–399.

204. Bailey DS, Freedman AR, Price SC, Chescoe D, Ciclitira PJ. Early biochemical responses of the small intestine of coeliac patients to wheat gluten. *Gut.* 1989; 30:78–85.

205. Barresi G, Tuccari G, Tedeschi A, Magazzu G. Lectin binding sites in duodenojejunal mucosae from coeliac children. *Biochemistry.* 1988; 88:105–112.

206. Katz AJ, Falchuk ZM, Strober W, Swachman H. Gluten-sensitive enteropathy: Inhibition by cortisol of the effect of gluten protein in vitro. *N Engl J Med.* 1976; 295:131–135.

207. Shiner M. Present trends in coeliac disease. *Postgrad Med J.* 1984; 60:773–778.

208. DeLuca F, Astori M, Pandullo E, et al. Effects of a gluten-free diet on catch-up growth and height prognosis in coeliac children with growth retardation recognized after the age of 5 years. *Eur J Pediatr.* 1988; 147:188–191.

209. Paré P, Douville P, Caron D, Lagacé R. Adult celiac sprue: Changes in the pattern of clinical recognition. *J Clin Gastroenterol.* 1988; 10(4):395–400.

210. Hall RP. Dietary management of dermatitis herpetiformis. *Arch Dermatol.* 1987; 123:1378A–1380A.

211. McNeish AS. Coeliac disease: Duration of a gluten-free diet. *Arch Dis Child.* 1980; 55:110–111.

212. Kumar PJ, Harris G, Colyer J, Clark ML, Dawson AM. Is a gluten-free diet necessary for the treatment of coeliac disease? *Gastroenterology.* 1985; 88(5):1459.

213. Montgomery AMP, Goka AKJ, Kumar PJ, Farthing MJG, Clark ML. Low gluten diet in the treatment of adult coeliac disease: effect on jejunal morphology and serum anti-gluten antibodies. *Gut.* 1988; 29:1564–1568.

214. Weyman-Daum M. Milk-free, lactose-free, and lactose-restricted diets. In: Chiaramonte LT, Schneider AT, Lifshitz F, eds. *Food Allergy: A Practical Approach to Diagnosis and Management.* New York: Marcel Dekker, Inc; 1988:401–420.

215. Savaiano DA, Kotz C. Recent advances in the management of lactose intolerance. *Contemporary Nutr.* 1988; 13:9,10. General Mills Nutrition Department Newsletter.

216. MacDonald I. Carbohydrates. In: Shils ME, Young VR, eds. *Modern Nutrition in Health and Disease.* Philadelphia: Lea & Febiger; 1988:38–51.

217. Lifshitz F. Food intolerance. In: Chiaramonte LT, Schneider AT, Lifshitz F, eds. *Food Allergy: A Practical Approach to Diagnosis and Management.* New York: Marcel Dekker, Inc; 1988:3–21.

218. Scrimshaw NS, Murray EB. The acceptability of milk and milk products in populations with a high prevalence of lactose intolerance. *Am J Clin Nutr.* 1988; 48(4)(suppl):1083–1159.

219. Villar J, Kestler E, Castillo P, Juarez A, Menendez R, Solomons NW. Improved lactose digestion during pregnancy: A case of physiologic adaptation? *Obstet Gynecol.* 1988; 71(5):697–700.

220. Perlow W, Baraona E, Lieber CS. Symptomatic intestinal disaccharidase deficiency in alcoholics. *Gastroenterology.* 1977; 72:680–684.

221. Keshavarzian A, Iber F, Dangleis MD, Cornish R. Intestinal-transit and lactose intolerance in chronic alcoholics. *Am J Clin Nutr.* 1986; 44:70–76.

222. Skala HW, Prchal JT. Presenile cataract formation and decreased activity of galactose enzymes. *Arch Ophthalmol.* 1980; 98:269–273.

223. Ziegler EE, Fomon SJ. Lactose enhances mineral absorption in infancy. *J Pediatr Gastroenterol Nutr.* 1983; 2:288–294.

224. Birge SJ, Keutmann HT, Cuatrecasas P, Whedon GD. Osteoporosis, intestinal lactase deficiency and low dietary calcium intake. *N Engl J Med.* 1967; 276:445–448.

225. Newcomer AD, Hodgson SF, McGill DB, Thomas PJ. Lactase deficiency: prevalence in osteoporosis. *Ann Intern Med.* 1978; 89:218–220.

226. Allen LH. Calcium bioavailability and absorption. *Am J Clin Nutr.* 1982; 35:783–808.

227. Griessen M, Cochet B, Infante F, et al. Calcium absorption from milk in lactase-deficient subjects. *Am J Clin Nutr.* 1989; 49:377–384.

228. Martini MC, Bollweg GL, Levitt MD, Savaiano DA. Lactose digestion by yogurt ß-galactosidase: influence of pH and microbial cell integrity. *Am J Clin Nutr.* 1987; 45:432–436.

229. Onwulata CI, Rao DR, Vankineni P. Relative efficiency of yogurt, sweet acidophilus milk, hydrolyzed-lactose milk, and a commercial lactase tablet in alleviating lactose maldigestion. *Am J Clin Nutr.* 1989; 49:1233–1237.

230. Bourlioux, P. Pochart P. Nutritional and health properties of yogurt. *World Rev Nutr Diet.* 1988; 56:217–258.

231. Martini MC, Smith DE, Savaiano DA. Lactose digestion from flavored and frozen yogurts, ice milk, and ice cream by lactase-deficient persons. *Am J Clin Nutr.* 1987; 46:636–640.

232. Lerebours E, Ndam CN, Lavoine A, Hellot MF, Antoine JM, Colin R. Yogurt and fermented-then-pasteurized milk: effects of short-term and long-term ingestion on lactose absorption and mucosal lactase activity in lactase-deficient subjects. *Am J Clin Nutr.* 1989; 49:823–827.

233. Hitchins AD, McDonough FE. Prophylactic and therapeutic aspects of fermented milk. *Am J Clin Nutr.* 1989; 49:675–684.

234. Gendrel D, Dupont C, Richard-Lenoble D, Gendrel C, Chaussain M. Feeding lactose intolerant children with a powdered fermented milk. *J Pediatr Gastroenterol Nutr.* 1990; 10(1):44–46.

235. McDonough FE, Hitchins AD, Wong NP, Wells P, Bodwell CE. Modification of sweet acidophilus milk to improve utilization by lactose-intolerant persons. *Am J Clin Nutr.* 1987; 45:570–574.

236. Duxbury DD. Liquid enzyme provides economical milk sugar sweetness replacement—potential solution to lactose intolerance problem. *Food Processing.* 1989; 50:77–78.

237. Efficacy of exogenous lactase for lactose intolerance. *Nutr Rev.* 1988; 46(4):150–152.

238. Martini MC, Savaiano DA. Reduced intolerance symptoms from lactose consumed during a meal. *Am J Clin Nutr.* 1988; 47:57–60.

239. Lee CM, Hardy CM. Cocoa feeding and human lactose intolerance. *Am J Clin Nutr.* 1989; 49:840–844.

240. Bergoz R. Trehalase malabsorption causing intolerance to mushrooms—Report of a probable case. *Gastroenterology.* 1971; 60(5):909–912.

241. Madzǎrovová-Nohejlova J. Trehalase deficiency in a family. *Gastroenterology.* 1973; 65:130–133.

Chapter 8

Adverse Food Reactions: Relationship to Arthritis and Migraine

Judy E. Perkin

Adverse food reactions, and in some instances, food allergies, have been proposed to be etiological factors in certain diseases or disorders. This chapter will review the current evidence related to the role of diet in the etiologies and treatment of arthritis and migraine headache.

ARTHRITIS AND OTHER DISORDERS OF CONNECTIVE AND JOINT TISSUE

Prior to exploring the potential role of food allergy, or adverse reaction, in the etiology of arthritis and other joint or connective tissue disorders, it is important to appreciate the vast array of clinical entities encompassed by these general terms. Table 8-1 summarizes major subcategories of joint and connective tissue disorders that have been studied from a dietary perspective. This review attempts to distinguish these entities to the extent present research permits. (A discussion of gout is not included in the present chapter and readers are referred to other sources for a review of diet related to this disorder.)

Rheumatoid arthritis has been most extensively studied in terms of a potential connection with food allergy or adverse food reaction. It should also be noted that a specific form of arthritis described as food hypersensitivity induced has been postulated to exist.[1,2,3] This arthritis type is described by Denman et al[2] and Zussman[3] as a form of arthritis seen in the presence of other allergy manifestations such as urticaria. Arthritis may also be seen in conjunction with gastrointestinal diseases such as Crohn's disease and ulcerative colitis.[2]

Basic research on mast cells gives theoretical basis for a potential involvement between food allergy and inflammatory rheumatic disorders. It is

171

Table 8-1   Major Subcategories of Arthritis or Connective Tissue and Joint Disorders (Relevant to Dietetics)

Subcategory	Definition
Rheumatoid Arthritis (Also known as chronic inflammatory arthritis)	A chronic systemic joint disease of unknown etiology, characterized by inflammation in joints and synovial membranes with bone atrophy and rarefication.
Osteoarthritis (Also known as degenerative arthritis)	A degenerative noninflammatory joint disease, characterized by synovial membrane alterations, bone hypertrophy, and cartilage degeneration.
Behçet's syndrome	A chronic disease of unknown etiology with joint problems seen in some cases. The disease is characterized as an inflammatory disorder of small blood vessels.
Henoch-Schönlein syndrome (Also known as Schönlein-Henoch disease or allergic purpura)	A type of nonthrombocytopenic purpura associated with vasculitis of unknown etiology. Arthritis is one component of the characteristic symptom complex that also includes urticaria, erythema, and symptoms related to the gastrointestinal and renal systems.
Kashin-Bek disease (Also known as osteoarthritis deformans endemica)	A chronic degenerative disease of the spine and joints believed to be related to consumption of grain contaminated with *Fusarium sporotrichiella*.
Palindromic rheumatism	A type of rheumatic disorder with no irreversible joint changes, but characterized by intermittent pain in and around the joints.

known that mast cells are found in synovial tissue, and mediator substances of mast cells (eg, histamine and leukotrienes) have the ability to influence inflammation.[4] Malone and Metcalfe[4] further point out the clinical presentation and course of diseases such as palindromic rheumatism are consistent with processes related to degranulation of mast cells in synovial tissue. These same researchers in 1988 developed a rat model for the study of IgE-dependent mast cell-mediated arthritis.[5]

Published human studies to date have not been definitive. Hunder and McDuffie[6] demonstrated increased levels of IgE in only 4 of 16 arthritis patients studied, and Peskett et al,[7] studying 40 children with juvenile chronic arthritis, found that IgE production in these individuals did not seem to be abnormal.

Research on arthritogenic properties of antigens using the Old English rabbit as an animal model is being proposed as an experimental design that can shed light on arthralgia (or joint pain) sometimes seen in conjunction with human food allergies. Because the disorder in rabbits is transient and not associated with IgM rheumatoid factor, some do not consider these experiments as relevant to rheumatoid arthritis etiology.[8] Panush et al,[9] however, do suggest that New Zealand white rabbits or Old English rabbits might be useful in the study of dietary-related arthritis.

The etiology of rheumatoid arthritis remains unknown, with food allergies being postulated as only one of many potential causative entities. It is best to say at the outset that the role of food allergy or adverse reaction to food in the etiology of arthritis is currently theoretically supported by suggestive clinical observation and research, but not by conclusive data. Many reports in this area have problems with lack of clarity in diagnosis classification, failure to use a blind experimental design, and/or failure to use adequate controls.[10] Other problems plaguing arthritis-diet research include the phenomenon of spontaneous improvement,[11] the high rate of placebo response in patients with rheumatoid arthritis,[12] the uncertainty as to whether currently defined diseases such as rheumatoid arthritis have single or multiple etiologies,[13] and the small numbers of patients studied.

Interest in the role of diet in rheumatoid arthritis is not new.[14] Zeller,[15] in 1949, published a paper on this subject, following up on earlier suggestive reports by Turnbull[16,17] and Lewin and Taub.[18]

Panush[19] has theorized that diet may play a role in the etiology of rheumatoid arthritis through two mechanisms, one or both of which may be involved in a clinical case. The first proposed mechanism is through a delayed hypersensitivity (or allergic) response (not IgE mediated), and the second is that diet in an as yet undefined way may affect inflammation or immune functions. Panush[20] has also speculated that selective IgA deficiency, hypogammaglobulinemia, or other factors associated with enhanced food antigen uptake from the gut may play a role. [Bjarnason et al,[21] using a ^{51}Cr-EDTA (edetic acid) absorption test, did find intestinal abnormalities associated with use of nonsteroidal anti-inflammatory drugs by rheumatoid arthritis patients, but Rooney et al[22] did not find intestinal abnormalities in a sample of seven arthritis patients.] Additional theories related to the diet-arthritis connection focus on alterations in prostaglandin synthesis.[23] Theories related to postulated mechanisms are summarized in Table 8-2.

Panush et al,[24] in 1983, published the results of a study testing the efficacy of a popular diet—the Dong diet—purported to help alleviate symptoms of rheumatoid arthritis. The diet calls for elimination of red meat, food additives, fruit, milk products, selected spices, alcohol, vinegar, chocolate, nuts, and carbonated beverages.[25] The 10-week study conducted with 26 subjects was a double-blind, controlled, randomized trial. The 11 patients following the Dong diet were found to have mean intakes from foods and beverages below the RDA for the following nutrients: calcium, magnesium, zinc, thiamin, riboflavin, folacin, vitamin B_6, and pantothenic acid. Clinical im-

Table 8-2   Mechanisms Theorized by Which Diet May Influence Arthritis or Other Joint Disease

- Food allergy
- Food intolerance
- Changes in intestinal absorption
- Alterations of immune system functioning
- Alterations of prostaglandin and leukotriene synthesis
- Changes in body weight

provement in rheumatoid arthritis related to the diet was not demonstrated by this study. Improvement was similar in treatment and placebo groups.[24]

Denman et al,[2] also in 1983, published the results of a study designed to test the efficacy of selected dietary restrictions on clinical manifestations of rheumatoid arthritis. No rationale in the research report was provided for choice of foods excluded. Foods eliminated were red meats, eggs, dairy products, food colorings and preservatives, chocolate, and selected baked goods. A major problem of this study was the inability to elicit compliance with the restricted diet for a sufficient period. Of the 18 subjects enrolled in the study, 13 (72%) did not follow the diet for more than 2 months. Tests to measure disease status showed no difference pre- and post-treatment for the five subjects who did follow the diet for more than five months.

Ratner et al[26] studied the effect of eliminating dairy products and beef on the course of rheumatoid arthritis and psoriatic arthritis in 15 women and 8 men. This research group reported that 7 women (6 with seronegative rheumatoid arthritis and 1 with seronegative psoriatic arthritis) ceased to be symptomatic within 3 to 4 weeks after initiation of the test diet. Provocation with dairy foods elicited recurrence of symptoms. (Testing was not conducted in a blind fashion.) All of the women responding positively to the diet were determined to be lactase deficient. Antibody testing results were described as not being definitive. The authors speculated that arthritis may be seen as one manifestation of allergy to cow's milk protein. They further speculated that lactase deficiency may potentiate arthritis by affecting permeability of the intestine.

Panush et al[13] published results of an inpatient clinical research center study of a female patient who demonstrated signs and symptoms compatible with the diagnosis of rheumatoid arthritis. The prospective partially blind study contrasted symptomatology experienced while on the patient's customary diet versus trials of fasting, elemental diet, and elemental diet plus capsules of placebo (D-xylose) or lyophilized foods (lettuce, carrot, chicken, beef, rice, and milk). Both the elemental diet only and fasting trials were accompanied by improvement in symptoms. For example, on the patient's customary diet, she experienced about 30 minutes of stiffness each morning. During the 3-day fast and 2-day elemental diet only, the patient experienced no morning stiffness. Challenge with milk evoked clinical symptoms similar to those observed on the customary diet. Measurement of joint tenderness index and grip strength was significantly affected in a deleterious manner in association with the milk challenge. Measurements of serum IgE did not vary significantly during study phases. Slight increases in IgG antimilk were noted, as were sporadic elevations in circulating immune complexes. The patient also had abnormally high mononuclear cellular reactivity to milk. Skin tests demonstrated mild reaction to milk. The authors concluded milk played a role in the arthritic symptoms of this patient. They felt either the patient suffered from milk allergy with arthritis as a manifestation or the patient had rheumatoid arthritis exacerbated by milk protein.

A single-blind outpatient study of 53 subjects (10 male and 43 female) conducted by Darlington et al[12] correlated clinical improvement in symptoms of rheumatoid arthritis with dietary therapy. Specifics of the tested dietary regimen were not given in the research report, but therapy appeared to have consisted of withdrawal of potentially offending foods with reintroduction of foods by families at greater than 4-day intervals. Subjects were randomly divided into two groups after a 2-week washout period. One group was placed on 6 weeks of the diet therapy, and the other group received placebo therapy for 6 weeks followed by 6 weeks of diet therapy. Both groups exhibited improvement in parameters such as pain and erythrocyte sedimentation rate. Although weight loss occurred during this study, weight loss was not necessarily related to positive clinical response. The research group concluded dietary restrictions may benefit some patients.

Inglis,[27] in 1987, proposed that contamination of milk with bacterial lipopolysaccharide may induce arthritis. He further speculated that milk fat may enhance absorption of this lipopolysaccharide. These speculations have yet to be confirmed.

Carini et al[28] were able to induce joint symptoms by food challenge in 10 patients. Symptoms appeared 12 to 48 hours after challenge. When examining total IgE levels on an individual level, however, there was no association with joint symptoms. A subgroup of six patients was assessed for the presence of IgG anti-IgE autoantibodies. Three patients exhibited autoantibodies that peaked 24 hours after food challenge. Although the authors admit the biological relevance of IgG anti-IgE autoantibodies to allergic disease is at present unknown, they postulate that IgG anti-IgE autoantibody may first bind to IgE and subsequently bind to mast cells with resultant release of inflammatory substances.

Panush[20] reported in 1988 that his research group had studied a total of 15 patients who had participated in double-blind food challenges. Three were reported to have symptoms related to challenge. The Panush group speculated that perhaps a small percentage (five or less) of patients with rheumatoid diseases have food reaction with an immunological basis.

Beri et al[29] published a study of 27 patients with rheumatoid arthritis designed to evaluate the usefulness of dietary exclusion of selected components. The diet was designed to progress from a few foods to a variety. The initial 2 weeks of the diet allowed only fruits, vegetables, oils, and sugar. Only 14 of the 27 patients completed this initial dietary phase, and ultimately only 3 patients followed the diet for as long as 10 months. Ten of the 14 who did get past phase 1 were reported to have some clinical improvement. The small sample size and lack of compliance make this study difficult to interpret. Nutritional adequacy of the regimen was also questionable.

Anecdotal case reports of individual improvement related to dietary exclusion also appear in the literature. Lunardi et al[30] reported that cereal exclusion was associated with at least a 1-year disease remission in a patient with rheumatoid arthritis.

Fasting and consuming only defined formula diets have been shown by some to be beneficial in reducing arthritis symptoms.[10,31] These strategies, however, do not represent acceptable long-term dietary alternatives, although some have used improvement seen with fasting to fortify the argument that arthritis may be related to adverse food reaction. Condemi[10] points out that a number of physiological changes associated with fasting may reduce inflammation.

Vegetarian diets have also been tried as part of arthritis therapies. Although these diets do not appear to influence the disease process, some persons report subjective improvement.[32,33] Wolman[33] suggests that patients following such a regimen may need supplements of zinc, calcium, and vitamins B_{12} and D.

In addition to dietary exclusion, fasting, and vegetarian diets, diet and arthritis studies have also focused on potential relationships with specific nutrients. Biochemical nutritional abnormalities that may be seen in patients with rheumatoid arthritis are shown in Table 8-3.[34]

Table 8-3 Biochemical Nutritional Status Abnormalities Observed in Rheumatoid Arthritis

- Decreased plasma histidine levels
- Increased urinary levels of xanthurenic acid, 3-hydroxyanthranilic acid, N-methyl-nicotin-amide, and 3-hydroxykynurenine (tryptophan metabolites)
- Decreased plasma iron
- Increased plasma ceruloplasmin and unbound copper
- Decreased serum zinc levels
- Decreased plasma and blood cell ascorbic acid levels

Zinc deficiency has been suggested to play a role in the etiology of rheumatoid arthritis.[23,24] Simkin[35] conducted a double-blind trial with 24 rheumatoid arthritis patients comparing the efficacy of zinc sulfate (660 mg/day divided in 3 doses) to placebo. Simkin[35] reported that while taking zinc all patients improved clinically, although no changes were found in serum levels of rheumatoid factor. Other studies to date have failed to support Simkin's findings.[34]

Decreased levels of serum histidine have also been studied. Some have linked low free-serum histidine levels to the worsening of rheumatoid arthritis.[36] It has been theorized that low-serum histidine levels may contribute to the process of gamma globulin aggregation in the synovial fluid.[36] Pinals et al[36] conducted a double-blind trial comparing the benefits of a 4.5 g/day supplement of L-histidine with placebo for a 30-week period. Both the histidine-treated group and the placebo group showed improvement in terms of decreased number of tender joints and hours of morning stiffness. The researchers did not feel their results warranted the recommendation that histidine supplementation be used in routine therapy for rheumatoid arthritis.

The role of selenium supplementation in rheumatoid arthritis treatment has been studied by Tarp et al.[37,38] Selenium was postulated to play a role in arthritis because of its role in the enzyme glutathione peroxidase as an antioxidant. (Peroxidation products in higher than normal amounts have been demonstrated in the serum and synovial fluid of rheumatoid arthritis patients.[38]) Selenium supplementation at levels of 256 μg/day for 26 weeks, however, has not proven helpful in alleviating arthritis symptoms.[38]

The potential benefit of the omega-3-fatty acids of fish oils for patients with rheumatoid arthritis is under investigation.[23,39-44] The theoretical basis for any potential omega-3-fatty acid benefit is its ability to generate prostaglandins of the E_3 series thought to be less inflammatory than prostaglandins of the E_2 series associated with intake of omega-6-fatty acids.[39]

In 1985, Kremer et al[39] conducted a 12-week double-blind controlled study of the effectiveness of a high polyunsaturated fat diet (1.4 to 1 polyunsaturated fatty acid (PUFA): saturated fat (SF) ratio) supplemented with 1.8 g eicosapentaenoic acid (EPA) in fish oil capsules, compared to a control group diet with a PUFA:SF ratio of 1 to 4 which was supplemented with placebo capsules (paraffin wax). Caloric intake was maintained so the mean body weights for the two groups did not change over the experimental period. At the end of the study period, the group receiving the high PUFA diet supplemented with fish oil had improvement in joint tenderness and morning stiffness. Concern has been expressed about the meaning of the results of this study because the design of the experiment manipulated the diet in two ways—PUFA:SF ratio and EPA.[40]

Cleland et al[42] contrasted 23 rheumatoid arthritis patients treated with 18 g/day of fish oil to 23 patients treated with olive oil in a double-blind, 12-week trial. Improvement in the fish oil group was noted both in terms of number of tender joints and grip strength. Both groups, however, showed improvement in some areas such as pain and morning stiffness.

Fish oil therapy has been demonstrated to induce macrophage changes that can decrease severity of symptoms in rheumatoid arthritis.[44] Results of biochemical studies and clinical studies indicate fish oils may be useful dietary agents to help decrease arthritis-associated inflammation. Fish oil capsules containing omega-3-fatty acids are an experimental therapy and should not currently be used in standard treatment. Patients can be encouraged to eat fishes containing omega-3-fatty acids with the explanation of potential anti-inflammatory benefits.[33]

While the role diet may play in terms of rheumatoid arthritis etiology or exacerbation is under investigation, it is known that dietary intakes of some patients may be inadequate. In Kowsari et al's[45] study of 24 rheumatoid arthritis patients, over two-thirds had inadequate intakes (less than 67% of the 1980 RDA) of zinc, vitamin E, and folacin as assessed by 3-day food records. Bigaouette et al[46] reported that dietary intakes of zinc, folic acid, vitamin B_6, and magnesium were low in 52 rheumatoid arthritis patients studied.

In order to properly assess the nutritional status of the patient with rheumatoid arthritis, the dietitian must appreciate the effects of disease and treatment. Reduced cutaneous hypersensitivity is commonly seen in these patients, but is believed to be unrelated to protein calorie malnutrition.[47] Total lymphocyte count is also of limited value in nutritional assessment of the arthritis patient because of treatment influence.[11] Levels of serum proteins (such as albumin and transferrin) may also be affected by disease, treatment, and hydration status.[11,48] Weight is considered to be the most accurate nutritional assessment measure for these patients.[11] Helliwell et al[49] have noted significant reductions in body mass index and triceps skinfold measures in patients with rheumatoid arthritis.

Nutrition-related problems associated with rheumatoid arthritis include xerostomia, Sjögren's syndrome, osteoporosis, osteomalacia,[11] and vitamin C deficiency.[50] The presence of xerostomia may indicate the need for foods high in moisture content and provision of cool fluids. Unsweetened lemon flavoring may be given as a salivary stimulant. Use of topical fluoride and restriction of dietary sucrose may also be helpful in order to prevent cavities. Vitamin D supplements (300 IU/day) may be given to patients with rheumatoid arthritis to aid in prevention of previously mentioned bone diseases.[11] Oral vitamin C (500 mg/day) has been used to treat deficiencies seen in conjunction with rheumatoid arthritis.[50]

Caloric requirements for rheumatoid arthritis patients may be determined using the Harris-Benedict formula to estimate basal energy expenditure (BEE). BEE should be multiplied by an activity factor of 1.2 (in the case of limited activity) or 1.3 (for the more active patient) and an injury factor of 1.14 to 1.35 when inflammation is present. During periods of remission, protein allotments of 0.5 to 1.0 g/kg/day are considered adequate with increased protein needs of 1.5 to 2.0 g/kg/day during inflammatory periods.[11]

Drug therapy used for rheumatoid arthritis may be associated with nutritional alterations.[11,51] Major drug-nutrient interactions are summarized in Table 8-4. Readers are also referred to the excellent discussion of Wolman[33] on this topic.

To summarize, while food restriction has been shown to be beneficial for selected rheumatoid arthritis patients, a definitive role for food allergy or adverse reaction has not been proven. Patients placed on restrictive experimental regimens need to be monitored and perhaps receive supplementation in order to ensure nutritional adequacy. Regimens that are too restrictive may not be practical alternatives for long-term management. Dietitians need to be familiar with and treat patients within currently acceptable guidelines.

Other joint diseases linked to diet include Kashin-Bek disease,[52] Behçet's syndrome,[53] and palindromic rheumatism.[54]

Kashin-Bek disease, first described in 1861, is a type of osteoarthritis believed to be related to consumption of cereals contaminated with the fungus *Fusarium sporotrichiella*. Areas of endemicity for Kashin-Bek syndrome described in the past have been the northern parts of China and Korea and eastern Siberia.[52]

Behçet's syndrome is a complex disease characterized by ulceration of the genitals, iritis, and stomatitis that may include arthritic symptoms. Marquardt et al[53] postulated that consumption of English walnuts may worsen the disease by inhibiting lymphocyte transformation.

Palindromic rheumatism (a type of intermittent arthritis) has been linked to consumption of sodium nitrate and peppermint by a dermatologist writing his own case history experience.[54]

Osteoarthritis has been linked to obesity,[23,35,45] but obesity is not believed to be causative.[34] Excess weight can create a strain on joints, and McCrae et al[23] note that patients with osteoarthritis in the knee are often obese. They also point out that patients with generalized osteoarthritis are often obese. Achieving or maintaining ideal body weight is considered an important part of therapy for osteoarthritis patients.[45]

Because arthritis is a painful, incurable disease, those with the disease often turn to nontraditional (or unproven) treatments for relief.[25,55] No specific diet or diets have been proven to be beneficial nor have nutrient deficiencies to date been proven as etiological factors.[25] Unproven dietary regimens may

Table 8-4   Drug-Nutrient Interactions Relevant to Rheumatoid Arthritis Treatment

Drug	Nutritional Implications
D-penicillamine	May cause inactivation of vitamin B$_6$[46] May be associated with chelation of cobalt, copper, magnesium, and zinc[46] May cause nausea, vomiting, stomatitis, anorexia, diarrhea, anemia, and proteinuria[11] May be associated with hypogeusia—usually of limited duration[11]
Prednisone	May be associated with increased excretion of calcium, zinc, and nitrogen in the urine[46] (calcium and vitamin D supplements may be used[34]) May cause nausea, edema, and ulceration. Edema may necessitate sodium restriction[11] May be associated with glucose intolerance, decreased serum potassium, and decreased total lymphocyte count[11]
Methotrexate	May induce alteration of folate metabolism and reduce liver folate stores.[46] Supplemental folate can affect drug's action[11] Daily supplementation of 1 mg of folic acid/day may be helpful during low-dose therapy[51]
Salicylates	May induce blood loss and gastrointestinal erosion with subsequent iron loss[46] May increase urinary excretion of vitamin C. Supplements may be needed[11]
Nonsteroidal anti-inflammatory agents	May be associated with salt and water retention and azotemia (in kidney disease patients)[34] May cause stomatitis, nausea, vomiting, and ulceration[11]
Antimalarial agents	May be associated with gastrointestinal side effects, anorexia, vomiting, nausea and diarrhea[11]
Gold	May cause protein excretion in the urine, diarrhea, and stomatitis[11] Associated with decreases in elevated plasma copper levels[34]

advocate toxic levels of nutrients or may advise elimination of food groups and encourage inadequate dietary intakes. Those promoting allergy or adverse food reaction as arthritis causes may be particularly prone to advocate elimination of many foods.[55] Fasting with or without enemas or colonic irrigations are other forms of unproven remedies that may be encountered.[25,55] Dietitians need to aid patients in identifying problem areas with diet and encouraging good dietary and weight management practices.

MIGRAINE

Migraine headache is a term often used to describe various types of vascular headaches.[10,55] Condemi[10] divides migraines or vascular headaches into four types, and Diamond et al[56] describe six types. The term migraine is a French version of a Greek word meaning half of the head. A general description of migraine is that the disorder is one in which there is intermittent headache accompanied by nausea, vomiting, and visual disturbances such as light flashes or blind spots. The headache pain is cited as being unilateral about 70% of the time.[56] Migraines can appear with a wide variety of clinical presentations,[57] and diagnosis of migraine may not always be accurate due to potential confusion with other disease states.

A high degree of placebo response associated with migraine treatment has been noted.[58] This should be borne in mind when assessing the efficacy of any proposed dietary therapy.

Some have advanced the hypothesis that migraine in selected instances may be related to food allergy.[59–61] Pinnas and Vanselow,[62] however, in a review of studies exploring the efficacy of elimination diets to treat migraine, point out that success with elimination diets may indicate adverse food reaction in some instances, but such successes do not indicate an allergic reaction with an immunological basis is necessarily involved. Medina and Diamond[63] measured serum IgE levels in migraine patients and found elevated levels in 5.7%, a level comparable to elevated levels in the general population. Diamond et al[64] point out that crossover prevalence of the two problems makes evaluation of association difficult. Based on prior research, these researchers noted that 15% of atopic individuals suffer from migraine and 20% of migraine patients have allergies. Egger et al,[65] in a recent trial designed to study the efficacy of oligoantigenic diets to treat children with migraine, could not correlate dietary response to either positive skin tests or elevated serum IgE levels. Mansfield et al,[58] however, found in 5 of 7 subjects that food provoked migraine and suggest that tests for IgE-related food allergy may be helpful in treatment. As Chapter 1 has summarized, current knowledge would indicate adverse food reaction rather than food allergy seems to be the mechanism by which a dietary component may serve as a migraine trigger. Results such as Mansfield's need further confirmation but deserve note. (Chapter 4 cites research to indicate that gut permeability may be increased in some persons who experience migraines.)

Adverse reactions to a variety of foods and chemicals have been linked to migraine. Chemicals often cited in this regard include tyramine and phenyl-ethylamine.[66]

Tyramine is an amino acid that has the ability to affect vasoconstriction and vasodilation. A defect in the ability to convert active tyramine to an inactive form is proposed to occur in some migraine patients.[56] Tyramine is cited as being found in such foods as sour cream, pickled herring, fermented cheeses, avocados, peanuts, and chicken livers.[55,66] The part of the food product eaten may affect tyramine content. In aged cheeses, for example, more tyramine is found near the rind.[67]

A recent article related to red wine and migraine cited the phenolic flavonoid content, rather than tyramine content, as being related to migraine etiology. Phenolic flavonoids cited were the catechins and anthocyanins.[68] Certain red wines have been noted to contain tyramine, notably sherry and Chianti, and in some instances have been cited as migraine triggers.[69]

Phenylethylamine is another compound believed to be a migraine trigger, with chocolate being a major source.[70] Sandler et al[70] studied phenylethylamine ingestion and linked it to headache induction 12 hours after ingestion. Moffett et al,[71] however, did not find chocolate to be a factor in migraine etiology. Schweitzer et al[72] found low levels of phenylethylamine in chocolate and suggested that if chocolate does serve as a migraine trigger, it would be only in those very sensitive to low levels of this chemical.

Nitrates are also cited as potentially being involved in migraine etiology. There is a case report of a 58-year-old man who was studied because he developed headaches approximately 30 minutes after consuming foods containing nitrites such as frankfurters and bacon. Sodium nitrite (10 mg in aqueous solution) was used to experimentally induce headache in this individual.[73]

Consumption of alcoholic beverages may precipitate migraine in susceptible individuals.[56] Alcohol is a vasodilator.[74]

Vitamin A toxicity is an infrequent cause of migraine, but one that is of particular concern to the dietitian.[66] Raskin and Appenzeller[74] reported migraines associated with supplementation at the level of 25,000 IU/day in 6 individuals.

Restriction of monosodium glutamate is advised in the diet of the patient with migraine.[74] Chinese restaurant syndrome, which may include headache, is discussed extensively in Chapter 7, dealing with adverse food reactions.

Aspartame, also discussed in Chapter 7, is being called a potential migraine trigger by some. Lipton et al[75] found migraine patients at the Montefiore Medical Center Headache Unit reported aspartame three times more frequently as a headache precipitant than did other headache patients. Johns[76] and Koehler and Glaros[77] also linked aspartame consumption to selected cases of migraine.

One proposed mechanism by which foods may be linked to migraine causation involves monoamine oxidase. In the gut, monoamine oxidase is postulated to act as a barrier to vasoactive substances. A deficit of monoamine oxidase could theoretically allow for more uptake of food chemicals with vasoactive properties.[67] Sandler et al[70] and Glover et al[78] have reported some migraine patient populations have low platelet levels of monoamine oxidase. Tyramine and phenylethylamine are monoamine oxidase substrates.[66,74] Glover et al,[79] in a more recent publication, indicate a link between monoamine oxidase deficiency and migraine has yet to be proven because there is considerable overlap in ranges of enzyme activity between patients and controls.

Another proposed mechanism by which diet may play a role involves the enzyme phenolsulphotransferase P.[79] Low levels have been reported in migraine patients. The M form of the enzyme interacts with tyramine and noradrenaline.

Ice cream consumption has been linked to migraine in certain patients via another mechanism. Rapid cooling of the oral pharynx is believed to be responsible.[80]

Studies related to dietary manipulation and migraine have been limited. Egger et al,[65,81] in two studies, have noted some success with oligoantigenic diets followed for brief periods; however, the physiological mechanism or mechanisms responsible were not detailed. Salfield et al[82] studied two groups of children with migraine and contrasted a diet low in vasoamines and high in fiber to a high-fiber diet in which vasoamines were not restricted. Both groups of children demonstrated improvement with dietary manipulation that the researchers ascribed in most instances to a placebo effect. Mansfield et al[58] reported success of 13 subjects who followed a restrictive diet for 1 month. This same study used double-blind food challenge techniques to provoke migraine in 5 subjects and found increases in plasma histamine upon food challenge in 3 patients.

The placebo effect, small numbers of subjects, short duration of dietary trials, and limited use of double-blind challenges leave questions as to the value of dietary manipulation. Most practitioners seem to advocate avoidance of suspect foods. Use of double-blind challenge to confirm the relationship of food ingestion to migraine would seem to be desirable. Some patients may be avoiding foods unnecessarily, and citing food improperly as a trigger may delay recognition of the true trigger or triggers. Dietitians need to monitor dietary nutritional adequacy and nutritional status of these patients and help counsel avoidance when appropriate.

Weaver[83] and Swanson[84] have recently made the case for magnesium deficiency as a potential cause for some migraine cases and Weaver[83] has been using magnesium supplements as a migraine prevention measure. (The rationale for magnesium use is that it can lower thromboxane, enhance prostacyclin production, and is a vasorelaxant.) Dietitians should monitor further research in this area to see if it leads to use of magnesium in routine therapy. Chapter 4 reviews research related to the use of oral cromolyn in migraine treatment.

CONCLUSION

The role of adverse food reaction in the etiology of rheumatoid arthritis and migraine is a current area of study. A strong case does not exist for either condition to suggest an allergic mechanism. Food avoidance and nutrient supplementation may in some instances prove helpful, and dietitians need to aid patients in this area. Dietitians need to differentiate between proven and experimental therapies.

REFERENCES

1. Wojtulewski JA. Joints and connective tissue. In: Brostoff J, Challacombe SJ, eds. *Food Allergy and Intolerance.* London: Bailliere-Tindall/WB Saunders; 1987:723–735.

2. Denman AM, Mitchell B, Ansell BM. Joint complaints and food allergic disorders. *Ann Allergy.* 1983; 51:260–263.

3. Zussman BM. Food hypersensitivity simulating rheumatoid arthritis. *South Med J.* 1966; 59:935–939.

4. Malone DG, Metcalfe DD. Mast cells and arthritis. *Ann Allergy.* 1988; 61:27–30.

5. Malone DG, Metcalfe DD. Demonstration and characterization of a transient arthritis in rats following sensitization of synovial mast cells with antigen-specific IgE and parenteral challenge with specific antigen. *Arthritis Rheum.* 1988; 31(8):1063–1067.

6. Hunder GG, McDuffie FC. Hypocomplementemia in rheumatoid arthritis. *Am J Med.* 1973; 54:461–472.

7. Peskett SA, Platts-Mills TAE, Ansell BM, Stearnes GN. Incidence of atopy in rheumatic disease. *J Rheumatol.* 1981; 8(2):321–324.

8. Welsh CJR, Hanglow AC, Conn P, Coombs RRA. Comparison of the arthritogenic properties of dietary cow's milk, egg albumin and soya milk in experimental animals. *Int Arch Allergy Appl Immunol.* 1986; 80:192–199.

9. Panush RS, Webster E, Endo L, Searle M, Hammach S, Woodard JC. Food induced ("allergic") arthritis: A unique new model of inflammatory synovitis in rabbits. *Arthritis Rheum.* 1986; 29(suppl):S-33.

10. Condemi JJ. Unusual presentations. In: Chiaramonte LT, Schneider AT, Lifshitz F, eds. *Food Allergy: A Practical Approach to Diagnosis and Management.* New York: Marcel Dekker, Inc; 1988:231–254.

11. Touger-Decker R. Nutritional considerations in rheumatoid arthritis. *J Am Diet Assoc.* 1988; 88(3):327–331.

12. Darlington LG, Ramsey NW, Mansfield JR. Placebo-controlled, blind study of dietary manipulation therapy in rheumatoid arthritis. *Lancet.* 1986; 1:236–238.

13. Panush RS, Stroud RM, Webster EM. Food-induced (allergic) arthritis-inflammatory arthritis exacerbated by milk. *Arthritis Rheum.* 1986; 29(2):220–226.

14. Darlington LG. Does food intolerance have any role in the aetiology and management of rheumatoid disease? *Ann Rheum Dis.* 1985; 44:801–804.

15. Zeller M. Rheumatoid arthritis—Food allergy as a factor. *Ann Allergy.* 1949; 7:200–205,239.

16. Turnbull JA. The relation of anaphylactic disturbances to arthritis. *JAMA.* 1924; 82:1757–1759.

17. Turnbull JA. Changes in sensitivity to allergenic foods in arthritis. *Am J Digest Dis.* 1944; 15:182–190.

18. Lewin P, Taub SJ. Allergic synovitis due to ingestion of English walnuts. *JAMA.* 1936; 100:2144.

19. Panush RS. Nutritional therapy for rheumatic diseases. *Ann Intern Med.* 1987; 106(4):619–621. Editorial.

20. Panush RS. Possible role of food sensitivity in arthritis. *Ann Allergy.* 1988; 61:31–35.

21. Bjarnason I, So A, Levi AJ, et al. Intestinal permeability and inflammation in rheumatoid arthritis: Effects of nonsteroidal anti-inflammatory drugs. *Lancet.* 1984; 2:1171–1173.

22. Rooney PJ, Jenkins RT, Goodacre RL, Sivakumaran T. Gut permeability to small molecules in rheumatoid disease. *Clin Res.* 1983; 31(1):160A.

23. McCrae F, Veerapen K, Dieppe P. Diet and arthritis. *Practitioner.* 1986; 230:359–361.

24. Panush RS, Carter RL, Katz P, Kowsari B, Longley S, Finnie S. Diet therapy for rheumatoid arthritis. *Arthritis Rheum.* 1983; 26(4):462–471.

25. Hawley DJ. Non-traditional treatments of arthritis. *Nurs Clin North Am.* 1984; 19(4):663–672.

26. Ratner D, Eshel E, Schneeyour A, Teitler A. Does milk intolerance affect seronegative arthritis in lactase-deficient women? *Isr J Med Sci.* 1985; 21:532–534.

27. Inglis TJ. Dietary lipopolysaccharides as arthritogenic antigen? *Lancet.* 1987; 1:274. Letter.

28. Carini C, Fratazzi C, Aiuti F. Immune complexes in food-induced arthralgia. *Ann Allergy.* 1987; 59:422–428.

29. Beri D, Malaviya AN, Shandilya R, Singh RR. Effect of dietary restrictions on disease activity in rheumatoid arthritis. *Ann Rheum Dis.* 1988; 47:69–72.

30. Lunardi C, Bambara LM, Biasi D, et al. Food allergy and rheumatoid arthritis. *Clin Exp Rheumatol.* 1988; 6:423–424. Letter.

31. Panush RB, Panush RS. Diet, food, and arthritis patients. In: Ahmed P, ed. *Coping with Arthritis.* Springfield, Ill: Charles C Thomas; 1988:181–187.

32. Skoldstam L. Fasting and vegan diet in rheumatoid arthritis. *Scand J Rheumatol.* 1986; 15:219–223.

33. Wolman PG. Arthritis. In: Gines DJ, ed. *Nutrition Management in Rehabilitation.* Rockville, Md: Aspen Publishers, Inc; 1990:245–269.

34. Bollet AJ. Nutrition and diet in rheumatic disorders. In: Shils ME, Young VR, eds. *Modern Nutrition in Health and Disease.* Philadelphia: Lea & Febiger; 1988:1471–1481.

35. Simkin PA. Oral zinc sulphate in rheumatoid arthritis. *Lancet.* 1976; 1:539–542.

36. Pinals RS, Harris ED, Burnett JB, Gerber DA. Treatment of rheumatoid arthritis with L-histidine: a randomized, placebo-controlled, double-blind trial. *J Rheumatol.* 1977; 4(4):414–419.

37. Tarp U, Overvad K, Thorling EB, Graudal H, Hansen JC. Selenium treatment in rheumatoid arthritis. *Scand J Rheumatol.* 1985; 14:364–368.

38. Tarp U, Hansen JC, Overvad K, Thorling LB, Tarp BD, Graudal H. Glutathione peroxidase activity in patients with rheumatoid arthritis and in normal subjects: effects of long-term selenium supplementation. *Arthritis Rheum.* 1987; 30(10):1162–1166

39. Kremer JM, Michalek AV, Lininger L, et al. Effects of manipulation of dietary fatty acids on clinical manifestations of rheumatoid arthritis. *Lancet.* 1985; 1:184–187.

40. Podell RN. Nutritional treatment of arthritis—can alterations in fat intake affect disease course? *Postgrad Med.* 1985; 77(7):65–72.

41. Darlington LG. Do diets rich in polyunsaturated fatty acids affect disease activity in rheumatoid arthritis? *Ann Rheum Dis.* 1988; 47:169–172.

42. Cleland LG, French JK, Betts WH, Murphy GA, Elliott MJ. Clinical and biochemical effects of dietary fish oil supplements in rheumatoid arthritis. *J Rheumatol.* 1988; 15(10):1471–1475.

43. Cathcart ES, Gonnerman WA, Leslie CA, Hayes KC. Dietary n-3 fatty acids and arthritis. *J Int Med.* 1989; 225(suppl 1):217–223.

44. Magaro M, Altomonte L, Zoli A, et al. Influence of diet with different lipid composition on neutrophil chemiluminescence and disease activity in patients with rheumatoid arthritis. *Ann Rheum Dis.* 1988; 47:793–796.

45. Kowsari P, Finnie SK, Carter RL, et al. Assessment of the diet of patients with rheumatoid arthritis and osteoarthritis. *J Am Diet Assoc.* 1983; 82(6):657–659.

46. Bigaouette J, Timchak MA, Kremer J. Nutritional adequacy of diet and supplements in patients with rheumatoid arthritis who take medications. *J Am Diet Assoc.* 1987; 87(12):1687–1688.

47. Emery P, Panayi G, Symmons P, Brown G. Mechanisms of depressed delayed-type hypersensitivity in rheumatoid arthritis: the role of protein energy malnutrition. *Ann Rheum Dis.* 1984; 43:430–434.

48. Burnham R, Russell AS. Nutritional status in patients with rheumatoid arthritis. *Ann Rheum Dis.* 1986; 44:788–791. Letter.

49. Helliwell M, Coombes EJ, Moody BJ, Batstone GF, Robertson JC. Nutritional status in patients with rheumatoid arthritis. *Ann Rheum Dis.* 1984; 43:386–390.

50. Oldroyd KG, Dawes PT. Clinically significant vitamin C deficiency in rheumatoid arthritis. *Br J Rheum.* 1985; 24:362–363.

51. Morgan SL, Baggott JE, Vaughn WH, et al. The effect of folic acid supplementation on the toxicity of low-dose methotrexate in patients with rheumatoid arthritis. *Arthritis Rheum.* 1990; 33(1):9–18.

52. Nesterov AI. The clinical course of Kashin-Bek disease. *Arthritis Rheum.* 1964; 7(1):29–40.

53. Marquardt JL, Snyderman R, Oppenheim JJ. Depression of lymphocyte transformation and exacerbation of Behçet's syndrome by ingestion of English walnuts. *Cell Immunol.* 1973; 9:263–272.

54. Epstein S. Hypersensitivity to sodium nitrate: a major causative factor in case of palindromic rheumatism. *Ann Allergy.* 1969; 27:343–349.

55. Wolman PG. Management of patients using unproven regimens for arthritis. *J Am Diet Assoc.* 1987; 87(9):1211–1214.

56. Diamond S, Freitag FG, Solomon GD, Millstein E. Migraine headache—Working for the best outcome. *Postgrad Med.* 1987; 81(8):174–183.

57. Certain foods provoke migraine. *Nutr Rev.* 1984; 42(2):41–42.

58. Mansfield LE, Vaughn TR, Waller SF, Haverly RW, Ting S. Food allergy and adult migraine. Double-blind and mediator confirmation of an allergic etiology. *Ann Allergy.* 1985; 55:126–129.

59. Wilson CW, Kirker JG, Warness H, O'Malley M. The clinical features of migraine as a manifestation of allergic disease. *Postgrad Med J.* 1980; 56:617–621.

60. Grant EC. Food allergies and migraine. *Lancet.* 1979; 1:966–969.

61. Monro J, Brostoff J, Carini C, Zilka K. Food allergy in migraine. Study of dietary exclusion and RAST. *Lancet.* 1980; 2:1–4.

62. Pinnas JL, Vanselow NA. Relationship of allergy to headache. *Res Clin Stud Headache.* 1976; 4:85–95.

63. Medina JL, Diamond S. Migraine and atopy. *Headache.* 1976; 15:271–273.

64. Diamond S, Praeger J, Freitag DO. Diet and headache: Is there a link? *Postgrad Med.* 1986; 79(4):279–286.

65. Egger J, Wilson J, Carter CM, Turner MW, Soothill JF. Is migraine food allergy? A double-blind controlled trial of oligoantigenic diet treatment. *Lancet* 1983; 2:865–869.

66. Perkin JE, Hartje J. Diet and migraine: a review of the literature. *J Am Diet Assoc.* 1983; 83:459–463.

67. Raskin NH. Migraine. *West J Med* 1975; 123:211–217.

68. Littlewood JT, Glover V, Davies PTG, Gibb C, Sandleu M, Rose FC. Red wine as a cause of migraine. *Lancet* 1988; 1:558–559.

69. Gershwin ME, Ough C, Bock A, Fletcher MP, Nagy SM, Tuft DS. Grand rounds: adverse reactions to wines. *J Allergy Clin Immunol* 1985; 75(3):411–420.

70. Sandler M, Youdim MBH, Hanington E. A phenylethylamine oxidising defect in migraine. *Nature.* 1974; 250:335–337.

71. Moffett AM, Swash M, Scott DF. Effect of chocolate in migraine: A double-blind study. *J Neurol Neurosurg Psych.* 1974; 37:445–448.

72. Schweitzer J, Friedhoff AJ, Schwartz R. Chocolate, beta-phenylethylamine, and migraine re-examined. *Nature.* 1975; 257:256.

73. Henderson WR, Raskin NH. "Hot dog" headache: Individual susceptibility to nitrite. *Lancet* 1972; 2:1162–1163.

74. Raskin NH, Appenzeller O. Headache: An overview in headache. In: Smith LD, ed. *Major Problems in Internal Medicine, XIX.* Philadelphia: WB Saunders; 1980:1–27.

75. Lipton RB, Newman LC, Cohen JS, Solomon S. Aspartame as a dietary trigger of headache. *Headache.* 1989; 29:90–92.

76. Johns JR. Migraine provoked by aspartame. *N Engl J Med* 1986; 315:456. Letter.

77. Koehler SM, Glaros A. The effect of aspartame on migraine headache. *Headache.* 1988; 28:10–13.

78. Glover V, Sandler M, Grant E, et al. Transitory decrease in platelet monoamine oxidase activity during migraine attacks. *Lancet* 1977; 1:391–393.

79. Glover V, Littlewood J, Sandler M, Peatfield R, Petty R, Rose R. Biochemical predisposition to dietary migraine: The role of phenolsulphotransferase. *Headache.* 1983; 23:53–58.

80. Raskin NH, Knittle SC. Ice cream headache and orthostatic symptoms in patients with migraine. *Headache.* 1976; 16:22–25.

81. Egger J, Carter CM, Soothill JF, Wilson J. Oligoantigenic diet treatment of children with epilepsy and migraine. *J Pediatr.* 1989; 114(1):51–58.

82. Salfield SAW, Wardley BL, Houlsby WT, et al. Controlled study of exclusion of dietary vasoactive amines in migraine. *Arch Dis Child.* 1987; 62:458–460.

83. Weaver K. Magnesium and migraine. *Headache.* 1990; 30(3):168. Letter.

84. Swanson DR. Migraine and magnesium: Eleven neglected connections. *Perspect Biol Med* 1988; 31(4):526–557.

Chapter 9

Food Allergies and Related Adverse Reactions to Foods: A Food Science Perspective

Steve L. Taylor

Only a few individuals in the population are allergic to any particular food, but a rather wide variety of foods are implicated in these adverse reactions. If food companies attempted to exclude all possible allergenic foods from the marketplace, the range of available food choices would become extremely limited. In addition, only a comparatively few individuals would benefit from each exclusion. Thus, food companies should not become overly concerned about allergic reactions to specific foods and food ingredients while making decisions on the formulation of new food products. The onus for the avoidance of the foods eliciting these individualistic adverse reactions falls on the allergic consumer. However, food companies must provide sufficient information to these patients and their physicians and dietitians, so effective avoidance can be achieved. Sufficient information can often be provided on the label of the food product, but the labeling must be in the clearest possible terms. Label reading by allergic patients is a key to avoiding the offending food or food ingredient. Food companies occasionally have greater responsibilities in cases where a food is marketed as hypoallergenic or being free of some particular food or food ingredient. In these situations, the food companies must be absolutely certain their label claims are correct. In this chapter, the nature of the substances in foods causing food allergies and other adverse reactions to foods are examined, the effects of processing and preparation on these substances are explored, and the construction of effective avoidance diets is considered.

THE NATURE AND CHEMISTRY OF THE OFFENDING SUBSTANCES IN FOODS

In IgE-mediated food allergies, the provoking allergens are usually naturally occurring proteins found in food.[1-4] In theory, any food containing

189

proteins and any protein in foods have the potential to cause sensitization and, upon subsequent exposure, allergic reactions in susceptible individuals. However, some proteinaceous foods such as peanuts and eggs are much more likely to elicit allergic reactions than other high-protein foods such as beef and pork. The most common foods causing IgE-mediated allergic reactions are legumes (peanuts and soybeans in particular), crustacea (shrimp, crab, lobster, and crayfish), cow's milk, eggs, fish, mollusks (clams, oysters, and scallops), tree nuts, and wheat. Allergies to milk, eggs, peanuts, and soybeans predominate in infancy and early childhood. Peanut and soybean allergies can persist into adulthood, while milk and egg allergies are likely to disappear. Some food allergies, such as those to crustacea, are much more prevalent among adults because children do not consume these foods. While factors such as the frequency of consumption, exposure dose, and age at exposure are likely to play some role in the development of allergic reactions, some foods simply seem to be more inherently capable of eliciting these adverse reactions than others. (Chapter 3 reviews major food allergens.)

While few allergenic food proteins have been purified and characterized, it is apparent some proteins are more likely to trigger IgE-mediated reactions than others. Obviously, the immunogenicity of the naturally occurring proteins in a particular food will have a great effect on the likelihood of allergic reactions to that food.[5] Even in common allergenic foods, some of the constituent proteins are allergens while others are not. The major factors affecting the likelihood of allergic sensitization to a particular food protein are the characteristics of the protein itself. The protein must be capable of stimulating IgE production, and food proteins appear to vary in this respect. The degree of perceived foreignness of the protein to the host may affect the immunogenicity of the protein.[5] Complex proteins with numerous antigenic determinants may be perceived as being more foreign than smaller proteins with few antigenic determinants.[5] Allergenic food proteins have certain characteristics in common. Because histamine release from the mast cells requires the allergen to bridge two IgE antibody molecules on the surface of the mast cell membrane, allergens must have two or more IgE-binding sites or allergenic determinants.[6] Allergens must also be the appropriate size to allow such bridging between the IgE-antibody molecules. Most allergens fall in the molecular weight range of 10,000 to 70,000, which must be ideal for bridging.[6] Some food allergens are much larger, but may be partially hydrolyzed to the appropriate size during digestion. A molecular weight of 10,000 probably represents the lower limit for the induction of an immunogenic response, although smaller peptides and other molecules could act as haptens. The upper limit of 70,000 may be only partially dictated by the bridging requirement. Intestinal permeability is another critical factor that is likely to be determined to some extent by the size of the allergen. Proteins in excess of a molecular weight of 70,000 are unlikely to be efficiently absorbed through the intestinal mucosal membranes, thus unlikely to have access to the lymphocytes generating allergen-specific IgE. The molecular shape of the protein is also likely to be important, but this factor has not been carefully studied. The three-dimensional structure of most food allergens is unknown.

Allergenic proteins or protein fractions have been partially purified from shrimp, peanuts, soybeans, green peas, rice, cottonseed, and tomatoes, but the identity of these allergens remains to be determined.[1,5] The major allergens in cow's milk have been identified as casein, ß-lactoglobulin, and α-lactalbumin, the major proteins in cow's milk.[1,7,8] Several minor allergens also exist in cow's milk.[8] The major allergens in egg whites are ovalbumin, ovomucoid, conalbumin (ovotransferrin), and ovomucin, the most common proteins in egg whites.[9-12] Egg yolks also appear to contain several allergens, including apovitellenin I, apovitellenin VI, and phosvitin.[12,13] The allergenic determinants in these identified allergens in cow's milk and eggs are not known, although some preliminary efforts have been made to isolate and characterize the allergenic determinants of egg ovalbumin.[14] The most well-characterized food allergen is allergen M from codfish.[2,5] Allergen M has been purified to homogeneity and is known to contain 113 amino acid residues and 1 glucose moiety, to have a molecular weight of 12,238, and to have an isoelectric point of 4.75.[15] The structure of the IgE-binding determinants is also known, and allergen M contains several IgE-binding sites.[16,17] Allergen M is a sarcoplasmic protein belonging to a group of proteins known as parvalbumins. The structure-function relationships of allergen M are much better understood than those for other food allergens.

An improved understanding of the nature and chemistry of these naturally occurring food allergens would be very helpful in the design of hypoallergenic foods and construction of safe and effective avoidance diets. The removal or destruction of these proteins is not easily accomplished until the identity and characteristics of these proteins are known.

While IgE-mediated allergic reactions are better understood than other forms of immunologically mediated food allergies, it is quite possible other immunological mechanisms account for certain adverse reactions to foods. However, because the existence of these forms of food allergy remains in some question, the nature of the substances in foods responsible for these illnesses has not been carefully investigated. One exception may be celiac disease or gluten-sensitive enteropathy. While the mechanism of celiac disease remains a mystery, a currently popular theory is celiac disease results from an immunocytotoxic reaction mediated by the intestinal lymphocytes.[18] Celiac disease is a malabsorption syndrome triggered in sensitive individuals by the ingestion of wheat, rye, barley, or oats. The naturally occurring gliadin fraction of wheat and the related prolamin fractions of rye, barley, and oats are responsible for this adverse reaction.[1,19] (See Chapter 7.)

Other types of adverse reactions to foods do not involve abnormal responses by the immune system. These illnesses fall into a variety of categories, including anaphylactoid reactions, metabolic food disorders, and idiosyncratic or idiopathic reactions.[1,20] The anaphylactoid reactions are thought to be caused by naturally occurring substances in foods, although these substances have not been identified. The most common metabolic food disorder is lactose intolerance, which is also caused by a naturally occurring constituent of foods, lactose. By definition, the mechanisms of the idiosyncratic reactions are unknown. For the most part, the foodborne substances eliciting these reactions are also unknown. Often, the association between the symptoms and specific foods has not been carefully established. A few idiosyncratic reactions have been attributed to naturally occurring substances such as the role of chocolate and cheese in migraine headaches, although the cause-and-effect role of these foods in these syndromes is uncertain. (See Chapter 8.) Some food additives cause well-documented idiosyncratic reactions. Examples include sulfites as a cause of asthma, tartrazine as a cause of hives, and aspartame as a cause of hives. A variety of other idiosyncratic reactions have been attributed to food additives, but convincing evidence of these associations remains to be provided.[1]

EFFECT OF PROCESSING AND PREPARATION

Most allergenic food proteins retain their allergenicity through various food processing treatments.[5] If they did not, then food allergies would not be a very important problem. While these proteins may be modified by various processes, they tend to retain their allergenic activities. In comparison to other food proteins, food allergens tend to be more heat stable, acid stable, and resistant to digestion.[21,22] These allergenic proteins must be able to reach their sites of action, the intestinal mucosa and beyond, in an immunogenic form.[5] The resistance of these proteins to physical and chemical modification provides limited options to the food scientist who may wish to destroy these allergens during processing. Usually, the functional properties of the food and its nutritional value will be destroyed before the allergenic activity of these proteins.

Most allergenic food proteins are remarkably heat stable, but a few exceptions do exist. The allergens in apples, potatoes, and carrots are heat labile, for example.[23] Individuals with allergies to these foods would usually be sensitive to the raw product, but not to the cooked or processed product.

Some exceptions may exist, especially with respect to potatoes. Other heat-labile allergens are found in coffee beans,[24] shrimp,[25] peanuts,[26] and rice.[27] Shrimp and peanuts also contain heat-stable allergens that are responsible for the reactions of sensitive individuals to processed shrimp and peanuts. However, the potent allergens in coffee beans that are responsible for considerable occupational allergy among coffee workers are apparently destroyed by roasting.[24] The cocoa bean allergen is destroyed by processing the cocoa beans into chocolate, but it is unknown whether the heat treatment alone is responsible for this reduction in allergenicity.[28]

In contrast, the most common allergenic foods contain heat-stable allergenic proteins. The allergens in cow's milk, egg whites, peanuts, soybeans, shrimp, and codfish are known to be heat stable.[21] For example, heat processing has little effect on the allergenicity of cow's milk; the major allergens retain their allergenicity at temperatures of 100°C and above.[21,29] The allergenicity of whey can be reduced by heat treatments of 100° to 115°C for 30 min.[30-32] However, the nutritional quality of the milk is substantially reduced by such extensive heat treatments.[33] Vitamins and lysine are destroyed, while lactulose and new, uncharacterized antigens are produced. While heat-treated whey may offer some hope as an ingredient in hypoallergenic formulae,[32] some of the lost nutritional quality must be restored, the absence of active residues of allergenic proteins must be ensured, and the possibility of formation of other toxic factors must be avoided. Condensation, evaporation, drying, pasteurization, and other common technological processes have no effect on the allergenicity of cow's milk.[34] Thus, the heat processes so common in the food industry and food preparation seem to have little impact on the allergenic food proteins.

Proteolysis is another process that may modify allergenic food proteins. This process was evaluated mostly from the standpoint of assessing the effects of digestion on food allergens until recently. Spies and coworkers[35-37] demonstrated new antigens could be produced by pepsin hydrolysis of ß-lactoglobulin and other milk proteins. They speculated that these hydrolysates may account for adverse reactions to milk in individuals with negative skin tests to intact milk proteins. Haddad et al[38] and Schwartz et al[39] produced protein fragments by partial digestion with pepsin or pepsin and trypsin from ß-lactoglobulin that were able to bind to IgE from patients with cow's milk allergy. Schwartz et al[39] failed to find any subjects who reacted to the ß-lactoglobulin digests, produced by pepsin hydrolysis according to Spies et al,[35-37] that did not also react to native, intact cow's milk proteins. In contrast, Haddad et al[38] did identify several patients (6 of 10 subjects) whose IgE reacted only with the ß-lactoglobulin digests. Despite such results, attempts have been made to use proteolysis as a means to produce hypoallergenic infant formulae. The initial attempts were quite successful because they were based on completely hydrolyzed casein. This ingredient is produced by chemical hydrolysis and is essentially a mixture of amino acids with a few small peptides. Mixtures of amino acids would not be predicted to have immunogenic activity, and completely hydrolyzed casein has negligible antigenicity and allergenicity by comparison to cow's milk.[8,40-42] Alternative infant formulae based on hydrolyzed casein such as Nutramigen® and Pregestimil® have enjoyed many years of safe use. These hypoallergenic formulae based on hydrolyzed casein also are useful in preventing the development of cow's milk protein intolerance in infants suffering from bouts of gastroenteritis.[43] However, these complete hydrolysates are not especially palatable for some infants. As a result, interest has developed in the use of partially hydrolyzed whey proteins as ingredients for hypoallergenic infant formulae. The hydrolysis of whey with α-chymotrypsin resulted in a hydrolysate with diminished allergenicity as determined by IgE binding.[44] A 60-min digestion with α-chymotrypsin led to a 7.5% degree of hydrolysis which was about 5 times less effective in binding to IgE than untreated whey. Clearly, this product would retain sufficient allergenic activity to cause adverse reactions in sensitized infants. A tryptic hydrolysate of whey protein has been produced that is not immunogenic to sensitized guinea pigs.[45] Unfortunately, this product has not been evaluated in humans, and its degree of allergenicity cannot be safely predicted from animal studies only. Nestle-Carnation has recently released a formula (first described as hypoallergenic) based on partially hydrolyzed whey protein that has elicited some adverse reactions in sensitized infants. The partial proteolysis of cow's milk or whey proteins does not appear to completely eliminate all of the allergenic activity of these proteins. The development of alternative formulae based on such processes should be approached with considerable caution. (*Editor's Note:* The Nestle-Carnation product mentioned is no longer being marketed using the term hypoallergenic.)

In theory, hydrolysates or partial hydrolysates from less allergenic food proteins should create fewer problems in the development of alternative infant formulae or other hypoallergenic processes. However, such hydrolysates have not been investigated thus far. Hydrolyzed peanut protein was unable to bind to IgE from the sera of peanut-allergic individuals.[46] Pepsin hydrolysis of ovalbumin destroyed its antigenicity, while trypsin hydrolysis and cyanogen bromide cleavage had little effect on this allergen.[14] Allergen M from codfish can be destroyed by proteolysis.[47]

Few other food processes have been evaluated for their effect on the allergenicity of food proteins. Homogenization of milk has no effect on its allergenicity.[48,49] The processing of peanuts into peanut butter or various types of peanut flours had no effect on the ability of peanut proteins to bind to IgE.[46] Chemical modification of the lysyl, tyrosyl, tryptophyl, or arginyl side chains of codfish allergen M or removal of two calcium ions from this protein diminished its allergenicity.[50] Polymerization of codfish allergen M with carbodiimide cross-linking also strongly reduced its immunochemical reactivity.[50] Carboxymethylation of ovalbumin resulted in some decrease in its ability to bind to IgE.[14] These chemical treatment processes would not necessarily be recommended as food processes, but demonstrate the potential for chemical modification of allergens. The heat-labile allergen in apples is also unstable during storage[51] and is inactivated by enzymatic browning.[52] The removal of allergens during food processing also has some potential, but this option has not been very thoroughly explored. For example, ß-lactoglobulin, a primary cow's milk allergen, can be removed from whey selectively by a FeCl$_3$ precipitation.[53] However, this treatment does not remove α-lactalbumin, which is also allergenic. The extraction of edible oils from peanuts, soybeans, and sunflower seeds removes all traces of protein from these products, and these oils are not allergenic to individuals with allergies toward those foods.[54-56]

With respect to individualistic adverse reactions to foods other than IgE-mediated food allergies, processing and preparation can play a significant role in some cases in lowering the risk of an adverse reaction. With lactose intolerance, several options exist. Lactose-hydrolyzed milk is available in certain markets or can be prepared at home. The lactose-hydrolyzed milk available in the marketplace has some limitations in acceptance because of its sweet taste, but it is effective in the treatment of lactose intolerance.[57] The addition of ß-galactosidase to milk at the time of ingestion is also effective.[58,59] The enzyme presumably retains its activity *in vivo* and hydrolyzes the ingested lactose in the gut. Several dairy products, most notably yogurt, are better tolerated by lactose-intolerant individuals than other dairy products.[60,61] Yogurt contains active ß-galactosidase, which is able to digest lactose *in vivo*.[60,62] Some brands of yogurt contain higher levels of ß-galactosidase activity than others; therefore, these brands are more easily tolerated by lactose-intolerant individuals.[63]

With the various food idiosyncrasies caused by food additives, such as sulfite-induced asthma, tartrazine-induced urticaria, and aspartame-induced urticaria, substitute food products that do not contain the additive in question are usually available. In the case of sulfites, numerous strategies have been employed to reduce or eliminate the need for sulfites in various food products.[64] In the specific case of the use of sulfites on fresh fruits and vegetables to prevent enzymatic browning, several alternatives now exist.[64] With celiac disease, little progress has been made in removing or inactivating the responsible proteins, but substitute food formulations are readily available.[65]

CONSTRUCTION OF SAFE AND EFFECTIVE AVOIDANCE DIETS

Selective avoidance diets are the most common mode of treatment for food allergies and related individualistic adverse reactions to foods. For example, if an individual is allergic to peanuts, that individual is simply instructed to avoid peanuts. When successfully implemented, these diets can be quite effective. However, successful avoidance of the offending food(s) or food ingredient(s) is not always a simple task. The patient must assume a large part of the responsibility for the construction and maintenance of a safe and effective avoidance diet. Yet, these patients are often poorly prepared to accept this responsibility. It requires enormous attention to detail. These patients often do not recognize the seriousness of their task. However, in some instances, the decisions can literally mean the difference between life and death. The patients frequently need to obtain more knowledge about food composition, sources of ingredients, and definition of terms appearing on food labels. Several questions must be posed during the construction of a safe and effective avoidance diet.

- Do tolerance levels exist for the offending food or food ingredient?
- Will exposure to small quantities of the offending substance elicit an adverse reaction or increase the degree of sensitization?
- Will all foods or ingredients made from the offending food pose a threat to health?
- Are there any likely hidden sources of exposure to the offending food?
- Will cross-reactions occur between closely related foods or between foods and other environmental substances?

Tolerance levels do exist for all food allergies and related food sensitivities. However, in the case of IgE-mediated food allergies, the tolerance levels for the offending food protein are so low they can be considered to be zero for all practical purposes. Some individual variability will certainly occur in the degree of tolerance for the offending food, even in cases of IgE-mediated food allergies. Gerrard and Shenassa[66] identified two types of cow's milk allergy in infants: one type was characterized by a very low tolerance level, while the other type was triggered only by ingestion of large doses of cow's milk. In addition, many food allergies first noted in infancy will be outgrown within a few months or perhaps years.[67] Thus, infants will frequently display an increasing tolerance for the offending foods as they mature. Infants are much more likely to outgrow their sensitivities to certain foods such as cow's milk than to other foods such as peanuts.[67] Peanut allergy is rarely, if ever, outgrown.[68] In celiac disease, the degree of tolerance for the protein fractions of wheat, rye, barley, and oats is thought to be extremely low.[65] With metabolic food disorders such as lactose intolerance, tolerance levels do exist.[69] Many individuals with lactose intolerance can tolerate the amount of lactose in an 8-oz glass of milk.[20] Of course, the degree of tolerance for lactose can worsen over time as the activity of intestinal ß-galactosidase continues to decrease.

Tolerance levels also exist for many of the food idiosyncrasies such as sulfite-induced asthma. Some sulfite-sensitive asthmatics are known to tolerate certain sulfited foods, especially those foods having low residual sulfite levels.[70,71] In controlled challenge studies, sulfite-sensitive individuals demonstrate variable tolerances for potassium metabisulfite in capsules or acidic solutions ranging from 5 mg to 200 mg.[72,73] Other food idiosyncrasies have been studied in fewer patients than sulfite-induced asthma, but tolerance levels appear to exist in most cases where controlled challenge studies have been performed.

With IgE-mediated food allergies, exposure to trace amounts of the offending food can trigger an adverse, and sometimes serious, reaction. Yunginger et al[74] have reported several deaths among food-allergic individuals caused by inadvertent exposure to their offending foods. Some of these incidents appear to have been precipitated by relatively minor exposures to the offending food, although it was not possible post hoc to put together detailed accounts of these incidents. More frequently, less serious reactions will be triggered by ingestion of trace amounts of the offending food.[75] Most reports of such reactions are anecdotal.[1,76] However, practices in the food industry such as the use of minor amounts of unlabeled ingredients as "rework," use of the same processing equipment for more than one food, failure to adequately clean equipment between processes, and use of contaminated ingredients could lead to these types of adverse reactions. An example was the use of peanut butter processing facilities to process sunflower butter, which resulted in a contamination of the sunflower butter with peanut residues and reactions in several individuals.[75] Restaurant settings can pose a hazard to these individuals because items are not labeled, and the restaurant staff may not be sufficiently knowledgeable or caring to provide the correct information on the content of various menu items. In homes or restaurants, using the same utensils for cooking or serving several different foods can result in the contamination of one food with trace amounts of another. Using cooking oils in food service facilities for the preparation of more than one type of food may also result in contamination. One of the reported deaths[74] may have resulted from this type of situation. Occasionally, patients are their own worst enemies, attempting to remove the offending food from mixtures, such as peanuts from trail mix, before consumption: an ill-advised practice. Patients have also reportedly reacted when opening packages containing the offending food (perhaps due to exposure to dust composed of fines of the offending food) and cooking the offending food.[1,76] These reactions could be psychosomatic, but exposure to trace quantities of the offending food cannot be ruled out. Exclusively breastfed infants have developed food allergies ostensibly through exposure to food allergens in the breast milk occurring as a result of ingestion of the offending food by the nursing mother.[77–79] Peanuts, eggs, and cow's milk have been implicated in these reactions. Apparently, trace quantities of proteins from these foods find their way into breast milk in sufficient quantities to sensitize the infant and occasionally trigger adverse reactions. While breastfeeding is still a recommended practice for infants born to parents with histories of allergies, the nursing mothers may be well advised to avoid highly sensitizing foods such as peanuts during the nursing period. The avoidance of highly nutritious foods such as cow's milk by nursing mothers should probably not be recommended, partly because cow's milk allergy is usually a self-limited condition.

Trace quantities of the proteins from wheat, rye, barley, and oats can also trigger the symptoms of celiac disease in sensitive patients.[65] Like individuals with IgE-mediated food allergies, celiac patients must diligently attempt to remove all traces of the offending food from their diets. With both celiac disease and IgE-mediated food allergies, no one knows how much exposure is too much. Some variability is likely to exist between individual patients, but in the absence of established tolerance levels, complete avoidance is the most prudent advice. Individuals with other food sensitivities such as metabolic food disorders or food idiosyncrasies can usually tolerate trace amounts of the offending substances without experiencing an adverse reaction. It is not known if such exposures are capable of heightening the degree of sensitivity to the offending substance, although present evidence suggests this is unlikely in certain cases such as lactose intolerance.

If the presence of potentially hazardous residues of allergenic foods in other foods is to be controlled in the food processing industry, procedures must be developed allowing the specific and sensitive detection of these residues. These procedures could then be incorporated into quality assurance programs to ensure equipment cleaning, for example, has been adequate to prevent such contamination. Unfortunately, very few such tests are currently available for use in the food industry.

Immunological assays probably have the greatest potential for such applications. Immunoassays have been developed for the detection of soy protein residues in soy-based foods and food ingredients such as lecithin, margarine, and soy oil[80] and the detection of peanut protein residues in sunflower butter.[75] Several different immunoassays have been developed for the detection of wheat gliadin in the gluten-free foods marketed for celiac patients.[81–85]

Other assays such as electrophoretic techniques could also be used for this purpose, but would likely be less sensitive and specific. An example would be an electrophoretic method developed to detect hazelnut residues in chocolate products.[86] Further efforts in this area seem warranted. However, the availability of these procedures will not eliminate the possibility of the contamination of other foods with potentially hazardous allergenic residues in restaurant or home settings.

An additional concern of food-allergic patients is the degree of required selectivity for the construction of safe and effective avoidance diets. This issue is connected to the degree of tolerance for the offending food. For IgE-mediated food allergies where the tolerance levels are virtually zero and traces of the offending food can trigger adverse reactions, the patient must attempt to avoid all exposure to the offending food. The patient will usually be instructed to avoid the offending food in all forms. For example, the patient with IgE-mediated soybean allergy will be instructed to avoid all products derived from soybeans, including soybean oil, soy sauce, hydrolyzed vegetable protein, and soya lecithin.[76] However, we know the causative substances for these IgE-mediated reactions in exquisitely sensitive patients are certain protein components of the offending foods. Therefore, foods that do not contain intact protein may not trigger these adverse reactions. Some food products such as soybean, peanut, and sunflower oils contain no detectable protein and do not elicit adverse reactions in sensitive individuals.[54-56] Soya lecithin often contains residues of soybean protein.[80] Whether this residual protein would induce adverse reactions remains unknown, but caution should be exercised. Edible oils may occasionally contain residues of proteins,[80] especially if the oils have been used to cook the parent food.[55] Lactose, a common ingredient in many foods, may contain residues of cow's milk proteins and elicit allergic reactions in sensitive individuals.[87] In other foods, the proteins are partially or completely hydrolyzed. The situation with partially or completely hydrolyzed cow's milk proteins in eliciting adverse reactions in sensitive individuals was discussed earlier. In soy sauce or hydrolyzed vegetable protein, the proteins have been extensively hydrolyzed. However, the ability of soy-based hydrolysates to trigger allergic reactions in sensitive individuals has not been carefully evaluated. As noted earlier, hydrolyzed peanut protein does not bind to IgE from sensitive patients and may not be allergenic. The only method for carefully establishing the safety of foods or food ingredients with altered or diminished levels of protein is to conduct a controlled clinical challenge study with allergic patients. This has only been accomplished with the edible oils and, perhaps through long and successful experience, hydrolyzed casein. Even if a food or ingredient fails to elicit adverse reactions in these controlled challenge studies, concerns remain about the consistent removal or destruction of all of the residues of the allergenic proteins during typical processing. Also, with certain products such as the edible oils, there is some concern about recontamination of the products in home or food service settings. Similar concerns exist for celiac patients and foods prepared from wheat, rye, barley, and oats. Again, only foods with detectable residues of the protein fractions of these grains will be hazardous in all likelihood. However, the presence or absence of proteins in various ingredients and products made from these grains such as malt extract, wheat starch, or rye alcohol has not been carefully established. Therefore, the most prudent advice is to avoid all exposures to any products made from these grains.[65] Such concerns are not as important in the cases of metabolic food disorders or idiosyncratic reactions. Because some tolerance exists for the offending substance, the avoidance of all foods containing the offending material may not be necessary.

Hidden sources of the offending food or food ingredient can exist. Some examples have already been provided, such as the presence of milk proteins in lactose[87] and the presence of soy proteins in lecithin.[80] The inadvertent or intentional contamination of one food with residues of another is also a major concern. Many of the most serious allergic reactions to foods occur following the inadvertent consumption of the offending food, often from hidden sources.[74] While caution is advised, a listing of all possible hidden sources of food allergens would be impossible to compile. In the formulation of food products, care must be taken to avoid the presence of hazardous allergenic residues or to acknowledge the presence of such foods on the label of the food product.[21] Also, care should be exercised in the formation of new food products to avoid especially potent allergenic materials where alternatives exist. Obviously, many products would not be the same without the presence of peanuts, but their presence should be noted on the label. In a recent incident with a new potentially allergenic material (cottonseed protein), use of this material in a food product resulted in adverse reactions and cottonseed allergy.[88]

Cross-reactions can also occur between closely related foods, although no general statements can be made on this topic. Tremendous individual differences occur with respect to cross-reactions. In a few cases, cross-reactions are rather commonly encountered among individuals with a particular type of food allergy. Examples would include cross-reactions between different species of avian eggs[89] and between cow's milk and goat's milk.[90] As noted earlier, cross-reactions are also very common in celiac disease among wheat, rye, barley, and oats. However, with other IgE-mediated food allergies, cross-reactions are somewhat less common. With respect to crustacea, many individuals with crustacean allergy will be sensitive to all species, including shrimp, crab, lobster, and crayfish, but some individuals will be sensitive to only one or a few of the species.[91] In the case of seafood allergies, individuals are often counseled to avoid all seafood species even though cross-reactions between finfish, crustacea, and mollusks have not been reported.[76] This advice is probably unnecessary, although cross-reactions within the crustacean and finfish categories have been documented. With respect to finfish, many fish species contain parvalbumins with structural similarities to allergen M, which may explain the existence of frequent cross-reactions between species.[92,93] However, cross-reactions do not always occur among all finfish.[94] With some types of IgE-mediated food allergies, cross-reactions with closely related foods are rather uncommon. The best example would be with legumes. On a comparative basis, many more individuals have peanut allergy than have soybean allergy. Only a few patients with peanut allergy are also sensitive to soybeans or other legumes,[95] although numerous peanut-allergic subjects will have positive skin tests to other legumes.[95,96] Cross-reactions can also occur between environmental and food allergens. The best examples are between birch pollen and various fruits, vegetables, and tree nuts including hazelnut, carrot, and apple,[23,51,97] between mugwort pollen and celery,[98] and between watermelon and ragweed.[99] The phenomenon of cross-reactivity is complex and poorly understood. Consequently, generalized advice is difficult to provide.

CONCLUSION

Specific avoidance diets are the best method available presently for the treatment of food allergies and sensitivities. However, these diets should be formulated so the patients can experience the widest possible array of foods within the necessary limits. Often, specific avoidance diets are too strict. However, with the present state of information, it is often not possible to provide individual patients with specific answers to many of their questions. The improved formulation of avoidance diets will require improved diagnosis of food allergies and sensitivities, additional research on critical questions such as the inactivation of allergens or the existence of cross-reactivity, and trained dietitians to assist patients with the formulation of safe and effective avoidance diets. In cases where incomplete information exists, the best advice is often conservative advice, especially for patients with histories of life-threatening or severe reactions.

REFERENCES

1. Taylor SL, Nordlee JA, Rupnow JH. Food allergies and sensitivities. In: Taylor SL, Scanlan RA, eds. *Food Toxicology: Perspectives on the Relative Risks.* New York: Marcel Dekker, Inc; 1989:255–295.

2. Lemanske RF Jr, Taylor SL. Standardized extracts, foods. *Clin Rev Allergy*. 1987; 5:23–36.

3. Taylor SL, Lemanske RF Jr, Bush RK. Chemistry of food allergens. *Comments Agr Food Chem*. 1987; 1:51–70.

4. Metcalfe DD. Food allergens. *Clin Rev Allergy*. 1985; 3:331–349.

5. Taylor SL, Lemanske RF Jr, Bush RK, Busse WW. Food allergens: structure and immunologic properties. *Ann Allergy*. 1987; 59:93–99.

6. Aas K. What makes an allergen an allergen. *Allergy*. 1978; 33:3–14.

7. Taylor SL. Immunologic and allergic properties of cow's milk proteins in humans. *J Food Proc*. 1986; 49:239–250.

8. Baldo BA. Milk allergies. *Aust J Dairy Technol*. 1984; 39:120–128.

9. Langeland T. A clinical and immunological study of allergy to hen's egg white, III: allergens in hen's egg white studied by crossed radio-immunoelectrophoresis (CRIE). *Allergy*. 1982; 37:521–530.

10. Hoffman DR. Immunochemical identification of the allergens in egg white. *J Allergy Clin Immunol*. 1983; 71:481–486.

11. Bleumink E, Young E. Studies on the atopic allergen in hen's egg. I. Identification of the skin reactive fraction in egg white. *Int Arch Allergy Appl Immunol*. 1969; 35:1–19.

12. Walsh BJ, Barnett D, Burley RW, Elliott C, Hill DJ, Howden MEH. New allergens from hen's egg white and egg yolk/in vitro study of ovocmucin, apovitellenin I and VI, and phosvitin. *Int Arch Allergy Appl Immunol*. 1988; 87:81–86.

13. Anet J, Back JF, Baker RS, Barnett D, Burley RW, Howden MEH. Allergens in the white and yolk of hen's egg. A study of IgE binding by egg proteins. *Int Arch Allergy Appl Immunol*. 1985; 77:364–371.

14. Elsayed S, Hammer ASE, Kalvenes MB, Florvaag E, Apold J, Vik H. Antigenic and allergenic determinants of ovalbumin. I. Peptide mapping, cleavage at the methionyl peptide bonds and enzymic hydrolysis of native and carboxymethyl OA. *Int Arch Allergy Appl Immunol*. 1986; 79:101–107.

15. Elsayed S, Bennich H. The primary structure of allergen M from cod. *Scand J Immunol*. 1975; 4:203–208.

16. Elsayed S, Apold J. Immunochemical analysis of cod fish allergen M: locations of the immunoglobulin binding sites as demonstrated by the native and synthetic peptides. *Allergy*. 1983; 38:449–459.

17. Elsayed S, Titlestad K, Apold J, Aas K. A synthetic hexadecapeptide derived from allergen M imposing allergenic and antigenic reactivity. *Scand J Immunol*. 1980; 12:171–175.

18. Kagnoff MF. Celiac disease: A model of an immunologically mediated intestinal disease. *Immunol Allergy Clin North Am*. 1988; 8:505–519.

19. Kasarda DD. The relationship of wheat protein to celiac disease. *Cereal Foods World*. 1978; 23:240–244, 262.

20. Taylor SL. Allergic and sensitivity reactions to food components. In: Hathcock JN, ed. *Nutritional Toxicology, II*. Orlando, Fla: Academic Press; 1987; 173–198.

21. Taylor SL. Food allergies. *Food Technol*. 1985; 39(2):98–105.

22. Taylor SL. Food allergy—the enigma and some potential solutions. *J Food Proc*. 1980; 43:300–306.

23. Dreborg S, Foucard T. Allergy to apple, carrot and potato in children with birch pollen allergy. *Allergy*. 1983; 38:167–172.

24. Lehrer SB, Karr RM, Salvaggio JE. Extraction and analysis of coffee bean allergens. *Clin Allergy*. 1978; 8:217–226.

25. Hoffman DR, Day ED, Miller JS. The major heat stable allergen of shrimp. *Ann Allergy.* 1981; 47:17–22.

26. Barnett D, Baldo BA, Howden MEH. Multiplicity of allergens in peanuts. *J Allergy Clin Immunol.* 1983; 72(1):61–68.

27. Shibasaki M, Suzuki S, Nemoto H, Kuroume T. Allergenicity and lymphocyte-stimulating property of rice protein. *J Allergy Clin Immunol.* 1979; 64(4):259–265.

28. Fries JH. Chocolate: A review of published reports of allergic and other deleterious effects, real or presumed. *Ann Allergy.* 1978; 41:195–207.

29. Hanson LA, Mansson I. Immune electrophoretic studies of bovine milk and milk products. *Acta Pediatr.* 1961; 50:484–490.

30. McLaughlan P, Anderson KJ, Widdowson EM, Coombs RRA. Effect of heat on the anaphylactic sensitizing capacity of cows' milk, goats' milk and various infant formulae fed to guinea pigs. *Arch Dis Child.* 1981; 56:165–171.

31. Kilshaw PJ, Heppell LMJ, Ford JE. Effects of heat treatment of cows' milk and whey on the nutritional quality and antigenic properties. *Arch Dis Child.* 1982; 57:842–847.

32. Heppell LM, Cant AJ, Kilshaw PJ. Reduction in the antigenicity of whey proteins by heat treatment: A possible strategy for producing a hypoallergenic infant milk formula. *Br J Nutr.* 1984; 51:29–36.

33. Heat-treated cow's milk remains allergenic. *Nutr Rev.* 1983; 41:96–97.

34. Moneret-Vautrin G, Humbert G, Alais C, Grilliat JP. Données récentes sur les propriétés immunoallergologiques des protéines laitières. *Le Lait.* 1982; 62:396–408.

35. Spies JR, Stevan MA, Stein WJ, Coulson EJ. The chemistry of allergens. XX. New antigens generated by pepsin hydrolysis of bovine milk proteins. *J Allergy.* 1970; 45:208–219.

36. Spies JR, Stevan MA, Stein WJ. The chemistry of allergens. XXI. Eight new antigens generated by successive pepsin hydrolyses of bovine ß-lactoglobulin. *J Allergy Clin Immunol.* 1972; 50(2):82–91.

37. Spies JR, Stevan MA, Stein WJ, Gordon WG. Chemistry of allergens. XXII. Isolation and characterization of three new antigens from the dialysates of six successive pepsin hydrolyses of ß-lactoglobulin. *Int Arch Allergy Appl Immunol.* 1975; 48:49–71.

38. Haddad ZH, Kalra V, Verma S. IgE antibodies to peptic and peptic-tryptic digests of beta-lactoglobulin: Significance in food hypersensitivity. *Ann Allergy.* 1979; 42:368–371.

39. Schwartz HR, Nerurkar LS, Spies JR, Scanlon RT, Bellanti JA. Milk hypersensitivity: RAST studies using new antigens generated by pepsin hydrolysis of beta-lactoglobulin. *Ann Allergy.* 1980; 45:242–245.

40. Bahna SL, Gandhi MD. Milk hypersensitivity. II. Practical aspects of diagnosis, treatment and prevention. *Ann Allergy.* 1983; 50:295–301.

41. Eastham EJ, Lichauco T, Grady MI, Walker WA. Antigenicity of infant formulas: role of immature intestine on protein permeability. *J Pediatr.* 1978; 93:561–564.

42. Gjesing B, Osterballe O, Schwartz B, Wahn U, Lowenstein H. Allergen-specific IgE antibodies against antigenic components in cow milk and milk substitutes. *Allergy.* 1986; 41:51–56.

43. Manuel PD, Walker-Smith JA. A comparison of three infant feeding formulae for the prevention of delayed recovery after infantile gastroenteritis. *Acta Paediatr Belg.* 1981; 34:13–20.

44. Asselin J, Amiot J, Gauthier SF, Mourad W, Hebert J. Immunogenicity and allergenicity of whey protein hydrolysates. *J Food Sci.* 1988; 53:1208–1211.

45. Pahud JJ, Monti JC, Jost R. Allergenicity of whey protein: its modification by tryptic in vitro hydrolysis of the protein. *J Pediatr Gastroenterol Nutr.* 1985; 4:408–413.

46. Nordlee JA, Taylor SL, Jones RT, Yunginger JW. Allergenicity of various peanut products as determined by RAST inhibition. *J Allergy Clin Immunol.* 1981; 68(5):376–382.

47. Aas K, Elsayed SM. Characterization of a major allergen (cod). Effect of enzymic hydrolysis on the allergenic activity. *J Allergy.* 1969; 44:333–343.

48. Poulsen OM, Hau J. Homogenization and allergenicity of milk—some possible implications for the processing of infant formulae. *N Eur Dairy J.* 1988; 53:239–242.

49. Host A. Cow's milk allergy in infants. *N Eur Dairy J.* 1988; 53:302–304.

50. Apold J, Elsayed S. The effect of amino acid modification and polymerization on the immunochemical reactivity of cod allergen M. *Molec Immunol.* 1979; 16:559–564.

51. Lahti A, Bjorksten F, Hannuksela M. Allergy to birch pollen and apple, and cross-reactivity of the allergens studied with the RAST. *Allergy.* 1980; 35:297–300.

52. Bjorksten F, Halmepuro L, Hannuksela M, Lahti A. Extraction and properties of apple allergens. *Allergy.* 1980; 35:671–677.

53. Kaneko T, Wu BT, Nakai S. Selective concentration of bovine immunoglobulins and α-lactalbumin from acid whey using FeCl$_3$. *J Food Sci.* 1985; 50:1531–1536.

54. Taylor SL, Busse WW, Sachs MI, Parker JL, Yunginger JW. Peanut oil is not allergenic to peanut-sensitive individuals. *J Allergy Clin Immunol.* 1981; 68(5):372–375.

55. Bush RK, Taylor SL, Nordlee JA, Busse WW. Soybean oil is not allergenic to soybean-sensitive individuals. *J Allergy Clin Immunol.* 1985; 76(2):242–245.

56. Halsey AB, Martin ME, Ruff ME, Jacobs FO, Jacobs RL. Sunflower oil is not allergenic to sunflower seed-sensitive patients. *J Allergy Clin Immunol.* 1986; 78(3):408–410.

57. Paige DM, Bayless TM, Huang SS, Wexler R. Lactose hydrolyzed milk. *Am J Clin Nutr.* 1975; 28:818–822.

58. Rosado JL, Solomons NW, Lisker R, et al. Enzyme replacement therapy for primary adult lactase deficiency: effective reduction of lactose malabsorption and milk intolerance by direct addition of ß-galactosidase to milk at mealtime. *Gastroenterology.* 1984; 87:1072–1082.

59. Barillas C, Solomons NW. Effective reduction of lactose maldigestion in preschool children by direct addition of ß-galactosidases to milk at mealtime. *Pediatrics.* 1987; 79:766–772.

60. Kolars JC, Levitt MD, Aouji M, Savaiano DA. Yogurt—an autodigesting source of lactose. *N Engl J Med.* 1984; 310:1–3.

61. Gallagher CR, Molleson AL, Caldwell JH. Lactose intolerance and fermented dairy products. *Cult Dairy Prod J.* 1977; 10(1):22–24.

62. Martini MC, Bollweg GL, Savaiano DA, Levitt MD. Lactose digestion by yogurt ß-galactosidase: Influence of pH and microbial integrity. *Am J Clin Nutr.* 1987; 45:432–436.

63. Wytok DH, DiPalma JA. All yogurts are not created equal. *Am J Clin Nutr.* 1988; 47:454–457.

64. Taylor SL, Higley NA, Bush RK. Sulfites in foods: uses, analytical methods, residues, fats, exposure assessment, metabolism, toxicity, and hypersensitivity. *Adv Food Res.* 1986; 30:1–76.

65. Hartsook EI. Celiac sprue: sensitivity to gliadin. *Cereal Foods World.* 1984; 29:157–158.

66. Gerrard JW, Shenassa M. Food allergy: two common types as seen in breast and formula fed babies. *Ann Allergy.* 1983; 50:375–379.

67. Bock SA. The natural history of food sensitivity. *J Allergy Clin Immunol.* 1982; 69(2):173–177.

68. Bock SA, Atkins FA. The natural history of peanut allergy. *J Allergy Clin Immunol.* 1989; 83(5):900–904.

69. National Dairy Council. Perspective on milk intolerance. *Dairy Council Digest.* 1978; 49:31–36.

70. Bush RK, Taylor SL, Busse W. A critical evaluation of clinical trials in reactions to sulfites. *J Allergy Clin Immunol.* 1986; 78(1):191–202.

71. Taylor SL, Bush RK, Selner JC, et al. Sensitivity to sulfited foods among sulfite-sensitive asthmatics. *J Allergy Clin Immunol.* 1988; 81(6):1159–1167.

72. Stevenson DD, Simon RA. Sensitivity to ingested metabisulfites in asthmatic subjects. *J Allergy Clin Immunol.* 1981; 68(1):26–32.

73. Taylor SL, Nordlee JA. Sensitivity to ingested sulfites. *ISI Atlas Sci Immunol.* 1988; 1:254–258.

74. Yunginger JW, Sweeney KG, Sturner WQ, et al. Fatal food-induced anaphylaxis. *JAMA.* 1988; 260:1450–1452.

75. Yunginger JW, Gauerke MB, Jones RT, Dahlberg MJE, Ackerman SJ. Use of radioimmunoassay to determine the nature, quantity and source of allergenic contamination of sunflower butter. *J Food Proc.* 1983; 46:625–628.

76. Taylor SL, Bush RK, Busse WW. Avoidance diets—How selective should we be? *N Engl Reg Allergy Proc.* 1986; 7:527–532.

77. Warner JO. Food allergy in fully breast-fed infants. *Clin Allergy.* 1980; 10:133–136.

78. Gerrard JW, Shenassa M. Sensitization to substances in breast milk: recognition, management, and significance. *Ann Allergy.* 1983; 61:300–302.

79. Van Asperen PP, Kemp AS, Mellis CM. Immediate food hypersensitivity reactions on the first known exposure to the food. *Arch Dis Child.* 1983; 58:253–256.

80. Porras O, Carlsson B, Fällström SP, Hanson LA. Detection of soy protein in soy lecithin, margarine, and, occasionally, soy oil. *Int Arch Allergy Appl Immunol.* 1985; 78:30–32.

81. Ciclitira PJ, Ellis HJ, Evans DJ, Lennox ES. A radioimmunoassay for wheat gliadin to assess the suitability of gluten free foods for patients with coeliac disease. *Clin Exp Immunol.* 1985; 59:703–708.

82. Freedman AR, Galfre G, Gal E, Ellis HJ, Ciclitira PJ. Monoclonal antibody ELISA to quantitate wheat gliadin contamination of gluten-free foods. *J Immunol Meth.* 1987; 98:123–127.

83. Skerritt JH, Smith RA. A sensitive monoclonal-antibody-based test for gluten detection: studies with cooked or processed foods. *J Sci Food Agric.* 1985; 36:980–986.

84. Skerritt JH. A sensitive monoclonal-antibody-based test for gluten detection: quantitative immunoassay. *J Sci Food Agric.* 1985; 36:987–994.

85. Skerritt JH, Diment JA, Wrigley CW. A sensitive monoclonal-antibody-based test for gluten detection: choice of primary and secondary antibodies. *J Sci Food Agric.* 1985; 36:995–1003.

86. Garrone W, Antonucci M, Bona U, Clementi S. Determination of hazelnut content by means of their protein fraction in chocolate bars, chocolates and milk containing spreads. *Lebensm Wiss Technol.* 1988; 21:76–82.

87. Kaminogawa S, Kumagai Y, Yamauchi K, Iwasaki E, Mukoyama T, Baba M. Allergic skin reactivity and chemical properties of allergens in two grades of lactose. *J Food Sci.* 1984; 49:529–530, 535.

88. Atkins FM, Wilson M, Bock SA. Cottonseed hypersensitivity: new concerns over an old problem. *J Allergy Clin Immunol.* 1988; 82(2):242–250.

89. Langeland T. A clinical and immunological study of allergy to hen's egg white. VI. Occurrence of proteins cross-reacting with allergens in hen's egg white as studied in egg white from turkey, duck, goose, sea gull, and in hen egg yolk, and hen and chicken sera and flesh. *Allergy.* 1983; 39:399–412.

90. Juntunen K, Ali-Yrkko S. Goat's milk for children allergic to cow's milk. *Kiel Milchwirt Forschungsber.* 1983; 35:439–440.

91. Waring NP, Daul CB, deShazo RD, McCants ML, Lehrer SB. Hypersensitivity reactions to ingested crustacea: clinical evaluation and diagnostic studies in shrimp-sensitive individuals. *J Allergy Clin Immunol.* 1985; 76(3):440–445.

92. Aas K. Studies on hypersensitivity to fish. Allergological and serological differentiation between various species of fish. *Int Arch Allergy.* 1966; 30:257–267.

93. Tuft L, Blumstein GI. Studies in food allergy. V. Antigenic relationships among members of fish family. *J Allergy.* 1946; 17:329–339.

94. Taylor SL, Bush RK. Allergy by ingestion of seafoods. In: Tu AT, ed. *Handbook of Natural Toxins, III, Marine Toxins and Venoms.* New York: Marcel Dekker; 1988:149–183.

95. Bernhisel-Broadbent J, Sampson HA. Cross-allergenicity in the legume botanical family in children with food hypersensitivity. *J Allergy Clin Immunol.* 1989; 83:435–440.

96. Barnett D, Bonham B, Howden MEH. Allergenic cross-reactions among legume foods—an *in vitro* study. *J Allergy Clin Immunol.* 1987; 79:433–438.

97. Halmepuro L, Vuontela K, Kalimo K, Bjorksten F. Cross-reactivity of IgE antibodies with allergens in birch pollen, fruits, and vegetables. *Int Arch Allergy Appl Immunol.* 1984; 74:235–240.

98. Vallier P, Dechamp C, Vial O, Deviller P. A study of allergens in celery with cross-sensitivity to mugwort and birch pollens. *Clin Allergy.* 1988; 18:491–500.

99. Enberg RN, McCullough J, Ownby DR. Antibody responses in watermelon sensitivity. *J Allergy Clin Immunol.* 1988; 82(5):795–800.

Chapter 10

Food Allergies and Adverse Food Reactions: An Anthropological Perspective

Leslie Sue Lieberman and Kathleen C. Barnes

This chapter on food allergies and adverse food reactions (AFR) is based on the review of a scant body of literature from nutritional and medical anthropology, nutritional geography, and epidemiology. Although the study of food habits, including food aversions, has been an active area of research among anthropologists since the 1940s work of the National Academy of Sciences and National Research Council's Committee on Food Habits,[1] virtually no attention has been paid to food allergies. Attention has focused on AFR and, particularly, on the worldwide problem of lactose intolerance and its relationship to biocultural variables promoting milk use or avoidance.

In this chapter, we discuss anthropological approaches to adverse food reactions and allergies and, when applicable, the sociopsychological and biocultural factors that explain these food-related behaviors and physiological responses. In the last section of this chapter, we focus on minority client and nutritionist or dietitian interactions. We discuss the problems arising in transcultural or cross-cultural therapeutic encounters, and we suggest a number of techniques for promoting more effective nutrition education and better adherence to recommended changes in diet and food-related behaviors.

A BIOCULTURAL PERSPECTIVE ON FOOD ALLERGIES AND INTOLERANCES

The paucity of data concerning food allergies and adverse food reactions in the archaeological and ethnohistorical records can be attributed to a number of reasons. First, allergic disease leaves no artifactual remains, so there is no physical evidence to be found in the archaeological record. There is scant evidence of foods and medicines. Infrequently, artwork on pottery vessels and walls depicts individuals with acute conditions (eg, smallpox), chronic diseases (eg, leprosy, leishmaniasis), traumatic injuries (eg, broken limbs), and malformations (eg, scoliosis).[2-4] Yet, none of these materials can be linked directly to allergy disease. Secondly, ethnohistorical records fail to report allergy because of its low prevalence in early historic populations and because food allergies, in particular, can be avoided after a single deleterious incident. Furthermore, high infant and childhood mortality rates due to malnutrition and infectious disease obscure secondary or confounding allergic symptoms. This situation continues to prevail in many developing countries.[5,6] An exception to the foregoing comment on the paucity of data is the case of lactose intolerance for which there are abundant ethnohistorical and biocultural data.[7-13]

The higher incidence of allergy (IgE-mediated hypersensitivity) among urban versus rural residents in developing countries has led researchers to search for immunological differences in these populations. Researchers found higher IgE titers among the rural inhabitants than among urban asthmatics and atopics.[14,15] Other researchers have identified higher titers in rural African children compared to European children.[16]

Most cases of nonsymptomatic, elevated IgE titers in developing countries have been attributed to chronic parasitic infections.[14-20] Parasitic infections are known to affect approximately one-third of the world's population.[21] The protective mechanism of IgE against parasitic infections is as follows: Upon penetration of the gut mucosa, an IgE-mediated response occurs in which worm-specific, IgE-sensitized mast cells, after contact with the worm antigen, degranulate and release mediators, such as histamine, that increase vascular permeability and eventually kill and expulse the worm.[21] Because exposure to gastrointestinal parasites is generally chronic, the protective response is continuous, and because all binding sites are occupied by worm-specific IgE, there is a decrease in circulating IgE available for binding to additional allergens, such as pollen, mites, or food. This process is referred to as the "mast cell saturation hypothesis," and is one explanation for the low prevalence of asthmatic and atopic symptomatology—despite elevated IgE titers—in parasite-infected populations.[14,15] The pleiotropic effect of IgE protection against biologically overwhelming parasitic infections is the reduction in immunological response to allergens.

In sum, parasitic infections and allergy disease are mutually exclusive.[15] Allergy is the result of an ecological transition from endemic parasitosis to improved hygienic conditions, reducing or eliminating parasitic exposure. This phenomenon is certainly recent in development, because for more than 90% of hominid history, humans have practiced a hunting and gathering or foraging form of subsistence and chronic parasitic infections were characteristic among these populations.[4,22-24] Parasitism continued to be a problem among higher-density, sedentary, early agriculturalists.[25,26]

Among contemporary populations, the incidence of IgE-mediated allergy to food varies by ethnic group and socioeconomic class. The most frequently incriminated foods are milk, fish, nuts, and egg.[27,28] It is theorized that in populations with a predisposition to a food allergy, the widespread consumption of that food will lead to an increased incidence of allergy. For example, it is not surprising the most common food allergy among a group of Thai children was to shrimp,[29] because fish and crustacea are common food items in Thai cuisine due to its geographical location. In contrast, it is unlikely shrimp would be the most common food allergen in a group of children from Kansas. Similarly, Moneret-Vautrin[30] reported that with the relatively recent introduction of soybean in the French diet, soy bean allergy is increasing and has become the third most common trophallergen (food allergen) among French children. With rapid, widespread introduction of new foods, we would expect to see a high incidence of allergies or AFR to these new allergens in populations not previously exposed. With long-term exposure to trophallergens, natural selection may operate to eliminate people with AFR, thereby reducing the incidence of allergic response and AFR.

Commonly eaten foods often contain toxic agents, but in such low quantities adverse reactions are generally few. In general, traditional methods of preparation and consumption eliminate the adverse effects of these foods. Knowledge of natural toxic agents is encyclopedic.[31] Both plant and animal foods that are generally considered unsafe (eg, many varieties of mushrooms and certain poisonous animals such as the pufferfish) are avoided completely and are not classified as edible foods. Other foods such as green potatoes have high levels of glycoalkaloids, including solanine in an unripe state, and are also eliminated from the diet. Many foods are treated through processing. For example, cassava or manioc may be fermented to hydrolyze the cyanogens or washed and dried to leach the cyanogenetic glycosides. Hemagglutinins and other toxic compounds are often destroyed by heating. Some foods, as noted elsewhere, affect only individuals who have particular susceptible genotypes and phenotypes. An example of this is the consumption of the fava bean by glucose-6-phosphate dehydrogenase (G6PD)-deficient individuals.

Hypersensitivity has been reported for a substance naturally produced in the processing or improper storage of certain fish.[32-34] Bryan[32] described cases of histamine poisoning in California following the consumption of Spanish mackerel and albacore that had been allowed to spoil. Similar occurrences were noted in Sri Lanka following the consumption of skipjack.[33] Fish consumption in Sri Lanka was particularly life-threatening in a number of individuals who were receiving isoniazid at the time of histamine poisoning; isoniazid is an inhibitor of histaminase, important in the metabolism of histamine.[33] Uragoda and Kottegoda[33] explain that although the altered taste of spoiled fish generally prevents its consumption, in some fish the taste may remain unaltered during the early period of spoilage. Although the population at risk for histamine poisoning is likely to be small, special consideration should be given to populations that regularly consume fish and live near or work on docks and oceanside markets.

In contrast, adverse food reactions may be genetic in nature, such as enzyme deficiencies. The epidemiological pattern of these diseases is more likely to be predicted by ethnicity than IgE-mediated food allergy or hypersensitivity. Favism is an example of a genetically based, yet non-IgE mediated, food intolerance. The consumption of the broad bean or fava bean (*Vicia fava*), widely produced and consumed throughout the Mediterranean and Middle East, produces a severe hemolytic anemia that is sometimes life-threatening in people who suffer from G6PD deficiency.[35-38] G6PD deficiency is an X-linked genetic condition that causes hemolysis of red blood cells due to a lack of the enzyme necessary for metabolism of erythrocytic glucose.[39] When the erythrocytes are exposed to oxidative foods and drugs (such as aspirin, quinine, vitamin K derivatives, and fava bean), the glucose level increases to the point of cell hemolysis.[39]

The etiology and manifestation of G6PD deficiency have been well documented.[37,38,40-42] G6PD deficiency is believed to have originated as a protective mechanism against falciparum malaria, because erythrocytes deficient in G6PD have a decrease in glutathione and malarial parasites are dependent on glutathione for maintaining parasitic protein synthesis.[38,40-42] Katz[38] concludes G6PD deficiency is the most common genetic disorder worldwide. Distribution of G6PD-deficient carriers is primarily circum-Mediterranean, but also includes Europe, the Middle East, northern and equatorial Africa, India, southern China, Southeast Asia, Indonesia, and New Guinea.[38] In the United States, G6PD deficiency affects approximately 1% to 2% of American whites and 10% to 15% of American blacks.[39] Katz[38] notes there are over 100 variants of the enzyme and the one found in the Mediterranean region exhibits the least enzymatic activity.

The genetically selective advantage of favism is that the consumption of fava beans by G6PD-deficient individuals enhances the antimalarial properties of G6PD deficiency.[36,40,41] Fava beans contain a number of active compounds that further oxidize glutathione.[41] However, extreme reduction of glutathione results in erythrocytic hemolysis, which initiates the favism crisis. Favism crisis is characterized by pallor, jaundice, weakness or fatigue, and hemoglobinuria, and onset of symptoms is usually within a few hours after consumption.[35]

In the circum-Mediterranean regions where fava beans have been cultivated possibly since Neolithic times[41,43] and, coincidentally, where there is a particularly high prevalence of G6PD deficiency, traditional methods of preparation (soaking, drying, and removing the skins) and cooking are used to reduce the toxicity of the fava bean.[41] Also, taboos exist that prohibit the consumption of fava beans by pregnant women and children.[43] Andrews[43] notes the Greeks felt a mixture of "respect and dread" about the bean, attributing a type of supernatural force to it, and beans were eaten most frequently during occasions associated with death. The development of an understanding of the fava bean in relation to hemolytic disease in the Mediterranean occurred over a long period of human history. In contrast, the international commercial exchange of food products and the widespread use of pharmacological products are recent phenomena that threaten the well-being of G6PD-deficient populations by offering them, often unknowingly, oxidative foods and drugs.

GLUTEN SENSITIVITY (CELIAC DISEASE): SENSITIVITY TO CEREAL GRAINS

Another example of an adverse food reaction due to a metabolic disorder is celiac disease (celiac sprue) or gluten-sensitive enteropathy. It has been suggested that celiac disease is an immunological abnormality, although possibly of a different type than IgE-mediated allergy.[44-48] There is at least an inherited genetic predisposition for celiac disease.[44,48] Support for an immunological basis includes an increase in the numbers of immunoglobulin-producing plasma cells and lymphocytes in the damaged mucosa, an increase in serum IgA, and decreased serum complement.[48]

Celiac disease is an adverse reaction to gluten, a prolamin found in cereals, particularly wheat,[49] but also found in rye, and to a lesser degree oats and barley.[44,47] Rice and buckwheat are considered nontoxic, while uncertainty exists for sorghum and millet.[47] Gluten-containing grains are also present in cakes, cookies, breads, crackers, cereals, pasta, and a number of other commercially prepared foods.[49] Celiac disease is characterized by malabsorption, and symptoms include diarrhea, steatorrhea, bloating, and weight loss.[49] If untreated, the disease may result in an iron-, B_{12}-, and folate-related anemia, as well as calcium deficiency.[49] In 95% of affected children, the disease is chronic.[48]

The theory that celiac disease, or gluten intolerance, is a result of the relatively late introduction of wheat in the human diet is supported by the fact that a gradient of haplotypes, B8 and DRW3, exists from Ireland toward the southeast to Israel,[44,48] which corresponds with the historical northwesterly spread of wheat consumption.[44,48] Both the HLA-B8 frequencies and the frequency of celiac disease are highest in the northwest of India, the fringe area of early cultivation of wheat, at least by 1000 BC, and toward the edge of Northern and Central Europe, the most recent cultivators of wheat.[47] Until the potato famine of the 1840s, wheat was not frequently consumed in Ireland, with the possible exception of the affluent Irish, in contrast to England and Wales, where it had been widely cultivated since the Roman occupation.[50]

Despite inconsistent reports from one country to another, celiac disease apparently occurs widely throughout Western and Eastern Europe, is rare in sub-Saharan Africa and the Far East, and possibly quite frequent in the Near East, the center of wheat domestication and a region where wheat is a significant dietary element.[47] It is generally agreed that incidence is highest in Ireland.[47,48,50,51] In Galway, Ireland, during an 11-year period, the incidence of celiac disease was 1 in 597 births.[48]

Simoons[47] notes medical research has ethnocentrically concentrated only on toxic cereals commonly consumed by Europeans and has failed to consider the cereals important to non-Westerners, especially sorghum, which is the fifth most commonly produced cereal worldwide. Special consideration should be given to persons at risk for celiac disease (ie, Irish-Americans, East Indians) when recommending cereal products in the daily diet. This is currently of particular concern because increasing the consumption of cereal for the purpose of increasing fiber intake has become a mania in American advertising. Consideration also should be given for the consumption of non-nutritious foods such as beer. Simoons[47] warned that in the United Kingdom beer is the principal barley product. The consumption of beer could be a health hazard for celiacs in Ireland.

As in the case of lactose intolerance, wheat-gluten tolerance may be seen as a genetotrophic adaptation to a relatively newly introduced nutritious food. The genes for wheat-gluten sensitivity would have been selected against over a number of generations because of decreased fertility of individuals with celiac disease. Conversely, those individuals tolerant of wheat gluten and also the gluten in rye and barley (Old World crops) would have had a selective advantage because of their ability to use these widely cultivated and nutritious staples. Further work is needed to establish the relationship between wheat-gluten sensitivity and genetic markers such as HLA-B8 in establishing confirmation for this hypothesis.

LACTOSE INTOLERANCE: AN EXAMPLE OF BIOCULTURAL ADAPTATIONS

Considerable confusion exists in the anthropological, public health, and nutrition literature regarding the multifaceted problem of milk intolerance. Allergic reactions to cow's milk is fairly common among human infants, estimated to be as high as 7%.[52] Milk proteins are the most common allergens in cow's milk; however, milk also may contain a number of contaminants such as ragweed or bacteria that can lead to allergic reactions in humans of all ages. However, milk intolerance related to lactase deficiency is far more common. Since the early 1960s, a number of studies have documented the worldwide existence of lactose intolerance among many divergent groups of people. Lactose intolerance is particularly high among traditional hunting and gathering groups, with levels exceeding 95% of the population. Intolerance levels are low (5% to 15%) among dairying populations of Northern Europe. Table 10-1 lists a number of populations by subsistence activities, the percentage of the population who are lactose tolerant, and the consumption rate of dairy products. The most extensive summary of results has been made by Simoons,[10-13] listing 197 population studies from around the world.

Although there is an abundance of reported materials on lactose intolerance, sometimes referred to as lactose malabsorption and lactase deficiency, there are a number of technical problems with these data. The first problem involves the diagnostic procedures that are used. In some instances, biopsies have been made. More commonly, a lactose tolerance test is used in which the subject is given an oral dose of at least 50 g of lactose (approximately the amount of lactose found in a quart of milk) and then the rise in blood glucose is followed over a period of several hours. A rise of less than 20 mg/100 mL of blood is considered indicative of lactose intolerance.[7] One modification of this test is to combine it with a glucose-galactose tolerance test. This method makes it possible to distinguish a defect in hydrolysis of lactose from a defect in absorption of one or both of these monosaccharides. Either capillary blood or venous blood may be used for these tests; capillary blood is preferred for field studies. Other techniques that have been used experimentally include the ingestion of radioactive-labeled lactose, a Clinitest based on testing the urine for sugars after ingestion of the lactose load, and the analysis of breath hydrogen at intervals after ingestion of lactose. Many studies have also relied on self-report of symptoms after the ingestion of fluid milk.

The second problem involves sampling. In general, the samples are not random samples of the population and are often opportunistic samples of people presenting with other disorders. Therefore, there may be a bias in favor of higher frequencies of lactose-intolerant individuals in these samples. In addition, the samples tend to be very small, some with as few as three individuals. The mean size of 108 samples listed by Harrison[7] was 68.8 people. However, 47 of the samples had 20 or fewer individuals. Particularly large samples came from Northern Europe. These articles by McCracken[9] and Harrison,[7] in particular, have brought lactose intolerance to the attention of cultural and biological anthropologists. They have also made an impact on applied anthropology, concerning the export of powdered milk and other milk-containing products as part of food-aid programs in the Third World.[52]

Table 10-1 Indicators of Genetic and Cultural Diversity in Lactose Absorption and Dairying

Category and Population Number	Population	Percentage of Lactose Absorbers	Total Milk Consumption (liters/person/year)	Cheese Production as Percent of Milk Production
Category 1	Hunters and Gatherers (traditionally lacking dairy animals)			
1	Eskimo of Greenland	15.1	0.00	—
2	Twa Pygmies of Rwanda	22.7	0.00	—
3	!Kung Bushmen	2.5	0.00	—
4	Bushmen of Botswana	8.0	0.00	—
	Average	12.6		
Category 2	Nondairying Agriculturalists			
5	Toruba	9.0	4.49	15.97
6	Ibo	20.0	4.49	15.97
7	Children in Ghana	27.0	0.64	11.95
8	Bantu of Zaire	1.9	0.23	37.44
9	Hausa	23.5	4.49	15.97
	Average	15.5		
Category 3	Recently Dairying Agriculturalists			
10	Kenyana (mainly Bantu)	26.8	67.51	0.30
11	Bantu of Zambia	0.0	8.78	12.11
12	Bantu of South Africa	9.7	92.11	10.22
13	Shi, Bantu of Lake Kivu Area	3.6	7.32	0.00
14	Ganda, other Bantu of Uganda	5.7	29.81	0.00
	Average	11.9		
Category 4	Milk-Dependent Pastoralists			
15	Arabs of Saudi Arabia	86.4	NA	NA
16	Nima Pastoralists	90.9	NA	NA
17	Tussi Pastoralists in Uganda	88.2	NA	NA
18	Tussi in Congo	100.0	NA	NA
19	Tussi in Rwanda	92.6	NA	NA
	Average	91.3		
Category 5	Dairying Peoples of North Africa and the Mediterranean			
20	Jews in Israel	40.8	203.38	40.09
21	Ashkenazi Jews	20.8	203.38	40.09
22	North African Sephardi	37.5	28.50	10.66
23	Other Sephardi	27.8	120.11	18.00
24	Iraqi Jews	15.8	38.27	38.45
25	Other Oriental Jews	15.0	71.10	33.79
26	Arab Villagers in Israel	19.4	203.58	40.09
27	Syrian Arabs	5.0	80.98	36.23
28	Jordanian Arabs	23.2	15.75	54.29
29	Arabs (Jordan, Syria, Morocco)	0.0	15.75	54.29
30	Other Arabs	19.2	80.98	36.25
31	Egyptian Fellahin	7.1	48.51	54.89

Table 10-1   continued

Category and Population Number	Population	Percentage of Lactose Absorbers	Total Milk Consumption (liters/ person/year)	Cheese Production as Percent of Milk Production
32	Greeks (mostly mainland)	52.1	181.09	48.84
33	Greek Cretans	44.0	181.09	48.84
34	Greek Cypriots	28.4	141.23	56.42
35	Ethiopians/Eritreans	10.3	21.85	5.40
	Average	38.8		
Category 6	Dairying Peoples of Northern Europe			
36	Danes	97.5	1032.82	9.92
37	Swedes	97.8	393.12	24.42
38	Finns	85.1	677.86	8.07
39	Northwest Europeans	87.3	283.32	15.01
40	French	92.9	580.28	21.18
41	Germans from Central Europe	85.5	390.18	23.02
42	Dutch (living in Suriname)	85.7	828.07	13.69
43	Poles (living in Canada)	71.4	516.57	15.37
44	Czechs (living in Canada)	82.4	391.49	20.19
45	Czechs (Bohemia and Moravia)	100.0	391.49	20.19
46	Spaniards	85.3	171.22	19.60
47	North Italians (Ligurians)	70.0	210.93	37.55
	Average	91.5		
Category 7	Groups of "Mixed" Ancestry (dairying and nondairying)			
48	Iru	61.5	29.81	0.00
49	Mutu	49.0	7.32	0.00
50	Mutu/Tussi mixed persons	45.5	7.32	0.00
51	Fulani/Hausa	33.3	4.49	15.97
52	Yoruba/European mixed	55.8	4.49	15.97
53	Nama Hottentots	30.0	81.63	0.01
54	Greenland Eskimo/European mix	62.0	21.56	—
55	Yemen Jews (mixed with Arabs)	55.6	203.58	41.97
56	Skolt Lapps in Finland	39.8	677.57	8.07
57	Mountain Lapps in Finland	62.7	677.57	8.07
58	Fisher Lapps in Finland	74.5	677.57	8.07
59	Mountain/Fisher Lapps	66.3	677.57	8.07
60	Rehoboth Besters	35.0	92.11	10.22
	Average	56.2		
Overall Average (all categories)		62.0*		

*This figure must be used with caution because Northern Europeans are greatly over-represented in the subsample.

Source: Durham WH (in press)[54]

Although we lack exact prevalence data for lactose intolerance, there is clearly an enormous range in lactose-absorbing abilities from 0% to 100% among those populations that have been investigated. There is also a clear geographical relationship between the high prevalence of lactose-intolerant groups in areas historically lacking dairy animals; conversely, adult populations with high levels of lactose tolerance are found in areas with a history of dairying.[10–13,53–55] Simoons[55] has clearly documented these relationships, showing that in the areas of Europe, Northern Asia, and North and South Africa, where domestication of dairy animals exceeds 8,000 to 10,000 years, populations have high levels of lactose tolerance. However, the practice of milking animals may be only 3,000-4,000 years old. It is generally accepted that dairying first developed in the Mesopotamian or Near East area around 3500 BC. Early evidence of milk use exists for the Near East, Egypt, and pastoral peoples of the Sahara earlier than 2000 BC. Spread of the milking habit to Eastern and Southern Africa, however, was delayed until late prehistoric time. Evidence of milking in Europe dates to about 2500 to 1500BC, although there is some evidence which is earlier. In the Indian subcontinent, the first good evidence of milking in Northern India dates from 1500 to 900 BC, spreading only later to South and East India. Southeast Asia and China have remained outside the milking area during most of history. These areas are illustrated in Figure 10-1.

The populations in category 5 in Table 10-1 contradict this positive association between traditional dairying societies and the high frequency of lactose absorption. These groups are primarily found near the equator to 40° north of the equator and include people in North Africa and the Mediterranean areas, such as Jews in Israel, Syrian Arabs, and Greeks. As indicated in Table 10-1, these people generally consume dairy products that are fermented with reduced lactose content. Yogurts, ghee, and cheeses are frequently consumed by these groups. Cheese production, as a percentage of milk, varies from 10% to well over 50% in many of these groups.[54] Therefore, these groups use a high proportion of low-lactose dairy products in their diets.

A number of explanations have been advanced concerning the etiology of lactase deficiency or lactose intolerance. The disease hypothesis suggests the differences in populations are secondary to diseases such as dysentery, protein calorie malnutrition, or the presence of other intestinal diseases or parasites. These conditions would damage the intestinal mucosa and, therefore, lead to lactose malabsorption. Although these malabsorption syndromes are well documented in the literature, they do not account for the widespread variations in lactose tolerance frequencies from population to population. This is particularly true when populations subjected to the same environmental pathogens show tremendous differences in their ability to utilize milk sugar.

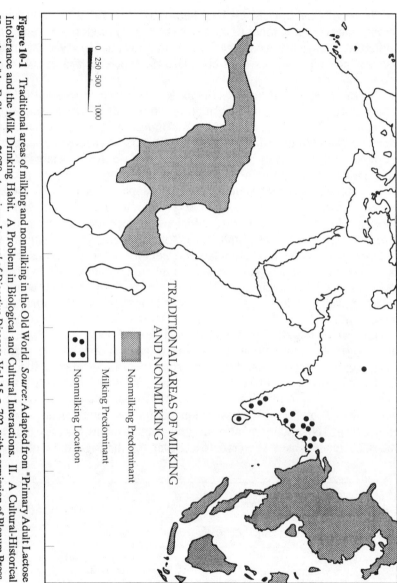

Figure 10-1 Traditional areas of milking and nonmilking in the Old World. *Source:* Adapted from "Primary Adult Lactose Intolerance and the Milk Drinking Habit. A Problem in Biological and Cultural Interactions. II. A Cultural-Historical Hypothesis" by F. Simoons, °1970, *American Journal of Digestive Diseases,* Vol. 15, p. 702, with permission of Plenum Press.

The second hypothesis involves dietary inhibition that holds that some groups may consume foods or drugs (possibly spicy foods or beetlenut) that inhibit lactase activity or damage the intestinal mucosa. However, the authors know of no studies that have correlated lactase deficiency with causal dietary elements.

The third hypothesis involves the induction of lactose production by the continued presentation and consumption of fluid milk. This postweaning and postchildhood consumption of milk would induce lactase activity in the intestine and keep the milk drinker a lactose absorber. However, experimental evidence indicates even prolonged exposure to milk in lactase-deficient subjects does not induce the production of lactase.[7]

The fourth and most widely held and supported hypothesis involves genetic selection for continued lactase production in adulthood. Most authors would contend that lactase sufficiency is dependent on a single gene with possibly three alleles (Table 10-2). Both the homozygous dominant and heterozygous states lead to adult lactose tolerance, whereas the homozygous recessive states can alternatively lead to infantile alactasia or adult lactase deficiency.[7,9,12,54] Individuals with primary congenital alactasia would be selected against unless an alternative low-lactose source to mother's milk were found.

Harrison[7] contends if persons with lactase sufficiency as adults had an average of 1% or more surviving offspring per generation for 400 generations (8,000 years) or approximately the time since the domestication of sheep and goats, the prevalence of lactose malabsorption in the population would decline from 90% to 16%. These percentages are consistent with those found worldwide (Table 10-1). The gene frequency for lactase sufficiency would go from 0.05 to 0.60 in 400 generations, if the selection intensity were 0.01. Thus, the selection intensity required to account for the high rates of lactose

---

Table 10-2 Lactase Deficiency

Single Autosomal Locus with 3 Alleles

Genotypes	Phenotypes
LL, L I_1, L I_2	Normal lactose tolerance
$I_1 I_1$	Primary adult lactase deficiency
$I_2 I_2$	Congenital alactasia
$I_1 I_2$	Lactase deficiency

L—Dominant Allele; I_1, I_2—Recessive Alleles

tolerance among Northern European and other dairying populations is not unreasonable. Furthermore, because populations that have not had historical evidence of the practice of dairying have high prevalences of lactase deficiency, it seems reasonable that the Western pattern of lactase sufficiency developed from the practice of drinking milk and not vice versa.

The question arises as to the exact nature of the selective pressures favoring the maintenance of lactase sufficiency and milk tolerance in adulthood.[54-56] The selective advantage of milk as a food lies not in the fact it is an excellent source of protein, fat, and carbohydrate, but in the fact it is also an excellent source of calcium. Most foods do not contain calcium, although they contain one or more of the other macronutrients. Both vitamin D and lactose enhance calcium absorption. When dietary vitamin D is low or when vitamin D synthesis is reduced because of low sunlight exposure, lactose hydrolysis may facilitate the absorption of calcium and counteract the development of the calcium deficiency diseases, rickets and osteomalacia.

Flatz and Rotthauwe[56] point out that reduced calcium absorption would lead to pelvic deformation among women, affecting their ability to bear children. Therefore, women with adequate calcium absorption would have a favorable reproductive advantage or differential. They would pass on the genes for lactase production to their offspring.

Loomis[57] documents the effects of rickets as a substantial contributor to childhood morbidity and mortality in Northern Europe. Both rickets and osteomalacia increase pelvic deformations and contribute to increased reproductive mortality among females. The ability to drink more milk and absorb more calcium, preventing rickets and osteomalacia, would be particularly advantageous where sunlight is limited as in cloudy Northern Europe. This hypothesis, however, does not account for the high lactose tolerance levels found in some African tropical populations with pastoral traditions or in some groups in the Arabian Peninsula where camel milk is a major source of nutrients.

The general consensus seems to be that the evolutionary hypothesis is correct, although some groups do not fit the model. In summary, it is the lactose-enhanced calcium absorption that has been selected for among humans, as well as in a number of other species. The more widely occurring sugars, such as fructose, glucose, and sucrose, do not show this effect of enhancing calcium absorption or genotrophic adaptations. Thus, there is a specific mechanism for selection favoring genes that enhance adequate calcium absorption when vitamin D is in short supply, either through diet or through endogenous manufacture on exposure to sunlight. Lactose intolerance or lactase deficiency represents one of the premier examples in nutritional anthropology involving the interaction of biological and cultural variables in the production of microevolutionary changes in populations.

ADVERSE REACTIONS TO FOOD ADDITIVES: CHINESE RESTAURANT SYNDROME AS AN EXAMPLE

Medical and nutritional anthropologists have become more concerned with adverse reactions to foods and food additives with the advent of wide distribution of new foodstuffs in developing countries. Many of these foodstuffs have been prepared, processed, and stored under conditions that are not permitted in the United States.

The following are some of the sources of AFR that have been documented and are due to food processing. For example, zinc poisoning can occur in zinc-coated (ie, galvanized) containers, such as pots, cans, and tubes, when their content is acidic (eg, lemonade, cooked apples, spinach, and tomatoes). This converts the zinc into soluble zinc salts. Copper poisoning can occur when copper pipes, containers, and cake decorators are used. Carbonated beverages, highly acidic foods, and cakes decorated with copper bands have been implicated in copper poisoning. Iron poisoning can occur with excessive dietary iron intake from iron pots. This has been found to be associated with beer and wine production.

There are also many instances of incidental and accidental toxic food additives. Among them are a number of insecticides, soil fumigants, rodenticides, detergents, solvents, and other products that are used to cultivate and process foods.[58]

There are a number of intentional food additives that have also been associated with adverse food reactions. Chinese restaurant syndrome has been associated with the ingestion of high quantities of MSG added to foods in Chinese restaurants. MSG is a natural flavoring enhancer. Nitrate poisonings have occurred due to processed meat and fish ingestion. High nitrate intake has also been associated with spinach and other plants when nitrates are used excessively in fertilization. The chemical emulsifier ME18 has been used in margarine and is known to have caused an intolerance referred to as "margarine disease."

Chinese restaurant syndrome was first reported in 1968 by Kwok,[59] who described a peculiar syndrome experienced by himself and other Chinese friends following the consumption of Northern Chinese food in a Chinese restaurant. Symptoms included generalized weakness and numbness behind the neck that radiated down the back and arms.[59] Additional symptoms have been reported, including headache, nausea, and occasionally abdominal pain,[60] as well as sudden tightening and numbness of the face.[61]

Kwok[59] hypothesized the etiology of the syndrome was related to the consumption of monosodium glutamate (MSG) seasoning, used liberally in Chinese restaurants, but not as frequently in private Chinese kitchens.[59] In 1981, Allen and Baker[60] confirmed two incidences of life-threatening asthma were the result of MSG consumption in Chinese restaurants.[60] While the typical Western diet consists of approximately 0.3 g of glutamate daily, up to 5 g are added to Chinese, Japanese, and Southeast Asian cuisine.[60] MSG is also present in bouillon cubes, and free glutamate occurs in mushrooms, tomatoes, and Parmesan cheese.[61]

Kwok[59] argued that Chinese-Americans do not typically prepare their own food with excessive amounts of MSG; in fact, Kwok and his Chinese friends only experienced the MSG-related syndrome in the restaurant environment. It is possible, by means of cultural assimilation, many Asian-Americans lessen the high content of MSG in their daily diet. Perhaps individuals most at risk for experiencing the Chinese restaurant syndrome are restaurant employees, who may regularly consume large quantities of MSG. As this example illustrates, when assessing an individual with questionable symptoms, the clinician should note *where* the food was consumed in addition to what was consumed.

Underwood[62] has suggested MSG sensitivity should be found in greater frequency among non-Asians, who have had recent exposure to MSG, compared to Asians with a long history of MSG use in their cuisine. In order to make the evolutionary argument of natural selection favoring genotypes with reduced MSG sensitivity or increased resistance to Chinese restaurant syndrome, a direct or indirect link must be made between MSG sensitivity and differential fertility. Hypersensitivity to MSG could lead to neurological disruptions and, hence, reduced fertility, so individuals with reduced sensitivity would have greater reproductive success. MSG hypersensitivity may have exerted a selection pressure favoring less sensitive individuals. This hypothesis needs to be tested.

FOOD HABITS AND ALLERGIES

Many anthropologists, as well as psychologists and nutritionists, have been interested in food-habit research. Lévi-Strauss in *Totem and Taboo*,[63] and Douglas,[64-65] in particular, have focused on the ideological and structural components of food preferences and aversions, while Marvin Harris and other materialists have focused on ecological and economic factors that govern food choices.[66,67] Although there are abundant anthropological data on food habits, very few studies have focused on the relationship between food avoidances and ideological prohibitions on food use and food allergies. One interesting study by Fischer et al[68] looked at the relationship between totems and allergy in the Caroline Islands in the South Pacific. They state potentially allergenic foods are chosen as totems, and allergies become activated by guilt over taboo violations. There is a common belief in many parts of Polynesia that eating one's totems causes skin disorders. On the island of Ponape, matrilineal clans and subclans have animal totems. These animals are often believed to have assisted an ancestor. These tabooed totem animals include shark, freshwater eel, and sting ray. In addition to the taboos on matriclan totem eating, many men and women indicate they will not eat their father's clan's totem. In some instances, the father's mother's clan's totem was considered to be even more dangerous to eat than one's own totem. Violating the totemic taboo in Ponape represents forbidden behavior toward a blood relative or close family. These feelings can be so strong, one informant reported, eating his father's totem fish was comparable to an act of sibling incest.

The consequences of eating tabooed foods vary from prenatal deformities from eating small bananas, deformed breadfruit, and runts of dog and pig litters to allergic symptoms with the violation of the eel and turtle taboo. Violations of fish totems often include the following symptoms: vomiting, headaches, swelling, and skin spots.

However, many people indicate they violate both their own totem and their father's matrilineal totem taboos in their consumption of foods. One man indicated he began to eat the totem animal because of food shortages during World War II, but has since continued to eat the animal in spite of the availability of other foods. The tabooed totems that are reported to cause allergic symptoms, namely fish and shellfish, are also those that cause symptoms in a number of other societies in which these animals are not tabooed. The authors then explain in psychoanalytic terms the association between psychological factors, namely guilt about violating prohibitions, and the production of allergic symptoms.[68] It is unfortunate not more anthropologists have been interested in pursuing these topics. We know very little about the epidemiology of allergy disease and the sociocultural, psychological, and biomedical contexts of food aversions and preferences.

As illustrated in the foregoing example, the psychodynamics of food selection involves both biomedical, as well as sociocultural, issues. Numerous variables have been examined in their relationship to food likes, preferences, and use.[69–71] Rozin, a psychologist at the University of Pennsylvania, has had a significant impact on the thinking of anthropologists concerning food preferences and aversions. The focus of his research has been primarily psychobiological, in which he has demonstrated a strong aversion to foods based on the coupling of distressful physiological effects, most notably nausea and vomiting, and its association with a particular food. He also has shown that in spite of physiological distress, such as the burning sensation accompanying the ingestion of chili peppers, individuals will tolerate and even enjoy this discomfort because eating hot chili peppers is a psychosocial marker of achieved adulthood. He also postulates the possibility of neuroendocrine responses in the release of pain-reducing endorphins in response to the burning distress of eating chili peppers.[69-71] Clearly, adverse reactions to foods based on toxic effects, enzyme deficiency, or allergic immune system responses are not always sufficient to ensure avoidance.

The assumption has been that food use reflects food preferences.[71] However, a number of sociocultural factors, particularly accessibility and economic considerations, can limit the use of foods that are preferred or liked. Furthermore, foods that are well liked may be avoided because of their association with health or religious ideology.

For example, there are the well-known religious prohibitions for Hindus concerning the consumption of beef and Moslems and Jews concerning the consumption of pork. The prohibition on pork consumption has been explained in terms of health (ie, trichinosis), economic, and ecological factors, but not allergic responses.[65-67] Other foods are not prohibited all the time, but may be avoided only under special conditions. The humoral (or hot and cold) theory of medicine in Haiti restricts the consumption of "cold" foods during the "hot" postpartum period, which may last up to three months.[72] The new mother must avoid foods such as pork, banana, sweet potato, and citrus fruits.[72] The anthropological literature has detailed descriptions of mediconutritional systems, yet no anthropologists to our knowledge have examined these systems of beliefs and behaviors in terms of allergy disease or adverse food reactions.

A Dietetic Practitioner's Guide to Cultural Beliefs, Attitudes, and Behaviors Concerning Food Allergies and Adverse Reactions

Dietitians encounter clients with different ethnic backgrounds, particularly in locations with new immigrants. Their exposure to new foodstuffs and new preparation and storage practices can lead to an increase in adverse reactions to food or food contaminants among foreign-born clients and their children. Special communication problems arise whenever the dietitian and client are of different ethnic backgrounds. In addition, age, gender, and socioeconomic status differences may present cultural barriers to communication even among individuals of the same racial or ethnic group.[73]

Appropriate communication with sensitivity to the ethnic beliefs, attitudes, and behaviors of the client is important in both diagnostic and therapeutic interactions and is vital in obtaining an accurate medical and dietary history. Because culture influences both the channels of communication and the content of the messages, it is important to be aware of your own, as well as your clients', cultural background. For example, eye-to-eye contact is important for Caucasian-Americans, but may be unacceptable for Hispanic-

and African-Americans, particularly if there is a status difference between speakers. While speaking, Anglos look away more frequently than blacks, but the opposite is true for listening behavior.[73] Because both verbal and nonverbal messages are filtered between two cultural screens, that of the dietitian and of the client, the intended message may be misinterpreted. Cross-cultural communication problems can lead to a lack of adherence to therapeutic diets or other prescribed changes in food-related behavior.[74]

A number of guidelines should be followed in establishing productive client-health provider interaction. These guidelines pertain not only to interactions with minority clients, but are applicable in all situations where medical information is being ascertained and therapeutic recommendations are being made. First, it is extremely important for the health care provider to establish a trusting and supportive relationship with the client. This demonstrates an interest in the patient and not simply an interest in the disease. Your manner should be warm and emphatic, conveying confidence and a knowledge of food-related allergies. A sense of hope and optimism should also be conveyed. Two of the attractive elements in traditional therapeutic encounters involve the trusting and friendly nature of the relationship, as well as the fact that the two individuals share a common knowledge. Both of these elements may be missing in interactions in the large and impersonal health settings in the United States. Therefore, it is most important to try to establish this relationship while obtaining information about the patient's health, dietary belief system, and behaviors. These data will be relevant to a successful therapeutic intervention. If you are not aware of the patient's belief system, then a series of questions can be used to ascertain the patient's conceptions about disease causality, problem priorities, and appropriate treatments.

Another hallmark of traditional medical encounters involves the use of the social support system and the family of the patient. The dietitian or nutritionist should, when possible, involve other family members, particularly if there is a major dietary change to be made. Because of language barriers, reading difficulty, and problems ensuing from more conceptually complex issues, often younger members of the family who have learned English in school will act as interpreters for older family members. Health care providers should be sensitive to any issues involving breach of appropriate interactions between the age and sex groups within this family context.

Because the avoidance of foods that cause adverse reactions is the primary and ongoing intervention, members of the family and/or the patient will have to be instructed in self-monitoring, including the ability to read package labels and ask about prepared foods or foods served in restaurants. You should provide lists of foods and products that may contain the foods or additives that are to be avoided. The use of exercises in reading labels and other ways of testing comprehension of the required dietary changes should be instituted in a friendly and helpful manner. If the proposed dietary changes will cause unpleasant side effects (for example, gas, constipation, diarrhea, changes in the taste of foods), then the dietitian should clearly explain what these side effects will be and how to offset them. You should ascertain the patient's view of the severity and implications of these side effects and whether or not there are traditional medicines that could be used to counteract these unpleasant effects.

Patient-related factors that will aid in adherence to new dietary behaviors should be assessed. Do the patient and his or her family understand these dietary changes, and can they carry them out in terms of access to the appropriate substitute foods? Will these changes create any family instability or disharmony regarding the types of foods that are prepared and served? Are there resources available to provide the appropriate foods and knowledge of the appropriate preservation and preparation techniques? Health care personnel often make assumptions that the environment is supportive of changes. However, the dietitian or nutritionist should carefully assess the probability of adherence to diets in the cultural setting of the patient or client. As much as possible, the client should be involved in planning and implementing the dietary change program and customizing the diets to follow the dietary behaviors and mediconutritional belief patterns. Changes should be simplified, yet achieve their effective end, and changes should be integrated into the lifestyle of the client.

The basic rule of effective patient-provider interactions is the more that is known about a patient's health, dietary beliefs, daily lifestyle, and patterns of behavior, the more effective and appropriate the dietary change effort will be, regardless of the patient's ethnicity. It is also important to keep in mind that although various ideological systems structure food choices, individual choice creates a great deal of latitude within the diets of members of all ethnic groups. Intraethnic variation is created by individual preferences and aversions.

A patient's mediconutritional beliefs and practices must be assessed with regard to food allergies and sensitivities. In many traditional medical systems, the balance of various elements is most important; when this is violated, good health is jeopardized. Fortunately, food ideological systems include a recognition of the relationship between food and particular symptoms of illness. Most of these systems also provide a therapeutic basis for intervening with appropriate food choices. In developing elimination diets, the nutritionist or dietitian must be aware of the appropriate categories of foods and their use within the individual's mediconutritional system.

Meichenbaum and Turk[75] suggest a number of questions for eliciting a patient's explanatory model of illness. For effective therapeutic interaction, it is important to understand the patient's mediconutritional model. The etiology can be assessed by questions such as "what do you call your problem?" and "what do you think has caused your problem?" It is also important to note the time and mode of onset of symptoms: "why do you think it started when it did?" with the ingestion of a particular food or a particular event. Pathophysiology might be assessed with such questions as "what does your sickness do to you?" and "how does it work?" The course of the illness, including the severity, could be assessed with "how severe are your symptoms when you ingest food x?" "how long do these symptoms last?" and "what are the chief problems that your food sensitivity has caused you?" In assessing treatment ideology, the dietitian or nutritionist may wish to ask "what kind of treatment do you think you should receive?" and "what are the most important results you expect from treatment?" In many cases of food aversions and sensitivity, avoidance of the food is the primary therapeutic advice. However, the client may need to have special dietary recommendations that are more complicated, as well as instructions in the use of medication.

Although diet therapy and herbal remedies are widely used across different ethnic groups, diet therapy plays a more important role in some ethnic groups than others. Many ethnic groups see dietary control as an integral part of good medical care. For example, among Hispanics, Asians, and Italians, theories of disease contain specific postulates about diet (for example, hot and cold, yin and yang, wet and dry theories, respectively).[76] Herbal remedies may be replaced by or used in conjunction with over-the-counter and prescription medicines (including the use of antihistamines and steroids for the control of allergic symptoms).

The dietitian or nutritionist should assess what kinds of dietary practices are currently in use. For example, if a mother suspects that her child may be allergic to milk, and herbal teas are then substituted for cow's milk-based formula, then the nutritionist should make appropriate recommendations for a more nutritious, but nonallergenic, substitute. The use of appropriate herbal teas may be encouraged along with the use of a new formula or breast milk. In short, awareness of culturally preferred modes of treatment and the inclusion of these behaviors when applicable can lead to increased compliance to standard dietary regimens.

Ethnically acceptable diets for allergies should reflect the ethnic food preferences of an individual. Therefore, diet lists of admissible foods should contain items that are typical to a particular ethnic cuisine and are acceptable substitutes for proscribed customary foods. Alternative methods of food preparation may also be included. Once there is agreement that a particular food or food substance is causing the undesirable symptoms, then alternatives should be selected among those that are appropriate both from a therapeutic perspective and the perspective of the patient. For example, a Puerto Rican mother may attribute her baby's rash to overconsumption of infant formula, which is classified as hot in the hot and cold system. In her attempts to restore balance to the baby, she will give the baby substances classified as cool, such as barley water, magnesium carbonate, or mannitol, or may switch to cow's milk. Cow's milk clearly would be contraindicated if the child is allergic to the cow's milk-based formulas. If possible, nursing should be recommended. If the patient adheres to the hot and cold system of classification, the dietitian or nutritionist should encourage the use of barley water and discourage the use of magnesium carbonate (a cathartic) or mannitol (a diuretic).[76,77] Soy-based formulas might be substituted, although recent evidence indicates many infants are also allergic to the soy proteins.[78]

Puerto Ricans and Other Hispanic-Americans

Very little has been written in the medical anthropology literature on the relationship between nutrition and allergies. In studies among Puerto Ricans, allergies have been ranked as a condition of high concern for populations in both Miami and New York.[76] While allergic symptoms tend to be reported more frequently for higher socioeconomic subgroups, the incidence of asthma has been reported more frequently for Puerto Ricans in the lower socioeconomic stratum.

Harwood[76,78] has written extensively on Puerto Rican health practices. He indicates that although the hot and cold theory is part of the culture repertoire of Puerto Ricans, Mexican-Americans, and Spanish-heritage Caribbean and Latin American populations, individuals vary in the degree to which they give credence to these theories. Even if they subscribe to the theory of a hot and cold dichotomy of diseases, food, and medications, individuals may classify these domains differently. Therefore, the nutritionist or dietitian must ascertain the belief system and behaviors of individual clients. You may state something such as "some of my patients say that blank (a food) or blank (a medicine) is either hot or cold. What do you think?"[74] Based on this information, the nutritionist or dietitian should propose dietary changes that are appropriate within the hot and cold framework.

For example, the typical diet of a Puerto Rican family contains milk and dairy products, particularly cheese, cereal grains, and eggs. Rice is traditionally an important part of the diet, and if gluten sensitivity is noted, rice substitutions can be made for wheat-based products. Milk and dairy products will be more difficult to replace if a true allergy exists. If lactose intolerance is a problem, then the dietitian might encourage cheese consumption over the consumption of fluid milk.

Tonics are considered to be a healthful part of the diet and recommended for children. These may be commercially manufactured or may be made at home as a type of eggnog. Again, if there is a sensitivity to eggs or milk, this type of tonic will have to be avoided and other tonics substituted. Because fruit juices are frequently consumed by both children and adults, they may be an appropriate substitute.

One of the potential areas of conflict in the etiology of allergies comparing the Western medical system to the hot and cold classification is that rashes, urticaria, and allergy-related eczema are considered to be hot, whereas asthma and other upper respiratory symptoms are considered to be cold. Therefore, these two sets of symptoms would be treated differently, and priority would have to be given to one set over the other.

Chinese and Other Asian-Americans

Among Chinese and other Asian groups a hot and cold system, conceptualized as yin and yang, exists. These two elements are complementary, and a balance must be achieved in the intake of particular foods to maintain health. As in the Hispanic classification system, a person's predisposition, constitution, and emotional and natural physiological states may also be classified as hot or cold.

Among Chinese-Americans, Koo[79] reports the notion of poison is very similar to the notion of allergy. Poison is a concept in traditional Chinese medicine, whereas allergy is a concept in modern Western medicine that has been adopted by Chinese-Americans. These concepts generally relate to foods that are considered to be irritating foods, causing a wide variety of undesirable symptoms.

The traditional Chinese diet is devoid of most dairy products; therefore, one does not see the typical children's allergies to milk. However, with acculturation, cow's milk and cheese have been added to the diet of Chinese-American children. These may cause an allergic response, as well as a response to the lactose content. Wheat intolerance may also be high because some areas of China have only recently adopted wheat cultivation. If there is an allergy to soy and soy products, it will be more difficult to eliminate these from the traditional Oriental diet. Soy sauce, as well as the bean curd and soy milk, may need to be eliminated from the diet, thereby removing both good sources of protein and a traditional flavoring component.[80] If an individual is found to be intolerant of soybean products, then the family should be alerted to the presence of soybean oils in prepared foods, as well as in such unlikely foods as soy oil-packed tuna fish. (Note: Soybean oil may not be a problem for soy-sensitive individuals. See discussion in Chapter 9.) In addition, many fishes are consumed, as well as fermented in fish sauce. Fermented products may lead to adverse food reactions in some people. The extensive use of MSG has been discussed previously and generally is not a problem among Orientals. Chinese herbal medicines and teas are frequently consumed, and the dietitian will want to inquire specifically about these traditional medicines.

SUMMARY

It is important to ascertain the food practices and food belief system of each client and particularly those of various ethnic groups. Ethnically specific diets should be developed and made available to physicians and dietitians. There is an abundant literature on dietary habits, mediconutritional beliefs, and practices for minority populations in the United States.[81-83] Unfortunately, little, if any, of the information has been used to develop appropriate therapeutic prescriptions for minority clients with allergies or food intolerances. The authors hope this chapter will serve as a catalyst for a more extensive and vigorous use of anthropological materials by nutritionists and dietitians and as an inspiration for anthropologists to pursue research on food allergies and adverse food reactions.

REFERENCES

1. National Academy of Food Sciences, Committee on Food Habits. *The Problem of Changing Food Habits.* Washington: National Academy of Food Sciences; 1943. National Research Council Bulletin No. 108, 1943.

2. Ackerknecht EH. Paleopathology. In: Kroeber AL, ed. *Anthropology Today.* Chicago: University of Chicago Press; 1953: 120–126.

3. Brothwell DR, Sandison AT. *Disease in Antiquity: A Survey of Diseases, Injuries and Surgery of Early Populations.* Springfield, Ill: Charles C Thomas, Publishers; 1967.

4. Cockburn TA. Infectious diseases in ancient populations. *Current Anthro.* 1971; 12:45–62.

5. Galway K, Wolff B, Sturgis R. *Child Survival Risks and the Road to Health.* Columbia, MD: Institute for Resource Development; 1987.

6. Corruccini RS, Kaul SS. The epidemiological transition and anthropology of minor chronic non-infectious diseases. *Med Anthro.* 1983; 7:36–50.

7. Harrison GG. Primary adult lactase deficiency: A problem in anthropological genetics. *Am Anthro.* 1975; 77:812–835.

8. Kretchmer N. Lactose and lactase. *Sci American.* 1972; 227(4):70–78.

9. McCracken RD. Lactase deficiency: An example of dietary evolution. *Current Anthro.* 1971; 12: 479–517.

10. Simoons FJ. Primary adult lactose intolerance and the milking habit: A problem in biological and cultural interrelations. I. Review of the medical research. *Am J Digest Dis.* 1969; 14:819–836.

11. Simoons FJ. Primary adult lactose intolerance and the milking habit: A problem in biological and cultural interactions. II. A cultural-historical hypothesis. *Am J Digest Dis.* 1970; 15:695–710.

12. Simoons FJ. The determinance of dairying and milk use in the Old World ecological, physiological, and cultural. *Ecol Food Nutr.* 1973; 2:83–90.

13. Simoons FJ. Dairying, milk use, and lactose malabsorption in Eurasia: A problem in cultural history. *Anthropos.* 1979; 74:61–80.

14. Godfrey RC. Asthma and IgE levels in rural and urban communities of The Gambia. *Clin Allergy.* 1975; 5:201–207.

15. Merrett TG, Merrett J, Cookson JB. Allergy and parasites: The measurement of total and specific IgE levels in urban and rural communities in Rhodesia. *Clin Allergy.* 1976; 6:131–134.

16. Johansson SGO, Mellbin T, Vahlquist B. Immunoglobulin levels in Ethiopian pre-school children with special reference to high concentrations of immunoglobulin E (IgND). *Lancet.* 1968; 1:1118–1121.

17. Aas K, Jebson JW. Studies of hypersensitivity to fish. partial purification and crystallization of a major allergenic component of cod. *Int Arch Allergy Appl Immunol.* 1967; 32:1–20.

18. Bazaral M, Orgel HA, Hamburger RN. The influence of serum IgE levels of selected recipients, including patients with allergy, helminthiasis and tuberculosis, on the apparent P-K titre of a reaginic serum. *Clin Exp Immunol.* 1973; 14:117–125.

19. Massicot JG, Cohen SG. Epidemiologic and socioeconomic aspects of allergic diseases. *J Allergy Clin Immunol.* 1986; 78(5, pt. 2):954–958.

20. Warrell DA, Fawcett IW, Harrison BDW, et al. Bronchial asthma in the Nigerian savanna region. *Quart J Med.* 1975;44:325–347.

21. Roitt IM, Brostoff J, Male DK. *Immunology.* St Louis: CV Mosby Co; 1989.

22. Gordon K. Evolutionary perspectives on human diet. In: Johnston FE, ed. *Nutritional Anthropology.* New York: Alan R. Liss; 1987: 3–37.

23. Dunn FL. Epidemiological factors: Health and disease in hunter-gatherers. In: Logan M, Hunt E, eds. *Health and the Human Condition. Perspectives on Medical Anthropology.* N. Scituate, MA: Duxbury Press; 1978: 107–118.

24. Polgar S. Evolution and the ills of mankind. In: Tax S, ed. *Horizons of Anthropology.* Chicago: Aldine; 1964: 200–211.

25. Armelagos GJ. Disease in ancient Nubia. *Science.* 1969;163: 255–259.

26. Cohen MN, Armelagos GJ, eds. *Paleopathology at the Origins of Agriculture.* New York: Academic Press; 1984.

27. Johansson SGO, Yman L. *In vitro* assays for Immunoglobulin E. *Clin Rev Allergy.* 1988; 6:93–139.

28. Pearson DJ. Food allergy, hypersensitivity and intolerance. *J Royal Coll London.* 1985; 19 (3):154–162.

29. Tuchinda M, Habanananda S, Vareenil J, Srimaruta N, Piromrat K. Asthma in Thai children: a study of 2000 cases. *Ann Allergy.* 1987; 59:207–211.

30. Moneret-Vautrin DA. Food antigens and additives. *J Allergy Clin Immunol.* 1986; 78 (5, pt. 2):1039–1046.

31. Committee on Food Protection, Food and Nutrition Board, National Research Council. *Toxicants Occurring Naturally in Foods.* 2nd ed. Washington, DC: National Academy of Sciences; 1973.

32. Bryan FL. Infections due to miscellaneous microorganisms. In: Riemann H, ed. *Food-Borne Infections and Intoxications.* New York, Academic Press; 1969: 224–290.

33. Uragoda CG, Kottegoda SR. Adverse reactions to isoniazid on ingestion of fish with a high histamine content. *Tubercle.* 1977; 58:83–89.

34. Wood CBS. How common is food allergy? *Acta Paediatr Scand.* 1986; 323(suppl): 76–83.

35. Belsey MA. The epidemiology of favism. *Bull World Health Org.* 1973; 48:1–13.

36. Bottini E, Lucarelli P, Agostino R, Palmarino R, Businco L, Antognoni G. Favism: Association with erythrocyte acid phosphatase phenotype. *Science.* 1971; 171:409–411.

37. Huheey JE, Martin DL. Malaria, favism and glucose-6-phosphate dehydrogenase deficiency. *Experientia.* 1975; 31:1145-1147.

38. Katz SH. Fava bean consumption: A case for the co-evolution of genes and culture. In: Harris M, Ross EB, eds. *Food and Evolution: Toward a Theory of Human Food Habits.* Philadelphia: Temple University Press; 1987: 133-159.

39. Luckmann J, Sorensen KC. *Medical-Surgical Nursing: A Psychophysiologic Approach.* 2nd ed. Philadelphia: WB Saunders Co; 1980.

40. Katz SH. Food, behavior and biocultural evolution. In: Barker LM, ed. *The Psychobiology of Human Food Selection.* Westport, CT: AVI; 1982: 171–188.

41. Katz SH, Schall JI. Fava bean consumption and biocultural evolution. *Med Anthro.* 1979; 3:459–476.

42. Bienzle U, Ayeni O, Lucas AO, Luzzatto L. Glucose-6-phosphate dehydrogenase and malaria. *Lancet.* 1972; 1:107–110.

43. Andrews AC. The bean and Indo-European totemism. *Am Anthro.* 1949; 51:274-292.

44. Strober W. Genetic and anthropologic factors in gluten-sensitive enteropathy. *Am J Phys Anthro.* 1983; 62:119–126.

45. Lessof MH. Food intolerance. *Proc Nutr Soc.* 1985; 44:121–125.

46. Saavedra-Delgado AM, Metcalfe DD. Interactions between food antigens and the immune system in the pathogenesis of gastrointestinal diseases. *Ann Allergy.* 1985; 55:694–702.

47. Simoons FJ. Celiac disease as a geographic problem. In: Walcher DN, Kretchmer N, eds. *Food, Nutrition and Evolution.* New York: Masson Publishers; 1981: 179–199.

48. McNicholl B, Egan-Mitchell B, Stevens FM, et al. History, genetics, and natural history of celiac disease gluten enteropathy. In: Walcher DN, Kretchmer N, eds. *Food, Nutrition and Evolution.* New York: Masson Publishers; 1981: 169–177.

49. Parker SL, Sussman GL, Krondl M. Dietary aspects of adverse reactions to foods in adults. *Can Med Assoc J.* 1988; 139:711–718.

50. Mylotte M, Egan-Mitchell B, McCarthy CF, McNicholl B. Coeliac disease in the west of Ireland. *Br Med J.* 1973 (1 Sept.):498–499. Letter.

51. O'Reilly D, Murphy J, McLaughlin J, Bradshaw J, Dean G. The prevalence of coeliac disease and cystic fibrosis in Ireland, Scotland, and England and Wales. *Int J Epidem.* 1974; 3:247–251.

52. Clein NW. Cow's milk allergy in infants. *Pediatr Clin North Am.* 1954; 1: 949–962.

53. Friedl J. Lactase deficiency distribution, associated problems and implications for nutritional policy. *Ecol Food Nutr.* 1981; 11:37–48.

54. Durham WH. Cultural mediation and adult lactose absorption. In: *Coevolution: Genes, Culture, and Human Diversity.* Stanford: Stanford University Press. In press.

55. Simoons FJ. The geographic hypothesis and lactose malabsorption: A weighing of the evidence. *Am J Dig Dis.* 1978; 23:963–980.

56. Flatz G, Rotthauwe HW. Lactose, nutrition and natural selection. *Lancet.* 1973; 2:76–77.

57. Loomis WF. Skin-pigment regulation of vitamin D biosynthesis in man. *Science.* 1967; 157:501–506.

58. Bryan FL. *Appendix Diseases Transmitted by Foods: A Classification and Summary.* Atlanta, US Dept Health and Human Services, Centers for Disease Control, HHS publication no. (CDC)81-8237, 1981.

59. Kwok RHM. Chinese restaurant syndrome. *N Engl J Med* 1968; 278:796. Letter.

60. Allen DH, Baker GJ. Chinese-restaurant asthma. *N Engl J Med* 1981; 305 (19):1154–1155. Letter.

61. Kenney RA, Tidball CS. Human susceptibility to oral monosodium L-glutamate. *Am J Clin Nutr.* 1972; 25: 140–146.

62. Underwood JH. *Biocultural Interactions and Human Variation.* Dubuque, IA: Wm C Brown Co; 1975.

63. Lévi-Strauss C. *The Raw and Cooked: Introduction to the Science of Mythology,* I. Chicago: University of Chicago Press; 1969.

64. Douglas M. *Purity and Danger.* London: Routledge and Kegan Paul; 1966.

65. Douglas M, Gross J. Food and culture: Measuring the intricacy of rule systems. *Soc Sci Info.* 1981; 20:1–35.

66. Harris M. *Good to Eat: Riddles of Food and Culture.* New York: Simon and Schuster; 1985.

67. Harris M, Ross E. *Food and Evolution toward a Theory of Human Food Habits.* Philadelphia: Temple University Press; 1987.

68. Fischer J, Fischer A, Mahony F. Totemism and allergy. *Int J Soc Psychiatry.* 1959; 5:33–40.

69. Rozin P. Human food selection: The interaction of biology, culture and individual experience. In: Barker LM, ed. *Psychobiology of Human Food Selection.* Westport, CT: AVI Press; 1981: 181–205.

70. Rozin P, Fallon AE. Psychological categorization of foods and non-foods: A preliminary taxonomy of food rejections. *Appetite.* 1980; 1:193–201.

71. Rozin P. Psychobiological perspectives on food preferences and avoidances. In: Harris M, Ross EB, eds. *Food and Evolution toward a Theory of Human Food Habits.* Philadelphia: Temple University Press; 1987: 181–205.

72. Wiese JC. Maternal nutrition and traditional food behavior in Haiti. *Human Org.* 1976; 35(2):193–200.

73. Atkinson DR, Morton G, Sue DW. *Counseling American Minorities: A Cross-Cultural Perspective.* 3rd ed. Dubuque, Ia: Wm C Brown; 1989.

74. Lieberman LS. Cultural sensitivity and problems of interethnic communication. *Direct Appl Nutr.* 1987; 1(1):6–7.

75. Meichenbaum D, Turk DC. *Facilitating Treatment Adherence: A Practitioner's Guidebook.* New York: Plenum Press; 1987.

76. Harwood A, ed. *Ethnicity and Medical Care.* Cambridge, MA: Harvard University Press; 1981.

77. Anderson JA, Sogen DD. *Adverse Reactions to Food.* Washington, DC: National Institute of Allergy and Infectious Diseases; 1984. US Dept Health and Human Services NIH 84-2442.

78. Harwood A. The hot-cold theory of disease-implications for treatment of Puerto Rican patients. *JAMA.* 1971; 216:1153-1158.

79. Koo CL. *Nourishment in Life: The Culture of Health in Traditional China.* Berkeley, Calif: Anthropology Dept, University of California; 1976. Thesis.

80. Rozin E. *The Flavor Principle Cookbook.* New York: Hawthorn; 1973.

81. Newman JM. *Melting Pot: An Annotated Bibliography and Guide to Food and Nutrition Information for Ethnic Groups in America.* New York: Garland Pub, Inc; 1986.

82. Wilson CS. Food habits: A selected annotated bibliography on sociocultural and biocultural aspects of nutrition. *J Nutr Educ.* 1973; 5(1)(suppl 1):38–72.

83. Wilson CS. Food—Custom and nurture: An annotated bibliography on sociocultural and biocultural aspects of nutrition. *J Nutr Educ.* 1979; 11(4)(suppl 1):212–264.

Chapter 11

Controversies in Food Allergy and Adverse Reactions

Judy E. Perkin

Because food allergy and adverse reactions to food are the subjects of genuine scientific controversy and inquiry, this area is also a fertile one for those promoting unproven etiologies, diagnostic techniques, and therapies.[1-4] The first chapter provided insight into the difficulty associated with terminology—ie, food allergy (immunologically mediated) versus adverse food reactions (nonimmunologically mediated with, in many instances, unknown mechanisms). Dr. Jordan Fink, past president of the American Academy of Allergy and Immunology, has estimated only a small percentage of the US population suffers from immunologically mediated food allergy. Yet despite this low number, a large variety of ills have been associated with foods and often in conjunction with the term "food allergy."[1]

Not only is allergy sometimes an inappropriate diagnosis, but controversial and unproven techniques for allergy diagnosis abound.[5] Problems in this area have been reviewed in Chapter 2, Part I. The present chapter covers areas of controversy not previously addressed or only briefly addressed.

CLINICAL ECOLOGY

Clinical ecology is an approach advocated by a subset of the medical and health community. The clinical ecology model promotes the theory that there are stress factors in the environment that can cause problems over time when low-level exposures to environmental antigens occur. The model also indicates changes in exposure may affect clinical symptoms and severity and that sensitivity to one or more environmental agents may induce sensitivity to others. Synthetic chemicals in foods and elsewhere are environmental factors considered to be important by clinical ecologists.[3,6-8] Diagnoses given by clinical ecologists (as outlined by Barrett) include total allergy syndrome, cerebral allergy, environmental illness, and 20th century disease.[3]

Clinical ecologists believe environmental sensitivity symptoms may occur in all parts of the body.[6] Clinical manifestations are reported to include altered intellectual functioning, asthma, bloating, constipation, cramps, diarrhea, drowsiness, eczema, fatigue, memory loss, irritability, headache, pain in the muscles and joints, mood alterations, nasal problems (congestion and running), frequent urination, itching of the nose and eyes, sneezing, swelling, tingling in the arms and legs, dark eye circles, and schizophrenia.[3,6] The major diagnostic test used by clinical ecologists is provocation and neutralization, a technique not considered standard by the medical community as a whole.[3]

Alteration of the diet is usually a component of clinical ecology therapy. The Executive Committee of the American Academy of Allergy and Immunology[7] has described dietary plans as being very limited in terms of food types allowed in many instances. Rotation of foods at 3- to 5-day intervals may be advocated, and avoidance of synthetic food chemicals may be attempted through avoidance of foods with artificial additives, such as flavorings or colorings.[7,8] Mold or yeast avoidance may also be suggested.[8] Food antigens in low doses may be given as part of neutralization treatment.[7,8] Vitamin and mineral supplementation may or may not be used.[8] The potentially restrictive nature of the diets that may be prescribed for patients by some clinical ecologists should be of concern to dietitians.

Terr,[8] in 1986, reviewed the cases of 50 patients who had been diagnosed by clinical ecologists as having environmental illness. Eight of the 50 were said to have no ascertainable clinical symptoms. Among the 50, no common pattern of laboratory or physical findings could be noted. Symptoms also did not appear to be related to duration of exposure. Terr[8] concluded his review of patients did not support the validity of clinical ecology and cautioned that use of this model could be associated with production of unreasonable patient fear and induce changes in living patterns that are unnecessarily restrictive.

Brodsky[9] conducted psychiatric evaluations of eight patients treated by clinical ecologists. Patients had diagnoses related to environmental illness or some form of chemical hypersensitivity. Common elements could be identified for these patients. Examples of these elements included gradual onset of symptoms, a history of unsubstantiated physical problems, a history of extensive searches for a physician who would provide a diagnosis of physical illness, and avoidances (as a part of treatment) that were life-changing. Brodsky[9] concluded that use of a clinical ecology practitioner would seem to appeal to individuals with chronic problems of a psychiatric nature. Stewart and Raskin,[10] after studying 18 patients, also concluded that patients with the clinical ecology diagnosis of 20th century disease were likely in actuality to have psychiatric problems.

Until more information is available, the clinical ecology approach remains unproven. Some patients who are following these treatments may be at risk both medically and nutritionally. Patients treated in this mode are best informed of its experimental nature.[7]

CANDIDIASIS HYPERSENSITIVITY

Candida albicans (commonly known as "yeast") is a fungus that normally resides in the human body, particularly the vagina, mouth, and gastrointestinal tract.[3] The *Candida* fungus can be infective in certain conditions. Some also believe it can be allergenic.[11-15] The Executive Committee of the American Academy of Allergy and Immunology[11] has stated that evidence supporting the existence of the candidiasis hypersensitivity syndrome leaves the diagnosis as yet unproven. The committee considers the diagnosis and treatment of candidiasis hypersensitivity to be experimental.

The idea that *Candida* can be an allergen is not new. Liebeskind[12] described 25 cases given this diagnosis in a 1962 report. Recent advocates of the idea that *Candida* hypersensitivity can exist have been Truss and Crook. Crook's book entitled *The Yeast Connection* has presented the concept to the public.[14]

Symptoms of candidiasis sensitivity are said to be multiple and may include constipation, diarrhea, bloating, fatigue, irritability, pain in the musculoskeletal system, skin problems (urticaria, psoriasis), mental problems (anxiety, depression), weight gain, impotence, infertility, and cystitis.[13] Kroker[15] has stated each *Candida* strain may contain 30 to 35 antigens, with polysaccharides on the cell surface being the major antigens present.

Dietary restrictions and nutritional supplements may be prescribed as part of the treatment for candidiasis hypersensitivity, and Kroker[15] has stated that dietary alteration is the major component of therapy. The diet prescribed is generally low in carbohydrate with variance in levels established for individual patients. Some patients are advised to avoid refined sugars, syrups, fruit juices, and milk. Others may be limited to a daily intake of 60 to 80 g of carbohydrate. Children may not be placed on carbohydrate restrictions. Kroker[15] has indicated carbohydrate cravings are characteristic of candidiasis hypersensitivity patients. The rationale for dietary restriction is that carbohydrates are considered the major nutrient source for the organism.

Yeast may or may not be restricted in the diets of those said to suffer from this malady. A diet incorporating both carbohydrate and yeast restriction may, however, be prescribed.[15]

The popularity of candidiasis hypersensitivity as a diagnosis has spawned the marketing of special products in health and natural foods stores. These include Cantrol, Candida Cleanse, Yeast Fighters, and Yeast Guard.[3] Barrett has asked the Food and Drug Administration (FDA) and the Federal Trade

Commission (FTC) to take action in regard to Cantrol, a product of Nature's Way Products, Inc. Cantrol supplements contain vitamin E, evening primrose oil, acidophilus, linseed oil, and other components (eg, pau d'arco).[16] Barrett[17] points out that some have said this product may also be promoted as a cancer cure because of its pau d'arco content (purported to be an anticancer herbal) and name.

Patients with the diagnosis of *Candida* hypersensitivity may also be advised to use other nutritional supplements. Those who promote the existence of this diagnosis say patients may be deficient in riboflavin, vitamin B_6, vitamin A, zinc, iron, magnesium, selected amino acids, and essential fatty acid.[15] Garlic supplements have been said to have antifungal action and may be used by some patients.[15]

Concern has been expressed over the drug therapy used to treat candidiasis hypersensitivity. Ketoconazole can be toxic to the liver and cause death.[3,18] Quinn and Venezio[18] describe a patient seen in their practice who had been given this drug to treat *Candida* hypersensitivity and developed transient hepatitis as a result.

Problems may also occur if a patient with mucocutaneous candidiasis is misdiagnosed as *Candida* hypersensitive. A case of this type of misdiagnosis in a child was described in a 1986 letter published in *The New England Journal of Medicine*.[19]

Dietitians need to consult current advisories from the government and professional societies (the American Medical Association, the American Academy of Allergy and Immunology, and the FDA) with regard to this topic. General guidelines given for dietary therapy could theoretically result in inadequate intakes of vitamin C and calcium in some patients. Severe carbohydrate restriction could result in ketosis. Nutritional supplements could be consumed in toxic quantities or may be an unnecessary expense for some patients. Investigation, using accepted ethical and scientific standards of research, is needed both with regard to this diagnosis and its dietary management.

FOOD AND BEHAVIOR

Food allergy or adverse food reactions have been commonly cited as being related to a variety of behavioral disorders. Prominent among these are hyperactivity, aggression, misbehavior, and poor learning abilities. Beliefs about food and behavior are not only present in the health and lay communities, but seem to be common among educators as well. McLoughlin and Nall[20] surveyed persons enrolled in university-level special education courses in one setting and found 91% believed dietary intake could adversely affect behavior and 86% believed consumption of certain foods or beverages could affect learning in a negative way.

Various mechanisms have been proposed for the relationship of food to behavior. These include allergy,[21,22] functional reactive hypoglycemia,[22] and adverse reactions (not immunologically mediated).[23] Other investigations have recently been conducted examining the relationship of diet to synthesis of serotonin, catecholamines, and acetylcholine.[24-26] Readers are referred to other sources for reviews of this latter area of inquiry.

Although allergy has been cited as a mechanism for adverse behavioral change, definitive evidence to implicate this mechanism is currently lacking. Atkins,[27] in an excellent review of the subject, summarizes major methodological problems in this area. Atkins discusses past research using open challenges that can have both experimenter and subject bias. Criteria used to define behavior change may be subjective. Wolraich[22] also provides a good review of this area and advocates further study using double-blind placebo challenges and objective behavioral measures.

The hypothesis that sugar allergy or intolerance is a cause of behavioral problems in children is currently unsubstantiated. In Wolraich's[22] review of retrospective, prospective, challenge, and dietary intervention studies, only two studies defined a small number of children with behavior problems related to sugar, and even these studies were cited as being unable to replicate their results. Mahan et al,[28] in testing 16 children whose behavior by parental report was defined to be adversely affected by sugar, found only 2 whose behavior deteriorated in controlled double-blind tests. Repeat double-blind challenges in these reactors failed to duplicate the initial results. Ferguson et al,[29] also using the double-blind challenges to study 100 children, did not find that sucrose (sugar) adversely altered behavior. In 1986, the Sugars Task Force of the FDA concluded that sugar consumption does not cause behavioral changes in normal individuals.[30]

One of the most widely known theories linking adverse food reaction to behavior problems and learning disabilities is the Feingold hypothesis enunciated in the mid-1970s.[23] Ben Feingold, MD, at that time associated with the Department of Allergy at the Kaiser-Permanente Medical Center in San Francisco, proposed that artificial food additives, specifically colors and flavorings, were related to learning disorders and hyperkinesis. He proposed a diet that eliminated these substances, as well as salicylates found naturally in foods and beverages.[23]

Although Feingold did not propose a specific mechanism for the hypothesized adverse reaction, several studies have investigated the effects of erythrosin B on neurotransmitter function to attempt to define a biochemical mechanism.[31-33] Results to date have not been definitive.

Harley et al,[34] in 1978, published the results of a dietary trial testing the effects of the Feingold diet versus control in 36 hyperactive males. No dietary effect on hyperactive behavior could be documented. A double-blind challenge experiment by Harley et al[35] published in the same year also concluded that behavior was not adversely affected by food additives. Other double-blind trials have also failed to document the relationship of hyperactivity or adverse behavior change to artificial coloring or flavor ingestion.[36,37] The results of a double-blind trial published in 1980 found that 20 out of 22 children did not react to artificial color challenge.[38] Levy et al[39] failed to link tartrazine to hyperkinesis in a double-blind crossover trial involving 22 hyperactive children.

In contrast to other studies, Conners et al[40] and Goyette et al,[41] using double-blind methodologies, concluded the Feingold (or Kaiser-Permanente) diet could alleviate symptoms of hyperactivity in selected children. Impairment in performance of laboratory learning tests was reported in hyperactive children receiving artificial food dye blend. This same study, however, did not note impairment in nonhyperactive children after food dye ingestion.[42] Egger et al[43] have reported some success in treating hyperkinetic children with an oligoantigenic diet.

In recent years, many have concluded that sufficient evidence does not exist to advocate a food additive- and salicylate-free diet to treat hyperactivity.[30,44,45] A small number of preschool children may be sensitive through a toxic, nonimmunologic mechanism and may benefit from dietary elimination of synthetic food colorings.[44] Lipton and Mayo,[45] writing in the *Journal of the American Dietetic Association*, concluded that the Feingold diet has no demonstrable detrimental effects and due to a placebo response may prove beneficial to certain individuals.

Psychological Aspects of Allergy and the Phenomenon of Pseudoallergy

There is no definitive evidence to suggest at present that food allergy per se causes psychological problems.[46] There is a belief, however, by some in both the medical and lay communities that such is the case. Those practicing clinical ecology, particularly, may advocate such a view.[47]

Allergy and mental problems may be indirectly linked through a variety of mechanisms. Hypoxia, associated with asthma, can induce mental changes. Drugs used to treat allergy may also have side effects involving the central nervous system. Examples of such drugs are antihistamines, corticosteroids, and decongestants. Persons can have psychologic reactions to their diagnosis of allergy with its associated physical problems and may develop mental problems such as anxiety or depression.[47]

In 1983, Pearson and Rix[48] published a study of 23 patients who believed they had food allergy. Only 4 were diagnosed as actually having allergy, and psychological symptoms were not reported by these patients when seeking treatment nor were psychological problems apparent upon testing. Some evidence of psychiatric disturbance was found in all of the unconfirmed food allergy (but multisymptomatic) patients in this series. Neurotic depression was the most common diagnosis in this group. This study would indicate some individuals with psychiatric problems may seek a diagnosis of food allergy.

Pearson[47] (in conjunction with Rix) has suggested the term pseudofood allergy to denote the erroneous belief that one suffers from food allergy. These investigators note many risks associated with such a belief, including adherence to restricted and potentially inadequate diets. They report some patients will go as far as restricting their diets to the point where only water is consumed.

VITAMIN SUPPLEMENTATION

Vitamin supplementation as a part of allergy treatment has been studied to a limited extent. Vitamin C (ascorbic acid) has been investigated to see if its use could prevent bronchospasm.[49–52] The results of these vitamin C studies do not support a role in standard therapy at this time.[53] Kline et al,[54] however, have tested the efficacy of vitamin C supplements in treating atopic dermatitis and have noted that slow-release vitamin C may be helpful.

Collipp et al,[55] in a double-blind study investigating 76 asthmatic children for 5 months, noted clinical improvement when using 200 mg of pyridoxine daily, as opposed to calcium lactate placebo. (All children in this study were taking concurrent medications such as bronchodilators and ephedrine.) These researchers postulate that asthmatic children may have a metabolic block in tryptophan metabolism. Supplementation levels of pyridoxine at the level of 200 mg/day have induced dependency when given for 33 consecutive days.[56] Dietitians need to be aware of this potential problem if working in a situation in which physicians are using pyridoxine as part of asthma treatment.

Dietitians should carefully evaluate claims that vitamin supplementation is a food allergy preventative or cure. Information to date does not support the majority of these claims, although there is evidence to suggest that vitamin C may be useful in treating atopic dermatitis.[54] Persons having a belief in the curative value of vitamins may be taking potentially toxic levels of nutrient supplements. Such individuals need to be identified and receive appropriate nutrition education.

CONCLUSION

The areas of food allergy and adverse food reaction are the focus of both controversy and promotion of unproven etiologies, diagnoses, and treatments. Dietitians need to be aware of the status of practice in these areas—ie, standard versus experimental. Dietitians need to be particularly concerned with promulgation of unproven therapies that could impact detrimentally on nutritional status.

REFERENCES

1. Thompson RC. Food allergies—separating fact from "hype." *FDA Consumer.* 1986; 20(5):25–27.

2. May CD. Food sensitivity: Facts and fancies. *Nutr Rev.* 1984; 42(3):72–78.

3. Barrett S. Unproven "allergies": an epidemic of nonsense. *Nutr Today.* 1989; 24(2):6–11.

4. Bock SA. Food sensitivity—a critical review and practical approach. *Am J Dis Child.* 1980; 134:973–982.

5. Grieco MH. Controversial practices in allergy. *JAMA.* 1982; 247(22):3106–3111.

6. California Medical Association Scientific Board Task Force on Clinical Ecology. Clinical ecology—A critical appraisal. *West J Med.* 1986; 144:239–245.

7. Executive Committee of the American Academy of Allergy and Immunology. Position statement—Clinical ecology. *J Allergy Clin Immunol.* 1986; 78(2):269–271.

8. Terr AI. Environmental illness—a clinical review of 50 cases. *Arch Intern Med.* 1986; 146:145–149.

9. Brodsky CM. "Allergic to everything": a medical subculture. *Psychosomatics.* 1983; 24(8):731–742.

10. Stewart DE, Raskin J. Psychiatric assessment of patients with "20th-century disease" ("total allergy syndrome"). *Can Med Assoc J.* 1985; 133:1001–1006.

11. Executive Committee of the American Academy of Allergy and Immunology. Position statement—Candidiasis hypersensitivity syndrome. *J Allergy Clin Immunol.* 1986; 78(2):271–273.

12. Liebeskind A. *Candida albicans* as an allergenic factor. *Ann Allergy.* 1962; 20:394–396.

13. James J, Warin RP. An assessment of the role of *Candida albicans* and food yeasts in chronic urticaria. *Br J Dermatol.* 1971; 84:227–237.

14. Crook WG. *The Yeast Connection: A Medical Breakthrough.* Jackson, TN: Professional Books; 1984.

15. Kroker GF. Chronic candidiasis and allergy. In: Brostoff J, Challacombe SJ, eds. *Food Allergy and Intolerance.* London: Bailliere-Tindall; 1987: 850–872.

16. Candidiasis promotion increases. *Nutr Forum.* 1986; 3(4):28.

17. Barrett S. Candidiasis hypersensitivity. *Nutr Forum.* 1987; 4(11):84–85.

18. Quinn JP, Venezio FR. Ketoconazole and the yeast connection. *JAMA.* 1986; 255(23):3250. Letter.

19. Haas A, Stiehm ER. The "yeast connection" meets chronic mucocutaneous candidiasis. *N Engl J Med.* 1986; 314:854–855. Letter.

20. McLoughlin JA, Nall M. Teacher opinion of the role of food allergy on school behavior and achievement. *Ann Allergy.* 1988; 61:89–91.

21. Rapp DJ. Food allergy treatment of hyperkinesis. *J Learn Disabil.* 1979; 12:608–616.

22. Wolraich ML. Sugar intolerance: Is there evidence for its effects on behavior in children? *Ann Allergy.* 1988; 61(Part II):58–62.

23. Feingold BF. Hyperkinesis and learning disabilities linked to artificial food flavors and colors. *Am J Nurs.* 1975; 75(5):797–803.

24. Wurtman RJ. Ways that food can affect the brain. *Nutr Rev.* 1986; 44(suppl):2–6.

25. Lovenberg WM. Biochemical regulation of brain function. *Nutr Rev.* 1986; 44(suppl):6–11.

26. Krassner MB. Diet and brain function. *Nutr Rev.* 1986; 44(suppl):12–15.

27. Atkins FM. Food allergy and behavior: Definitions, mechanisms, and a review of the evidence. *Nutr Rev.* 1986; 44(suppl):104–112.

28. Mahan LK, Chase M, Furukawa CT, et al. Sugar "allergy" and children's behavior. *Ann Allergy.* 1988; 61:453–458.

29. Ferguson HB, Stoddart C, Simeon JG. Double-blind challenge studies of behavioral and cognitive effects of sucrose-aspartame ingestion in normal children. *Nutr Rev.* 1986; 44(suppl):144–150.

30. International Food Information Council. Taking the hype out of hyperactivity. *Food Insight.* 1988; Winter:2–3.

31. Lafferman JA, Silbergeld EK. Erythrosin B inhibits dopamine transport in rat caudate synaptosomes. *Science.* 1979; 205:410–412.

32. Logan WJ, Swanson JM. Erythrosin B inhibition of neurotransmitter accumulation by rat brain homogenate. *Science.* 1979; 206:363–364.

33. Mailman RB, Ferris RM, Tang FLM, et al. Erythrosine (red no. 3) and its nonspecific biochemical actions: What relation to behavioral changes? *Science.* 1980; 207:535–537.

34. Harley JP, Ray RS, Tomasi L, et al. Hyperkinesis and food additives: Testing the Feingold hypothesis. *Pediatrics.* 1978; 61(6):818–828.

35. Harley JP, Matthews CG, Eichman P. Synthetic food colors and hyperactivity in children: A double-blind challenge experiment. *Pediatrics.* 1978; 62(6):975–983.

36. Mattes JA, Gittelman R. Effects of artificial food colorings in children with hyperactive symptoms: A critical review and results of a controlled study. *Arch Gen Psychiatry.* 1981; 38:714–718.

37. Thorley G. Pilot study to assess behavioral and cognitive effects of artificial food colours in a group of retarded children. *Dev Med Child Neurol.* 1984; 26:56–61.

38. Weiss B, Williams JH, Margen S, et al. Behavioral responses to artificial colors. *Science.* 1980; 207:1487–1489.

39. Levy F, Dumbrell S, Hobbes G, Ryan M, Wilton N, Woodhill JM. Hyperkinesis and diet— A double-blind crossover trial with a tartrazine challenge. *Med J Aust.* 1978; 1(2):61–64.

40. Conners CK, Goyette CH, Southwick DA, Lees JM, Andrulonis PA. Food additives and hyperkinesis: A controlled double-blind experiment. *Pediatrics.* 1976; 58(2):154–166.

41. Goyette CH, Connors CK, Petti TA, Curtis LE. Effects of artificial colors on hyperkinetic children: A double-blind challenge study. *Psychopharmacol Bull.* 1978; 14(2):39–40.

42. Swanson JM, Kinsbourne M. Food dyes impair performance of hyperactive children on a laboratory learning test. *Science* 1980; 207(28):1485–1487.

43. Egger J, Graham RJ, Carter CM, Gumley D, Soothill J. Controlled trial of oligoantigenic treatment in the hyperkinetic syndrome. *Lancet.* 1985; 1:540–545.

44. Ribon A, Subhash J. Is there any relationship between food additives and hyperkinesis? *Ann Allergy.* 1982; 48:275–278.

45. Lipton MA, Mayo JP. Diet and hyperkinesis—an update. *J Am Diet Assoc.* 1983; 83(2):132–134.

46. Pearson DJ, Rix KJB. Psychological effects of food allergy. In: Brostoff J, Challacombe SJ, eds. *Food Allergy and Intolerance.* London: Bailliere-Tindall; 1987: 688–708.

47. Pearson DJ. Psychologic and somatic interrelationships in allergy and pseudoallergy. *J Allergy Clin Immunol.* 1988; 81(2):351–360.

48. Pearson DJ, Rix KJB. Food allergy: How much is in the mind? A clinical and psychiatric study of suspected food hypersensitivity. *Lancet.* 1983; 1:1259–1261.

49. Cockcroft DW, Killian DN, Mellon JJA, Hargreave FE. Protective effect of drugs on histamine-induced asthma. *Thorax.* 1977; 32:429–437.

50. Kreisman H, Mitchell C, Bouhuys A. Inhibition of histamine-induced airway constriction negative results with oxtriphylline and ascorbic acid. *Lung.* 1977; 154:223–229.

51. Kordansky DW, Rosenthal RR, Norman PS. The effect of vitamin C on antigen-induced bronchospasm. *J Allergy Clin Immunol.* 1979; 63(1):61–64.

52. Schachter EN, Schlesinger A. The attenuation of exercise-induced bronchospasm by ascorbic acid. *Ann Allergy.* 1982; 49:146–151.

53. Furukawa CT. Nondietary management of food allergy. In: Chiaramonte LT, Schneider AT, Lifshitz F, eds. *Food Allergy: A Practical Approach to Diagnosis and Management.* New York: Marcel Dekker, Inc; 1988: 365–375.

54. Kline G, Strem EL, Williams ML, Frick OL. Ascorbic acid therapy for atopic dermatitis. *J Allergy Clin Immunol.* 1989; 83(1):196.

55. Collipp PJ, Goldzier S, Weiss N, Soleymani Y, Snyder R. Pyridoxine treatment of childhood bronchial asthma. *Ann Allergy.* 1975; 35:93–97.

56. McCormick DB. Vitamin B$_6$. In: Shils ME, Young VR, eds. *Modern Nutrition in Health and Disease.* Philadelphia: Lea & Febiger; 1988: 376–382.

General Guidelines for Management of Cow's Milk Allergy

GENERAL GUIDELINES

1. Ensure dietary adequacy because diets eliminating cow's milk proteins may be low in calcium, protein, vitamin D, vitamin A, and riboflavin. Supplements of calcium particularly may be warranted.[1,2]

2. Food components on labels that may indicate cow's milk protein presence are butter, buttermilk, casein, caseinate, cheese, cottage cheese, cream, curds, whey, custard, cow's milk, nonfat milk, milk solids, milk chocolate, lactalbumin, lactoglobulin, sodium caseinate, and sour cream.[1-3] Persons should avoid consumption of the above items. (Examples of milk presence in food products are shown at the conclusion of this section.)

3. Major food categories to be avoided by the milk-allergic individual include:

   - dairy products (such as milk, ice cream, yogurt, cream, cheeses)
   - cow's milk-based formulas and supplements
   - beverages made with milk (such as malted milk, cocoa, hot chocolate, eggnog, and Yoo-hoo Chocolate Flavored Drink,® Ovaltine,® General Foods International Coffees® (sodium caseinate), Slender,® Ultra Slim Fast,® Sego Lite,® Nutrament,® and Go®)
   - bread, crackers, cereals, cookies, and other flour products made with cow's milk protein ingredients
   - candies and desserts made with milk or milk products (eg, puddings, custards, many cakes, cream pies, doughnuts)
   - margarine (if it contains milk protein) and butter
   - vegetables and pastas prepared with milk or milk products

- gravies, sauces, soups, and salad dressings made with milk or butter or other milk protein sources (eg, white sauce (béchamel), Florentine sauce, Mornay sauce, sauce Dijonnaise, and Hungarian sauce)
- meats prepared with butter or milk
- cold luncheon meats containing milk proteins
- scrambled eggs or egg-substitute products with milk components
- meat substitutes made with milk or milk protein products
- spreads made with sodium caseinate, nonfat milk solids, and/or whey, and nondairy creamers with milk protein[1-4]

Nondairy coffee creamers, dried sauces, gravy mixes, sour cream alternatives, and imitation cheeses may contain milk protein ingredients. Careful label reading is advised.

4. The designation "parve" means a product does not contain milk.[1]

5. Many packaged entree, vegetable, and salad mixes contain milk products and should be avoided.

6. Simpleese® (fat substitute) contains milk protein and should not be consumed.[5]

REFERENCES

1. Weyman-Daum M. Milk-free, lactose-free, and lactose-restricted diets. In: Chiaramonte LT, Schneider AT, Lifshitz F, eds. *Food Allergy: A Practical Approach to Diagnosis and Management.* New York: Marcel Dekker, Inc; 1988: 401–420.

2. Dong FM. *All about Food Allergy.* Philadelphia: George F Stickley Co; 1984.

3. The American Dietetic Association. *Food Sensitivity—A Resource Including Recipes.* Chicago: The American Dietetic Association; 1985.

4. Rombauer IR, Becker MR. *Joy of Cooking.* Indianapolis: Bobbs-Merrill Co, Inc; 1931.

5. Wardlaw G. *Fat Replacements.* December 1, 1989 (unpublished handout).

EXAMPLES OF MILK PROTEIN SOURCES IN FOOD PRODUCTS

Bars/Cookies/Tarts

- Carnation Breakfast Bars—Chocolate Chip® (calcium caseinate, nonfat milk)
- Keebler Chocolate Fudge Creme Filled Cookies® (whey)
- Keebler Deluxe Graham Fudge Covered Graham Crackers® (whey)
- Keebler E.L. Fudge Sandwich Cookies® (whey)
- Keebler Grasshopper Chocolaty Cookies with Mint Creme® (whey)

- Keebler Iced Animal Cookies® (whey)
- Keebler Rainbow Chips Deluxe® (whey)
- Kellogg's Pop Tarts®—Frosted Brown Sugar, Cinnamon, Frosted Chocolate Fudge, and Frosted Chocolate Vanilla Creme (whey)
- Little Debbie Coconut Cakes® (whey)
- Little Debbie Figaroos® (whey)
- Nabisco Brown Edge Wafers® (whey and butter)
- Nabisco Cameo Creme Sandwich® (sodium caseinate, whey, skim milk)
- Nabisco Deviled Food Cakes® (nonfat milk)
- Nabisco Oreo Chocolate Sandwich Cookies® (whey)
- Sunshine Chip-O-Lotomus Cookies® (dairy whey)
- Sunshine Fig Bars® (dairy whey)
- Sunshine Fudge Family Bears Creme Filled Sandwich Cookies® (dairy whey)

Breads/Cereals

- B & M New England Style Brown Bread—Raisin® (whey and buttermilk)
- Country Hearth Light Wheat Bread® (cultured whey, dairy whey)
- General Mills Cinnamon Toast Crunch® (nonfat milk)
- General Mills Golden Grahams Cereal® (nonfat milk)
- Kellogg's Cocoa Krispies Cereal® (nonfat dry milk)
- Kellogg's Special K Cereal® (whey and calcium caseinate)
- Nabisco Zwieback Teething Toast® (lactalbumin and butter)
- Quaker Honey Graham Oh's Cereal® (whey, sodium caseinate)
- Post Fruit & Fibre Cereal® (whey)
- Post Honey Bunches of Oats with Almonds® (whey)

Candies

- Andes Daydreams Creme de Menthe Milk Wafers® (nonfat dry milk and milk)
- Baby Ruth® (buttermilk solids, milk, skim milk)
- Butterfinger® (buttermilk solids, skim milk)
- Tootsie Rolls (condensed skim milk and whey)
- Whopper's Malted Milk Candy® (whey and malted milk)

Crackers

- Lance Peanut Butter Malt Crackers® (whey)
- Nabisco American Classic Crackers—Dairy Butter (butter and whey)
- Nabisco Better Cheddars Snack Thins® (cheddar cheese)
- Nabisco Cheese Tid-Bit Crackers® (cheddar cheese and whey)
- Pepperidge Farm Cheddar Cheese Goldfish® (cheddar cheese, pasteurized processed cheddar cheese)
- Pepperidge Farm Original Goldfish® (nonfat milk and butter)
- Sunshine Cheez-It Snack Crackers® (skim milk cheese)

Dips

- Kraft Avocado Dip® (sodium caseinate and whey protein concentrate)
- Kraft French Onion Dip® (sodium caseinate and whey protein concentrate)
- Kraft Green Onion Dip® (sodium caseinate and whey protein concentrate)

Egg Substitutes

- Morningstar Farm's Cholesterol Free Real Egg Product Scramblers® (calcium caseinate and nonfat milk)

Meats

- Oscar Mayer Honey Loaf® (dried whey and calcium caseinate)
- Oscar Mayer Pickle and Pimento Loaf® (dried whey and calcium caseinate)

Pancake Mixes

- Aunt Jemima Buttermilk Complete Pancake and Waffle Mix® (dried buttermilk, dried whey, sodium caseinate)

- Aunt Jemima Complete Pancake and Waffle Mix® (dried whey and sodium caseinate)
- Mrs. Butterworth's Buttermilk Complete Pancake and Waffle Mix® (buttermilk powder, whey powder, powered nonfat dry milk, and sodium caseinate)

Note: The above listings are only examples. Readers are also advised to confirm contents by reading the package labels or contacting the manufacturer.

General Guidelines for Management of Soy Allergy

GENERAL GUIDELINES

1. Avoid obvious sources of soy in the diet—tofu (soybean curd), soybeans, soy grits, soy flour, soy formulas, soy granules, soy milk, soy sauce, miso, and tempeh.[1,2]

2. Do not eat meats or other products containing hydrolyzed vegetable protein, textured vegetable protein, or vegetable protein. Soy protein may be included.[1]

3. Do not eat products containing lecithin[2] or soy lecithin.[1]

4. Check the labels of the following product categories that may contain soy, and avoid those containing soy:
   - baked goods
   - candies
   - cereals
   - cheese substitutes
   - coffee replacements
   - commercial fruit products
   - commercial vegetable products
   - desserts
   - meats (that may have soy additives such as cold cuts, sausage, hamburger)
   - milk or cream replacements
   - pastas
   - sauces

- soups
- vegetable oil sprays[1]
5. Avoid cold-pressed soybean oils or other soybean oil products that contain residual soy proteins. (Many soybean oils are now believed to be nonallergenic.[3])

REFERENCES

1. Dong FM. *All about Food Allergy.* Philadelphia: George F Stickley Co; 1984.
2. The American Dietetic Association. *Food Sensitivity—A Resource Including Recipes.* Chicago: The American Dietetic Association; 1985.
3. Bush RK, Taylor SL, Nordlee JA, Busse WW. Soybean oil is not allergenic to soybean sensitive individuals. *J Allergy Clin Immunol.* 1985;76:242–245.

EXAMPLES OF SOY PROTEIN SOURCES IN FOOD PRODUCTS

Bread/Muffins

- Pepperidge Farm Blueberry Muffins® (lecithin)
- Sara Lee Oat Bran Muffins® (lecithin)
- Roman Meal Bread® (soy flour)

Cake Mixes

- Betty Crocker Golden Pound Cake Mix® (isolated soy protein)
- Duncan Hines Yellow Cake Mix® (soy protein isolate)

Candies/Cookies/Bars

- Carnation Breakfast Bars—Peanut Butter with Chocolate Chip® and Chocolate Chip® (soy protein isolate)
- Hershey's Milk Chocolate® (soya lecithin)
- M & M Mars Milky Way® (soy protein and soy lecithin)
- M & M Mars Snickers® (soy protein and soy lecithin)
- M & M Mars 3 Musketeers® (soy protein and soy lecithin)

Cereals

- Nabisco Honey Teddy Grahams Breakfast Bears Graham Cereal® (soy lecithin)
- Post Oat Flakes® (soy flour)
- Quaker Honey Graham Oh's® (soy protein)
- Quaker Life High Protein Toasted Oat Cereal—Cinnamon and Regular® (soy flour)

Cooking Spray

- Pam No-Stick Cooking Spray® (natural lecithin)

Frozen Dessert

- Tofulite All Natural Non-Dairy Frozen Dessert® (tofu, soy lecithin)

Meats and Meat Substitutes

- Betty Crocker BAC* Os Bacon Flavor Chips® (defatted soy flour and soybean oil)
- Le Menu Veal Parmigiana® (soy flour used in cooked breaded veal pattie)
- Morningstar Farms Cholesterol Free Breakfast Links® (soy isolate and concentrate)
- Morningstar Farms Cholesterol-Free Breakfast Strips® (textured soy concentrate)

Pancake Mixes

- Aunt Jemima Buttermilk Complete Pancake and Waffle Mix® (soy flour)
- Aunt Jemima Lite Buttermilk Complete Pancake and Waffle Mix® (soy protein concentrate and lecithin)

Sauces/Toppings

- Heinz 100% Natural Thick and Rich Barbeque Sauce® (powdered soy sauce)
- Heinz Worcestershire Sauce® (soy sauce)
- Kikkoman Stir-Fry Sauce® (soy sauce)
- London Pub Original Steak and Chop Sauce® (fermented soy protein)
- McCormick Salad Toppings® (textured soy flour, soy nuts, soy oil, and hydrolyzed vegetable protein)
- Smucker's Chocolate Fudge Topping® (lecithin)
- Texas Best Barbeque Sauce—Sweet and Sour® (soy sauce)

Soups

- Campbell's Cream of Celery Soup® (soy protein isolate)
- Campbell's Cream of Chicken Soup® (soy protein isolate)

Note: The above listings are only examples. Readers are also advised to confirm contents by reading the package labels or contacting the manufacturer.

General Guidelines for Management of Egg Allergy

GENERAL GUIDELINES

1. Avoid obvious egg sources in the diet (such as scrambled eggs, omelettes, timbales, souffles, custards, egg noodles, and eggnog).

2. Check product labels for eggs or egg proteins and avoid these products. In addition to being listed as eggs, egg white, dried egg yolk, or egg powder, the presence of egg may be indicated by the terms livetin, ovomucin, ovomucoid, ovoglobulin egg albumin, ovovitellin, vitellin, and globulin.[1,2]

3. Avoid sauces with eggs (such as hollandaise, Béarnaise, Foyot, and Newburg).[3]

4. Baked products may contain eggs because eggs help create and maintain product structure. Check labels of commercial baked goods to ensure they are egg-free and use egg-free baked goods recipes.[1,3]

5. Ovaltine® sold in the United States does not need to be avoided by the egg-allergic individual. (This product is traditionally listed as a must to avoid.) According to the manufacturer, the product has not contained egg since 1960. Certain European versions of this product do contain eggs, and those purchasing the product overseas are advised to read the label and avoid consumption in the event of egg content.[4]

6. Egg substitute products are generally made with egg white and should be avoided. Check labels.

7. Mayonnaise contains egg and should be avoided.

8. Avoid eating fats in which eggs have been fried.[2]

9. Check cookbooks for products to substitute for eggs. Egg Replacer® marketed by Ener-G-Foods is designed for baking.[1] Substitution mixtures usually involve combining wheat flour, oil, baking powder, and

milk or water.[5] Baking powder may contain egg derivatives and content needs to be checked closely.[1,2,5]

10. Egg may be present in root beer, wine, and coffee. Check on the processing methods for these products.

11. Major product categories to avoid or scrutinize for egg presence include:
    - beverages or formulas potentially containing egg or powdered egg[5]
    - cheese products made with egg[5]
    - baked goods made with egg or baking powder[1,3]
    - vegetable dishes prepared with egg (such as scalloped corn, potato pancakes, Duchess potatoes, and sweet potato puffs)[3,5]
    - candies made with egg (such as divinity and nougat)[3,5]
    - fritters made with egg[3]
    - meats made with egg (such as meat loaf or meats with egg in the breading)
    - salads with egg (such as Caesar salad) or salads with mayonnaise[5]
    - salad dressings and sandwich spreads
    - ice creams, cream pies, and other egg-containing desserts
    - pastas made with egg
    - soups with egg such as egg drop, egg noodle, and won ton soup[2] and soups with egg garnishes such as hard-cooked eggs, liver dumplings, or cheese balls[3]

12. Simpleese® (fat substitute) contains egg protein and should not be consumed.[6]

REFERENCES

1. The American Dietetic Association. *Food Sensitivity: A Resource Including Recipes.* Chicago: The American Dietetic Association; 1985.

2. Dong FM. *All about Food Allergy.* Philadelphia: George F Stickley Co; 1984.

3. Rombauer IS, Becker MR. *Joy of Cooking.* Indianapolis: The Bobbs-Merrill Co, Inc; 1931.

4. Bryan R. Sandoz Nutrition Sales Representative. Personal communication, February 1990.

5. Greenberg LE, Moses NS. Egg-free and corn-free diets. In: Chiaramonte LT, Schneider AT, Lifshitz F, eds. *Food Allergy: A Practical Approach to Diagnosis and Management.* New York: Marcel Dekker, Inc; 1988: 441–452.

6. Wardlaw G. *Fat Replacements.* December 1, 1989 (unpublished handout).

EXAMPLES OF EGG PROTEIN SOURCES IN FOOD PRODUCTS

Baked Goods

- Little Debbie Coconut Cakes® (egg whites)
- Nabisco Zwieback Teething Toast® (eggs and egg whites)
- Sara Lee All Butter Cinnamon Rolls® (fresh whole eggs)
- Sara Lee Individual Cheese Danish® (fresh whole eggs)

Candies

- Brach's Silkies Jelly Nougat® (egg whites)
- Mars Bar® (egg whites)
- Snickers Candy Bar® (egg whites)
- 3 Musketeers Candy Bar® (egg whites)

Cookies

- Keebler E.L. Fudge Rich Fudge Covered Buttery Cookies® (eggs)
- Keebler Magic Middle Cookies® (eggs)
- Keebler Pecan Sandies Cookies® (eggs)
- Little Debbie Figaroos® (eggs)
- Nabisco Almost Home Oatmeal Raisin Cookies® (eggs)
- Nabisco Almost Home Real Chocolate Chip Cookies® (eggs)
- Nabisco Giggles Vanilla Sandwich Cookies® (eggs)
- Nabisco Imported Danish Cookies® (eggs)
- Nabisco Lorna Doone Shortbread Cookies® (eggs)
- Nabisco Nilla Wafers® (eggs)
- Nabisco Nutter Butter Peanut Butter Sandwich Cookies® (eggs)
- Pillsbury's Best Oatmeal Raisin Cookies® (egg yolks and egg whites)
- Pillsbury's Best Sugar Cookies® (egg yolk and egg white)
- Sunshine Chip-O-Lotomus Cookies® (eggs)

- Sunshine Fig Bars® (eggs)
- Sunshine Golden Fruit Raisin Biscuits® (eggs)
- Sunshine Vanilla Wafers® (eggs)

Dumpling Mixes

- Knorr Bread Dumpling Mix® (egg yolk and egg white)
- Maggi Spaetzle Swiss Style Dumplings® (eggs)

Egg Substitutes

- Fleishmann's Egg Beaters® (egg white)
- Morning Star Farms Cholesterol-Free Real Egg Product—Scramblers® (egg white)

Pancake Mixes

- Aunt Jemima Buttermilk Complete Pancake and Waffle Mix® (dried whole eggs)
- Aunt Jemima Complete Pancake and Waffle Mix® (dried egg solid products, dried whole eggs, and egg yolks)
- Aunt Jemima Lite Buttermilk Pancake and Waffle Mix® (dried whole eggs and dried egg whites)

Salad Dressings/Spreads

- Bennett's Tartar Sauce® (egg yolk)
- Kraft Miracle Whip® (egg yolk)
- Kraft Sandwich Spread® (egg yolk)
- Kraft's Saucework's Tartar Sauce® (egg yolk)
- Wishbone Thousand Island Dressing® (egg yolk)

Note: The above listings are only examples. Readers are also advised to confirm contents by reading the package labels or contacting the manufacturer.

General Guidelines for Management of Wheat Allergy

GENERAL GUIDELINES

1. Avoid foods containing wheat flours, bran, cracker meal, graham flour, wheat germ, and wheat gluten.[1]
2. Avoid foods that contain malt or cereal extract. (Some patients who are wheat sensitive can eat these.[2])
3. Alternatives to wheat flour include rice flour, buckwheat flour, potato sauce, rye flour, oat flour, and barley flour.[1,2] (Reference 2 gives detailed instructions on quantities for substitution.)
4. Certain alcoholic beverages may contain wheat and should be avoided. These include beer, gin, and selected whiskeys.[2]
5. Check cereal boxes carefully. Some oat cereals, for example, contain whole wheat or wheat starch.
6. Other product categories to carefully check for wheat content include:
   - baked goods and baked good mixes
   - commercial chocolate and other candies
   - pancake/waffle mixes
   - cakes/pies, cookies
   - sauces/gravies
   - processed meats, breaded meats, and meat casseroles
   - pastas
   - salad dressings
   - soups[1]

REFERENCES

1. The American Dietetic Association. *Food Sensitivity: A Resource Including Recipes.* Chicago: The American Dietetic Association; 1985.
2. Dong FM. *All about Food Allergy.* Philadelphia: George F Stickley Co; 1984.

General Guidelines for Management of Corn Allergy

GENERAL GUIDELINES

1. Avoid obvious sources of dietary corn (fresh, frozen, or canned corn, corn chips, popcorn, hominy, and grits).

2. Check food labels for words that may indicate corn presence and avoid these foods. These terms include corn flour, cornmeal, cornstarch, corn sugar, corn dextrose, high fructose corn syrup, baking powder (with cornstarch), maize, vegetable gum, sorbitol, commercial glucose, modified food starch, and vinegar.[1,2] Some individuals may need to avoid these products. (Some such as corn syrup may contain minute quantities of corn protein, if any.)

3. Commercial baking powders may contain cornstarch and may need to be avoided. Examples are shown below:
   - Davis OK Baking Double Acting Powder® (cornstarch, sodium bicarbonate, calcium acid phosphate, and sodium aluminum sulfate)
   - Calumet Double Acting Baking Powder® (baking soda, cornstarch, sodium aluminum sulfate, calcium sulfate, and calcium acid phosphate)

4. Breads, cookies, cereals, and commercial dessert products may contain corn flour, cornmeal, corn syrup, or cornstarch. Labels should be checked carefully.

5. Gravies and sauces may be thickened with cornstarch and therefore should be avoided.

6. Traditional Mexican foods use corn as a major ingredient and may need to be avoided. Tamales and corn tortillas are examples. Masa harina is a corn flour product.

7. Heavy syrup (used with canned fruits) is usually corn syrup.

8. Luncheon meats and franks contain corn syrup or dextrose. (Kosher meats, however, are usually allowed on a corn-free diet.[2])

9. Most processed foods contain some type of corn products. Cooking at home with known ingredients may be important. Certain alcoholic beverages may contain corn and need to be avoided. These include beer, bourbon, vodka, and gin. (For a more complete listing, consult Reference 1.)

REFERENCES

1. Greenberg LE, Moses NS. Egg-free and corn-free diets. In: Chiaramonte LT, Schneider AT, Lifshitz F, eds. *Food Allergy: A Practical Approach to Diagnosis and Management*. New York: Marcel Dekker, Inc; 1988: 441–452.

2. Dong FM. *All about Food Allergy*. Philadelphia: George F Stickley Co; 1984.

Appendix F

Examples of Recipe Sources
for the Allergic Individual

PAMPHLETS

1. The American Dietetic Association. The Food Sensitivity Series. *Food Sensitivity: A Resource Including Recipes.* Chicago, IL: American Dietetic Association; 1985. (Note: Other titles in this series are excellent resources related to gluten and lactose intolerance.)
2. *Cooking with Isomil,*® Columbus, OH: Ross Laboratories; 1986.
3. *Cooking for People with Food Allergies.* US Department of Agriculture Human Nutrition Information Service. Washington, DC: Superintendent of Documents, Government Printing Office; 1988.
4. *The Mocha Mix® Non-Dairy Cookbook.*
   Write: Mocha Mix Non-Dairy Cookbook
   P.O. Box 9670
   Newport Beach, CA 92658
5. *The Quaker Oats Allergy Cookbook: Wheat, Milk, and Egg-Free Recipes.*
   Write: The Quaker Oats Company
   Merchandise Mart Plaza
   Chicago, IL 60654

BOOKS

1. Dong FM. *All about Food Allergy.* Philadelphia: George F Stickley Co; 1984.
2. Nonken PP, Hirsh, SP. *The Allergy Cookbook and Food Buying Guide: A Practical Approach to Cooking and Buying Food for People Who Are Allergic to Foods.* New York: Warner Books; 1982.

3. Thomas LL. *Cooking and Caring for the Allergic Child.* New York: Sterling Publishing Co; 1980.
4. Williams M. *Cooking Without.* Ambler, PA: Gimball Corporation; 1989.

Examples of Products Containing Aspartame

BEVERAGE MIXES

- Alba Fit 'n Frosty Reduced Calorie Dairy Shake Mix® (chocolate, vanilla, strawberry)
- Carnation Sugar Free Hot Cocoa Mix®
- Lipton Iced Tea Mix No Sugar, No Saccharin®
- Sugar Free Crystal Light®
- Sugar Free General Foods International Coffees®
- Sugar Free Kool Aid®
- Sugar Free Tang Breakfast Beverage Crystal®
- Weight Watcher's Hot Cocoa Mix®
- Weight Watcher's Orange Sherbet Artificially Flavored Shake Mix®

CEREALS

- General Mills Fiber One Cereal®

SNACK/DESSERT ITEMS

- Crystal Light Bars—Diet Frozen Drink Bars®
- Fudgsicle Sugarfree Fudge Pops®
- Jell-O Sugarfree Gelatin Dessert Mixes®
- Jell-O Sugarfree Pudding and Pie Filling Mixes®
- Royal Instant Sugarfree Pudding and Pie Filling Mixes®

- Royal Sugarfree Gelatin Dessert Mixes®
- Sugar-Free Eskimo Pies® (vanilla frozen dairy dessert)
- Weight Watcher's Black Forest Cake® (frozen)
- Weight Watcher's Chocolate Cake® (frozen)
- Weight Watcher's Chocolate Mousse® (frozen)
- Weight Watcher's Raspberry Mousse® (frozen)

SOFT DRINKS

- A & W Diet Creme Soda®
- A & W Diet Root Beer®
- Canada Dry Diet Ginger Ale®
- Diet Barq's Root Beer®
- Diet Cherry 7-Up®
- Diet Coke®
- Diet Crush®
- Diet Dr. Pepper®
- Diet Hires Root Beer®
- Diet Minute Maid Orange Soda®
- Diet Mountain Dew®
- Diet Pepsi®
- Diet Rite Cola®
- Diet 7-Up®
- Diet Slice Mandarin Orange®
- Diet Sprite®
- Diet Sunkist®
- Diet Wink®

SWEETENERS

(Information from Equal® Toll-Free Number: 1-800-323-5316)
- Equal® (35 mg aspartame per 1-g packet)
- Sugar Delight® (Sugar Delight® is 1% aspartame and 99% cane sugar) (20-22 mg aspartame per 2-g packet)

YOGURTS

- Dannon Light Yogurt®
- Light and Lively Fat and Cholesterol Free Yogurt®
- Light and Lively 100 Calorie Yogurt®
- Weight Watcher's Ultimate 90 Yogurt®
- Yoplait Light Yogurt®

Note: The above listings are only examples. Readers are also advised to confirm contents by reading package labels or contacting the manufacturer.

Examples of Products Containing Sulfites

CEREALS

- Kellogg's Fruitful Bran®
- Nabisco Blueberry Fruit Wheats®
- Post Fruit and Fibre® with Pineapple, Bananas, Coconut, and Oat Clusters

COOKIES/CRACKERS/TARTS

- Carr's Croissant Crackers®
- Nabisco American Classic Crackers—Dairy Butter®
- Nabisco Fig Newtons®
- Nabisco Frosted Toastettes Tarts® (blueberry)
- Nabisco Old Fashion Ginger Snaps®
- Nabisco Swiss Cheese Naturally Flavored Snack Crackers®
- Sunshine Golden Fruit Raisin Biscuits®
- Sunshine Vienna Fingers Sandwich Cookies®

DRIED FRUITS AND OTHER FRUIT PRODUCTS

- Real Lemon Lemon Juice from Concentrate®
- Sun Maid Dried Mixed Fruit®
- Sun Maid Fruit Bits®

ENTREES/VEGETABLES/PASTA

- Betty Crocker Hamburger Helper Cheeseburger Macaroni®
- Betty Crocker Hamburger Helper Lasagne®
- Betty Crocker Potato Buds Mashed Potatoes®
- Betty Crocker Suddenly Salad—Caesar®
- Betty Crocker Suddenly Salad—Classic Pasta®
- Hungry Jack Mashed Potatoes®
- Idahoan Mashed Potatoes®
- Kraft Pasta and Cheese—Cheddar Broccoli®
- Kraft Potatoes and Cheese—Scalloped®
- Pillsbury Real Cheese Sauce Scalloped Potatoes®

SOUP MIXES

- Borden's Chowder Starter—New England Style®
- Borden's Soup Starter—Beef Vegetable and Chicken Noodle®
- Borden's Stew Starter—Hearty Beef®
- Knorr Vegetable Soup and Recipe Mix®

MISCELLANEOUS

- Jell-O Cook'n Serve Coconut Cream Pudding and Pie Filling®
- Kitchen Bouquet for Meat & Gravy®
- Old El Paso Pickled Jalapeño Slices®

Note: The above listings are only examples. Readers are also advised to confirm contents by reading the package labels or contacting the manufacturer.

Examples of Products Containing Tartrazine (FD&C Yellow No. 5)

BERVERAGE MIXES

- Country Time Lemonade Mix®
- Gatorade Citrus Cooler Thirst Quencher®
- Gatorade Lemon-Lime Thirst Quencher®
- Golden Hawaiian Punch (Passion Fruit)®
- Lemonade Flavor Kool Aid®
- Mello Yello®
- Sugar Free Crystal Light Decaffeinated Iced Tea Mix®
- Sugar Free Crystal Light Iced Tea Mix®
- Sugar Free Crystal Light Lemon-Lime Mix®
- Sugar Free Crystal Light Lemonade Mix®
- Sugar Free Tang Orange Flavor®
- Tang Orange Flavor Breakfast Beverage Crystals®
- Wyler's Lemonade Crystals®

BREAD PRODUCTS/CAKE MIXES/CEREALS/COOKIES

- Betty Crocker Yellow Cake Mix®
- Duncan Hines Butter Recipe Golden Cake Mix®
- Duncan Hines Lemon Supreme Cake Mix®
- Duncan Hines Yellow Cake Mix®
- General Mills Trix®
- Jell-O Real Cheesecake Mix®
- Keebler Baby Bear Cookies®
- Keebler Chocolate Fudge Fudge Creme Filled Cookies®

- Keebler French Vanilla Creme Filled Cookies®
- Keebler Grasshopper Chocolaty Cookies with Mint Creme®
- Keebler Rainbow Chips Deluxe Cookies®
- Pillsbury Plus Artificial Lemon Cake Mix®
- Pillsbury Plus Yellow Cake Mix®
- Quaker Cap'n Crunch Crunch Berries®
- Quaker Crunchy Bran High Fiber Corn Cereal®
- Quaker Honey Graham Oh's Cereal®
- Quaker Life Toasted Oat Cereal® (regular and cinnamon)
- Ralston Batman Cereal®
- Ralston Breakfast with Barbie Cereal®
- Ralston Cookie-Crisp Chocolate Chip Sweetened Cereal®
- Royal Real Cheesecake Mix®
- Stella D'Oro Almond Toast®
- Stella D'Oro Anginetti®
- Stella D'Oro Anisette Toast®

CANDIES

- Andes Daydreams Creme de Menthe Mint Wafers®
- Butterfinger®
- Five Flavor Lifesavers®
- M & M's Peanut Chocolate Candies®
- M & M's Plain Chocolate Candies®

EGG SUBSTITUTES

- Fleischman's Egg Beaters®

FROSTINGS

- Betty Crocker Creamy Deluxe Lemon Frosting®
- Betty Crocker Creamy Deluxe Cream Cheese Frosting®

PACKAGED ENTREE AND VEGETABLE MIXES

- Betty Crocker Hamburger Helper Cheeseburger Macaroni®

- Betty Crocker Suddenly Salad Classic Pasta®
- Betty Crocker Tuna Helper Cheesy Noodles®
- Kraft Macaroni and Cheese Dinner—Original®
- Kraft Pasta and Cheese—Cheddar Broccoli®
- Kraft Potatoes and Cheese—Scalloped®
- Pillsbury Real Cheese Sauce Scalloped Potatoes®

SALAD DRESSING

- Wishbone Lite Less Oil Italian Reduced Calorie Dressing®

SAUCES/SYRUPS/TOPPINGS

- Smucker's Butterscotch Flavored Topping®
- Smucker's Pineapple Topping®
- Virginia Dare Creme de Menthe Syrup®

SNACKS/DESSERTS

- Del Monte Pudding Cups® (banana, butterscotch, chocolate, chocolate fudge, tapioca, vanilla)
- Iberia Flan Custard®
- Jell-O Americana Golden Egg Custard Mix®
- Jell-O Cook-N-Serve Pudding & Pie Filling® (coconut creme, lemon, vanilla)
- Jell-O No Bake Dessert Chocolate Mousse Pie Mix®
- Mrs. Smith's Thaw and Serve Banana Cream Pie®
- Mrs. Smith's Thaw and Serve Coconut Cream Pie®
- Pillsbury All Ready Pie Crusts®
- Royal Instant Sugarfree Butterscotch Pudding & Pie Filling®
- Royal Orange Gelatin Dessert®
- Royal Pistachio Instant Pudding & Pie Filling Mix®
- Sunkist Fun Fruits Assorted Real Fruit Snacks®

Note: The above listings are only examples. Readers are also advised to confirm contents by reading package labels or contacting the manufacturer.

Examples of Products Containing Benzoates

GENERAL

- Dips and spreads may contain benzoates.
- Jarred pickles and jalapeño peppers may contain benzoates.
- Candy products may contain benzoates.

FRUIT

- Royalette Salad Cherries®

SAUCES/SYRUPS

- Heinz 57 Sauce®
- Heinz Traditional Steak Sauce®
- Kikkoman Stir-Fry Sauce®
- Old El Paso Hot Taco Sauce®
- Virginia Dare Creme de Maraschino Syrup®
- Virginia Dare Creme de Menthe Syrup®

Note: The above listings are only examples. Readers are also advised to confirm contents by reading package labels or contacting the manufacturer.

Lactose Content of Common Food Items

≥ 35.0 g LACTOSE/100 g FOOD/BEVERAGE	g/100 g
• Buttermilk powder	49.0-50.0
• Condensed whey	38.5-39.0
• Dried acid whey	66.5-73.4
• Dry whole milk	35.9-38.4
• Modified solids whey	56.5-72.0
• Nonfat dry milk	50.0-52.3
• Sweet dry whey	73.5-74.5

10.0 TO 34.9 g LACTOSE/100 g FOOD/BEVERAGE	
• American cheese, pasteurized processed	1.8-14.2
• Evaporated milk (whole & skim)	9.7-11.0
• Sweetened condensed milk	10.0-16.3

<10.0 g LACTOSE/100 g FOOD/BEVERAGE	
• American cheese	1.6-5.2
• Brie cheese	0-2.0
• Butter	0.8-1.0
• Buttermilk	3.6-5.0

continues

275

<10.0 g LACTOSE/100 g FOOD/BEVERAGE

• Chocolate milk	4.1-4.9
• Cottage cheese, creamed	0.6-3.3
• Cottage cheese, uncreamed	0-3.5
• Cream cheese	0.4-2.9
• Half and half	4.0-4.3
• Human milk	6.2-7.5
• Ice cream	3.1-8.4
• Ice milk	7.6
• Light cream	3.7-4.0
• Low-fat milk (2%)	3.7-5.3
• Low-fat milk (1%)	4.8-5.5
• Mozzarella, part-skim, low-moisture cheese	0-3.1
• Neufchatel cheese	0.4-2.9
• Nonfat fluid milk	4.3-5.7
• Orange sherbet	0.6-2.1
• Parmesan cheese, grated	2.9-3.7
• Ricotta cheese	0.2-5.1
• Roquefort cheese	2.0
• Sour cream	3.4-4.3
• Whipping cream	2.8-3.0
• Whole cow's milk	3.7-5.1
• Yogurt, low fat	1.9-7.7
• Yogurt, whole milk	4.1-4.7

Source: Adapted from "The Acceptability of Milk and Milk Products in Populations with a High Prevalence of Lactose Intolerance" by N Scrimshaw and E Murray, 1988, *American Journal of Clinical Nutrition*, Suppl, 48(4): pp 1099–1104, © *Am J Clin Nutr,* American Society for Clinical Nutrition.

Index

A

Aas, K., 58
Adrenergic agents
  drug therapy and 70–71
  epinephrine and, 3, 69–71
Alcohol, 18–19, 148
  migraine and, 182
Alcoholism, 156
Alexander, J., 95–96
Allen, D. H., 220
Allergens. *See* Food allergens
Allergies. *See* Food allergies
Allergy assays (screening *in vitro*),
  21–22
American Academy of Allergy and
  Immunology, 234, 236
American Academy of Dermatology,
  88, 97–100
American Diabetes Association, 130
American Dietetic Association,
  130, 140
American Frozen Food Institute, 139

American Health, 131
Ana-Kit Insectsting Treatment Kit,
  32, 117
Anaphylaxis
  allergens and, 52, 63
  cromolyn and, 71
  diagnosis and, 15, 16, 26, 31
  emergency treatment and, 69, 117
  epinephrine and, 70
  food allergy analysis and, 9, 192
  food coloring and, 141
  passive cutaneous (PCA), 82
  sulfite and, 138
Anderson, G. H., 53
Andrews, A. C., 211
Angioedema, 141, 144
Animals, Polynesia and taboo, 222
Annals of Allergy, 134
Antihistamines
  blocking of skin test and, 26
  drug therapy and, 73–76
Antioxidants, 145

Note: *Page numbers in italics indicate material in tables or figures.*

Arthritis
basic research on, 171–73
diet and, 173–74
dietary restrictions (elimination
diets) and, 174–75, 176–78, 179–80
fish oils and, 177–78
food challenge and, 175–76
foods and, 173, 174, 175, 176
selenium and, 177
serum histidine levels and, 177
treatment and, 178–79
zinc deficiency and, 177
Arylsulfatase, 85
Asiatic ethnic groups, 228–29
Aspartame, 182
adverse reaction and, 129–34
dietitians and, 134
products containing, 263–65
Aspirin intolerance, 149
Association for Dressings and Sauces,
139
Asthma, 5, 118, 238, 239
baker's, 60
benzoates and, 144
breastfeeding and, 87, 90, 91,
92, 96
cromolyn and, 71
diet and, 197
dietitians and, 239
food additives and, 8
MSG and, 144
sulfites and, 134, 137, 139
Atkins, F. M., 56, 57, 237
Atopic disease
maternal influence in
breastfeeding and, 83–106
diet modification and,
106–109
prenatal sensitization and,
81–83
study implications for dietetic
practice and, 109–10
treatment of infants and,
118–119
Avoidance diets. See Diet
avoidance

B

Bahna, S. L., 53
Bailey, D. S., 152
Baker, G. J., 220
Barresi, G., 152
Barrett, S., 235–36
Baylis, J. M., 82
Behavioral complaints, 10
food and, 236–38
Behcet's syndrome, 179
Bennich, H., 24
Benzoates, 144–45
products containing, 273
Berger, H., 72
Beri, D., 176
Bernhisel-Broadbent, J., 52
BHA and BHT antioxidants, 145
Bill, K., 83
Biocultural perspective on food
allergies. See Food allergies,
biocultural perspective on
Birge, S. J., 157
Birx, D. L., 60
Bjarnason, I., 173
Bjorksten, B., 92
Blair, H., 90
Bock, S. A., 44, 56, 121
Bourlioux, P., 158
Bradstock, M. K., 131, 133
Breastfeeding
atopic disease and maternal influence
and, 83–106
treatment of infants and, 119–20
Brodsky, C. M., 234
Bronchitis, 91
Bryan, F. L., 209
Burks, A. W., 55
Burr, M., L., 97
Bush, R. K., 134
Businco, L., 52, 82, 85, 89, 92

C

Caffeine, 148
Candidiasis hypersensitivity, 235–36
Cant, A., 85, 86, 103, 104, 106

Carini, C., 175
Casein hydrolysates, 35–45
Cataracts, lactose and, 156
Celiac sprue, 149, 151–53
  biocultural perspective on, 211–12
  cross-reactions and, 200
  gliadin and, 191–92
Centers for Disease Control, 133
Cereal grain sensitivity. *See* Celiac
  sprue
Challenges
  dietitians and, 43–45
  double-blind placebo-controlled
    challenge (DBPCFC), 1, 10, 11, 15,
    19, 22, 23, 28–29, 31, 43, 117
  migraine and, 183
  sulfite and, 138
Chandra, R. K., 82, 90, 108
Cheema, P. S., 82
Children. *See also* Infants
  allergic reactions in, 1
  allergy as genetic characteristic and, 5
  epinephrine and, 70
  management of food allergies in,
    123–24
Chinese, 228–29
Chinese restaurant syndrome, 143–44,
  147
  biocultural perspective on, 220–21
  migraine and, 182
Chin, K. W., 147
Cimetidine, 74
Clancy, R., 141, 142
Cleland, L. G., 178
Clinical ecology approach, 233–35
Coca, A. F., 118
Cogswell, J. J., 95–96
Cole, D. E. C., 136
Colic, 8–9
Collipp, P. J., 239
Colostrum, 83, 84
Compliance, 124–25
Condemi, J. J., 176
Conners, C. K., 238
Contaminants, 145
Cook, W. G., 235

Coombs, R. R. A., 3
Cord blood (fetal), 82
Corn allergy, 60
  management of, 259–60
Corticosteroids, 76–78
Cow's milk allergy (CMA), 121, 155
  allergen analysis and, 52–55
  cromolyn and, 72
  dietitians and, 30–31, 36, 37
  guidelines for management of,
    243–47
  prenatal sensitization and, 82, 88
Criep, L. H., 142
Cromolyn
  migraine and, 183
  therapy and, 71–73
Crook, W. G., 30
Cross-reactivity, 51–52, 200–201
Cultural perspective on food allergies.
  See Food allergies, biocultural
  perspective on

D

Darlington, L. G., 175
David, T. J., 63, 141
Delayed reactions, 5, 18, 19
DeLuca, F., 153
Denman, A. M., 171, 174
Deoglas, H. M. G., 141
Dermatitis, 17, 18, 26, 239
  atopic, 5, 87, 88, 90–91, 92
  herpetiformis, 153–54
Dermographism, 26
Dexamethasone, 26
Diagnosis. *See also* Symptoms;
  Testing
  anaphylaxis and, 15, 16, 26, 31
  DBPCFC and, 15, 19, 22, 23, 28–29,
    31, 43
  diet avoidance and, 2, 10
  food allergy analysis and, 10–11
  food reaction history and, 16–21
  inappropriate and, 233
  medical complaints and, 16, 27–28,
    35

signs and symptoms and, 15, 16, 17, 32
true food allergies and, 15
Diaries. *See* Diet and symptom diaries
Dietary elimination regime, dietitians and, 32–33, 35–36, 42, 43
Diet avoidance
diagnosis and, 2, 10
food allergy and, 196–201
sulfite and, 138–39
treatment of infants and children and, 122–25
Dietitians
arthritis and, 178, 180
aspartame and, 134
asthma and, 239
Candidiasis hypersensitivity and, 236
CMA and, 30–31, 36, 37
cultural beliefs guide for, 223–27
dietary manipulation and, 36–42
diet and symptom diaries and, 18, 33–35
emergency devices and, 32
evaluating studies and, 101, 105–106
food allergy and food intolerance incidence and, 30–31
food allergy prevalence and, 30,31
food intolerance prevalence and, 30, 31
migraine and, 183
mold allergy and, 145
physical examination and medical history and, 31–32
research design and, 102, 109
sulfites and, 140
Diet programs, 10, 117
diagnosis and, 15–16
drug therapy and, 78
cromolyn and, 73
food allergens and, 62–63
maternal dietary intervention and, 109–10, 121
maternal influences studies and breast-feeding research and, 102–106
pregnancy and lactation and, 106–109
newborns and, 3

Diet and symptom diaries, 18
dietitians and, 33–35
Diagitalis purpurea (foxglove), 7
Diarrhea, 17, 40
Dohan, F. C., 150, 151
Dominguez, J., 61
Dong diet, 173
Dong, F. M., 145
Donnally, H. H., 103
Donovan, G. K., 55
Double-blind placebo-controlled challenge (DBPCFC). *See* Challenges
Douglas, M., 221
Drowsiness, antihistamines and, 74, 75, 76
Drugs, 117
epinephrine (injectable aqueous), 3
therapy and
adrenergic agents and, 70–71
antihistamines and, 73–76
corticosteroids and, 76–78
cromolyn and, 71–73
epinephrine and, 69–71
Dulton, A. M., 106

E

Ebkom's syndrome, 148
Eczema, 118
breastfeeding and, 81, 87, 88, 89–90, 91, 92, 93, 94, 95–97, 104, 108
Edwards, J. H., 59
Egger, J., 181, 183, 238
Eggleston, P. A., 121
Eggs, 59–60, 86–87, 121
breastfeeding and, 96, 97, 103, 104, 106, 108
management guidelines and allergy and, 253–56
Elimination diets. *See* Dietary elimination regime
Emergency situations
anaphylaxis and drug therapies and, 69
devices for, 32, 70, 117

dietitians and devices for, 32
epinephrine and, 69, 70
food allergy analysis and, 2–3, 11
Environmental factors
  allergic sensitivity and, 233–34
  celiac sprue and, 151–52
  food allergy and, 81, 86, 90
Enzyme-linked immunosorbent assay
  (ELISA), 24
Epilepsy Institute, 133
Epinephrine, 3
  drug therapy and, 69–71
Epi Pen Jr.-Autoinjector, 32, 70, 117
European Glutamate Manufacturers
  Association, 144
Exorphins (opioid peptides), 150–51

F

Falliers, C. J., 61, 62
Favism, 210–11
FDA Consumer, 139
Federal Trade Commission (FTC),
  236
Feingold, Ben, 237, 238
Ferguson, H. B., 131, 132, 237
Fergusson, D. M., 95, 96
Fink, Jordan, 233
Firer, M. A., 87
Fischer, J., 221
Fish, 200–201
  biocultural analysis and, 209–10,
  222
  food allergens and, 58
Fish poisoning, 147
Flatz, G., 219
Fomon, S. J., 157
Food additives
  adverse reaction to, 9, 140–42
  adverse reaction diagnosis and,
  10
  food intolerance and, 8
  terminology and, 3
Food allergens
  cross-reactivity and, 51–52
  dietary management and, 62–63
  identifying, 51

major
  bee pollen, 62
  citrus fruits, 61
  cow's milk, 52–55. *See also* cow's
    milk allergy (CMA).
  crustacea, 57–58
  eggs, 59–60
  exotic foods, 61–62
  fish, 58
  fruits, 58–59
  kola nut products, 61
  legumes, 55–57
  nuts and seeds, 57
  parenteral nutrition, 62
  spices, 61
  vegetables, 58–59
  wheat and other grains, 60
Food allergies
  biocultural perspective on
    archaeological and ethnohistorical
      records and, 207–208
    ethnic group and socioeconomic
      class and, 209
    favism and, 210–11
    food habits and, 221–29
    food processing and, 209–10
    genetics and, 210–11, 212,
    214–15
    lactose intolerance and, 212–19
    parasitic infection and, 208
    urban and rural people and, 208
  clinical ecology approach to,
    233–35
  clinical manifestations of, 9–10
  compliance and, 124–25
  delayed reaction and, 5, 18, 19
  diagnosis and, 10–11
  dietitians and, 30–31
  emergency situations and, 2–3, 11
  evaluating, 1–2, 10–11
  food processing and, 192–95, 200,
    209–10
  immune basis of, 3–4, 87
  mechanisms responsible for,
    7–9
  nature and chemistry of offending
    substances in, 189-92

prevalence of, 1, 30, 31, 189
psychiatric problems and, 234
terminology concerning, 2, 3
treatment of children and infants and, 117–24
types of, 1, 2, 3, 5–7
Food challenges. *See* Challenges
Food coloring. See Tartrazine (FD&C yellow #5)
Food contaminants, 145
Food and Drug Administration (FDA), 130, 134, 135, 136, 139, 140, 144, 236
ARMS of, 129
Sugars Task Force of, 237
Food intolerance
confused with allergy, 10, 17
dietitians and, 30–31
food additives and, 8
incidence of, 30, 31
mechanisms responsible for, 7–9
terminology and, 2, 3
as type of adverse reaction, 1
Foods
alcohol adverse action and, 148
allergenicity of, 5
arthritis and, 173, 174, 175, 176
behavior and, 236–38
breastfeeding and eggs and, 96, 97, 103, 104, 106, 108
cross-reactivity and, 51–52
delayed reaction and, 18, 19
exorphins and, 150, 151
food allergy in children and, 1
histamine and, 146
identifying sensitizing, 121
intolerance reactions and, 7, 8, 9
lactose and dairy, 154–55, 158–59
lectins and, 148, 149
major allergens and, 52–62
maternal influence and, 86–87
migraine headaches and, 9, 182, 183, 192
pregnancy and lactation and, 106–109
prolamins and, 151, 152, 154
psychological effects of, 238–39
sulfites and, 135–36, 139, 140

trehalose and, 160
tyramine and, 147
Food processing and preparation, 192–95, 200, 209–10
Food provocation and neutralization testing, 28–29
Food specific IgG antibodies and immune complex *in vitro* assays, 29
Food toxicity as mechanism of food intolerance, 7–8
Ford, P. P. K., 59
Formulas, 194, 227
analysis of, 36–42
breastfeeding and, 90, 91, 95, 105
milk-based, 36, 37
breastfeeding and, 90, 92, 93, 103, 104, 105, 106, 107, 108
soy-based, 36, 37, 55
breastfeeding and, 92, 93, 107
Foucard, T., 87
Foxglove, 7
Freedman, B. J., 137
Freier, S., 72
Fries, J. H., 56
Frick, O. L., 91

G

Gann, D., 143
Garrow, D., 96
Gastrointestinal tract infections, 84–85
Gell, P. G. H., 3
Gell and Coombs reactions, 4
Gendrel, D. 159
Generally Recognized as Safe (GRAS) list, 140, 144
Genetic factors. *See also* Maternal influences
biocultural aspects of, 210–11, 212, 214–215
celiac disease and, 151
children and, 5
food allergy and, 5
lactose intolerance and, 8
maternal influence and, 81, 109
treatment of infants and, 119
Genton, C., 141

Gerber, J. G., 141–42
Gerrard, J. W., 53, 87, 103, 104, 196
Ghadimi, H., 144
Gibson, A., 141, 142
Glaros, A., 132, 182
Glaser, J., 106
Gliadin, 151, 153
  celiac disease and, 191–92
Glover, V., 182–83
Goat milk, 37, 52
Goldin, J., 95
Gordon, R. R., 95
Goyette, C. H., 238
Grasberger, J. C., 151
Greenberg, M. A., 60
Griessen, M., 158
Grulee, C. G., 89
Gruskay, F. L., 89, 92
Guenther, D. M., 59
Gunnison, A. F., 136
Guyer, B. M., 91, 96

H

Haddad, Z. H., 193
Halpern, S. R., 94
Hamburger, R. N., 82, 87, 106, 107,
  108, 110
Hannuksela, M., 145
Harley, J. P., 238
Harris, Marvin, 221
Harrison, G. G., 213, 218
Harwood, A., 227
Hayfever, 29
Headache. *See also* Migraine headaches
  asparatame and, 131–32
  MSG and, 144
Heat process (food preparation), 193
Heizer, W. D., 130
Heiner, D. C., 53
Heiner's syndrome, 21, 27, 54
Helliwell, M., 178
Heredity. *See* Genetic factors
Hide, D. W., 91, 96
Hispanic-Americans, 227–28
Histaminase, 85

Histamine, 6, 9, 71, 73, 74, 146–47,
  190, 209
Hoffman, D. R., 59
Homogenization, 194–95
Hunder, G. G., 172
Hydrolysis, 194, 195
Hypoplasia, 153
Hypoxia, 238

I

Idiosyncratic (or ideopathic) reactions,
  192
IgE food allergen-specific assays, 24–26
IgE food antibody assays, 15
IgE immediate-reacting skin test, 22–24
  See also Skin tests
IgG antibody and immune complex
  assays, 29
Immune function testing, 29–30
Immune mechanism, 87
  as basis of food allergy, 3–4
  food reaction and, 1
Immunologic testing, 15, 19–21
Immunotherapy, 118
Infant formula. *See* Formulas
Infants. *See also* Children; Formulas
  CMA and, 53
  colic and, 8–9
  diet programs and, 3
  management of food allergies in,
    117–23
  oral allergy syndrome and, 58
  studies of adverse reactions in, 1
Inglis, T. J., 175
Inheritance. *See* Genetic factors
Intestinal tract (immature), 84

J

Jackson, P. G., 88, 92
Jacobsen, D. W., 136
Jakobsson, I., 121
Johansson, S. G. O., 24, 118, 119
Johns, J. R., 132
Johnstone, D. E., 106

Joint Council of Allergy and
  Immunology, 140
*Journal of the American Dietetic
  Association*, 238
Juto, P., 86, 92

K

Kaiser-Permanente Medical Center, 237
Kajosaari, M., 92
Kashin-Beck disease, 179
Katz, A. J., 54
Kaufman, H. S., 91
Kay, S. R., 150, 151
Kerr, G., 143
Kemp, A. S., 59
Kilshaw, P. J., 85, 86, 103, 104
Kjellman, N-IM, 118, 119
Kline, G., 239
Kochen, J., 134
Koehler, S. M., 132, 182
Koo, C. L., 228
Kottegoda, S. R., 209
Kotz, C. 158
Kovar, M. G., 97
Kowsari, P., 178
Kramer, M. S., 88, 94, 101, 102
Kreindler, J. J., 142
Kremer, J. M., 177
Kroker, G. F., 235
Kruesi, M. J. P., 131
Kulczycki, Jr., A., 133
Kumar, P. J., 154
Kumar, S., 144
Kunkel, R. S. 132
Kuzemko, J. A., 72
Kwok, R. H. , 220, 221

L

Lactose
  adverse reactions and, 154–60
  content in common food items, 275–76
Lactose intolerance, 192, 197
  biocultural perspective and, 212–19
  genetics and, 8

Lahti, A., 145
Lake, A. M., 105
Lawrence, R. A., 107
Lectins, 148–49
Leukocytoxic food test, 28
Levy, D. L., 150
Levy, F., 238
Lewin, P., 173
Liebeskind, A., 235
Lilja, G., 109
Lindberg, T., 121
Lipton, M. A., 238
Lipton, R. B., 132, 182
Lloyd-Still, J. D., 63
Loomis, W. F., 219
Lucarelli, S., 91

M

McCracken, R. D., 213
McDonough, F. E., 159
McDuffie, F. C., 172
McLoughlin, J. A., 236–37
Mahan, L. K., 237
Maher, T. J., 133
Malnutrition, 35
Malone, D. G., 172
Malone, M. H., 146
Mansfield, L. E., 72, 181, 183
Marsden, R. A., 85
Martini, M. C., 158, 159
Maternal influences. *See also* Genetic
  factors
  breastfeeding and atopic disease
  allergies in breastfed infants, and,
    102–06
  analysis of pros and cons of,
    97–102
  general analysis of, 83–89
  studies concerning
  it does not delay or prevent allergies,
    94–97
  it does prevent or delay allergies,
    89–94
  diet modification during pregnancy
  and lactation and, 106–109

prenatal sensitization and, 81–83
study implications for dietetic practice
and, 109–10
Matsumura, T., 82
Matthew, D. J., 90
Mayo, J. P., 238
Medical complaints, 16, 27–28, 35
food reaction history and diagnosis, 16–21
Medical history, 16, 31–32
Meggs, W. J., 138
Meichenbaum, D., 225
Merritt, R. J., 63
Metabolic food disorders, 192
Metcalfe, D.D., 146, 172
Methylprednisolone, 76
Methylxanthines, 35
Michel, F. B., 82, 106
Midwinter, R. E., 96
Migraine headaches, 8, 9. *See also*
Headaches
analysis of, 181–83, 192
cromolyn and, 71–72
Milk-based formulas. *See* Formulas
Milk-precipitant test, 27. *See also*
Testing
Miller, D. L., 82
Miller, J. R., 60
Miskelly, F. G., 93
Moffett, A. M., 182
Mold allergy, 145
Mold avoidance, 234
Molkhov, P., 72
Moneret-Vautrin, D. A., 209
Monosodium glutamate
adverse reaction to, 143–44
Chinese restaurant syndrome and,
143–44, 182, 220–21
food allergy analysis and, 8
migraine and, 182
Monroe, J., 72
Montefiore Headache Unit, 132, 182
Montgomery, A. M. P., 154
Moore, W. J., 93
Moroz, B., 94, 102
Murdoch, R. D., 142
Murphy, K. R., 60

Murray, A. B., 90
Murray, E. B., 156, 158

N

Nall, M., 236–37
Nasal manifestations, 9
National Academy of Sciences, 207
National Research Council, 207
National Restaurant Association, 139
Neuman, I., 142
Neurologic complaints, 10
Neutralizations and provocation testing,
28–29
Newcomer, A. D., 157
New England Journal of Medicine, 236
Nitrites, migraine and, 182
Nordlee, J. A., 56
Nutritional defects. *See* Maternal
influences, breastfeeding and atopic
disease

O

O'Connell, E. J., 51, 52
Octopamine, 147
Olaldi, S. 53
Oral allergy syndrome, 58
Oral desensitization, 118
Orgel, H. A., 87
Orofacial granulomatosis, 144
Ortolani, C., 58
Osborne, M., 150, 151
Osteoarthritis, 179. *See also* Arthritis
Osteoporosis, lactose and, 157–58

P

Palidromic rheumatism, 179
Panush, R. S., 173, 174, 175–76
Parasitic infections, 208
Pardridge, W. M., 131
Parenteral nutrition, 62
Pare, P., 153
Paroli, E., 151
Pauli, G., 59

Peanuts, 56–57
Pearson, D. J., 239
Perelmutter, L., 104
Peskett, S. A., 172
Peters, T., 96
Petterson, R., 138
Phenolsulphotransferase P, migraine
    and, 183
Phenylalanine, 129, 130,131
Phenylephrine, 147
Phenylethylamine as migraine trigger,
    182, 183
Photosensitivity, 141
Physical examination, 16,
    31–32
Pinals, R. S., 177
Pinnas, J. L., 181
Pittard, W. B., 83
Podell, R. N., 141
Polysaccharides as food allergens,
    51
Ponzone, A., 85, 89
Potkin, S. G., 150
Pouchart, P. 158
Pratt, H. F., 93, 96
Prchal, J. T., 156
Prednisone, 76
Prenatal sensitization. See Maternal
    influences
Prenner, B. M., 134
Prolamins, 151–54
Proteins, 51, 190–91, 192, 193, 198
Proteolysis, 193–94
Provocation and neutralization testing,
    28–29
Pseudoallergy, 239
Psoralens, 149
Psychiatric problems, 234
Psychological effects of foods,
    238–39
Puerto Rico, 227–28
Puri, S., 82

Q

Quinn, J. P., 236

R

Radioallergosorbent tests (RAST), 22,
    24, 31, 42. See also Testing
    prenatal sensitization and, 82, 104, 106
Randolf, T. G., 29, 30
Ranitidine, 74
Rapaport, J. L., 131
Raskin, J., 234
Raskin, N. H., 182
Ratner, D., 174
Recipe sources, 261–62
Respiratory reactions, 9
Respiratory syncytial virus, 94
Rheumatism, 179
Rheumatoid arthritis. See Arthritis
Rhinitis
    allergic, 90, 92
    chronic, 91
Rhinoconjunctivitis, 118
Rix, K. J. B., 239
Roberton, D. M., 53
Rollins, J. P., 29
Rooney, P. J., 173
Rosenhall, L., 142, 144
Rossi, P. 59
Rotthauwe, H. W., 219
Rozin, P., 222
Rural residents, 208
Ryan-Harshman, M., 133

S

Saarinen, U. M., 90–91, 92
Sachs, U. M., 51, 52
Salfield, S. A. W., 183
Salicylates, 149–50
Sampson, H. A., 44, 51–52, 88, 106
Sandler, M., 182
Sanford, H. N., 89
Savaiano, D. A., 158, 159
Savilahti, E., 85
Schiffman, S. S., 132
Schwartz, H. J., 137, 138
Schwartz, H. R., 193
Schweitzer, J., 182

Scrimshaw, N. S., 156, 158
Seizure, 133
Settipane, G. A., 137
Shannon, W. R., 103
Sheard, N. F., 84
Shenassa, M., 53, 87, 104, 196
Sher, T. H., 138
Shock, 19
   epinephrine and, 70
Simkin, P. A., 177
Simon, R. A., 136, 137, 138, 139
Simoons, F. J., 212, 213, 216
Simpson, K. R., 72
Sinatra, F. R., 63
Singh, M. M., 150,151
Skala, H. W., 156
Skin tests. *See also* Testing
   antihistamine and, 26
   diagnosis and, 15, 16, 18, 19, 22–24,
      26, 31, 43
   unproven, 27–30
Sodium cromoglycate. *See*
   Cromolyn
Somatic complaints, 10
Sonin, L., 138
Sorbitol, 35
Soy allergy management, 249–52
Soy-based formulas. *See* Formulas
Speer, F., 60, 61
Spies, J. R., 193
Sri Lanka, 209
Stegink, L. D., 131
Steinmetzer, R. V., 132
Stevens, J. J., 134
Stevenson, D. D., 142
Stewart, D. E., 234
Stintzing, G., 107
Strunk, R. C., 60
Stuart, C. A., 103
Sublingual provocation and
   neutralization testing, 29
Sulfites, 195, 197
   adverse reactions and, 134–40
   dietitians and, 140
   products containing, 267–68
Swanson, D. R., 183

Symptoms, 234. *See also* Diagnosis;
   Diet and symptom diaries
   aspartame reaction and, 133–34
   celiac disease and, 153
   citrus allergy and, 61
   CMA and, 53–54
   diagnosis and, 15, 16, 17, 32
   egg allergy and, 56
   fish allergy and, 58
   fish poisoning and, 147
   food allergies in infants and, 118
   fruit and vegetable allergies and,
      58–59
   legume allergy and, 56
   remission of, 121
   shrimp allergy and, 57–58
   trehalase deficiency and, 160

T

Tainio, V. M., 86
Tarp, U., 177
Tartrazine, (FD&C Yellow #5), 108,
   195
   food allergy analysis and, 8
   products containing, 269–72
Taub, S. J., 173
Taylor, B., 59, 96
Taylor, S. L., 135, 138
Terminology, 2, 3
Terr, A. I., 234
Testing. *See also* Diagnosis
   allergy assays (screening *in vitro*),
      21–22
   food provocation and neutralizing,
      28–29
   food-specific IgG antibodies and
      immune complex assays (*in vitro*), 29
   IgE food allergen-specific assays,
      24–26
   IgE food antibody assays, 15
   IgE immediate reacting skin test,
      22–24
   IgG antibody and immune complex
      assays, 29
   immune function testing, 29–30

immunologic testing, 15, 19–21
leukocytoxic food test, 28
milk preciptant test, 27
neutralization and provocation, 28–29
radioallergosorbent tests (RAST), 22,
    24, 31, 42
prenatal sensitization and, 82, 104, 106
skin tests
    antihistamine and, 26
    diagnosis and, 15, 16, 18, 19, 22–24,
    26, 31,43
    unproven, 27–30
Thailand, 209
Thickeners, 145
Tobey, N. A., 130
Torres-Pinedo, R., 55
Toxicity. *See* Food toxicity
Trehalose, 160
Turk, D. C., 225
Turnball, J. A., 173
Tyramine, 147
    migraine and, 181–82, 183

U

Udall, J. N., 84
Underwood, J. H., 221
Uradgonda, C. G., 146, 209
Urban residents, 208
Urticaria, 17, 18, 19, 53, 58, 60, 141,
    144, 148, 195

V

Valdivieso, R., 60
Vallier, R., 59
Van Asperen, P., P., 96
Vanselow, N. A., 181
Vasal eosinophilia, 90
Vaz, G. A., 73
Vegetarian diets, 176
Venezio, F. R., 236
Villar, J. ,156
Vitamin supplementation, 239
Voglino, G. F., 85

W

Waguet, J. C., 72
Walker, W. A., 84
Walton, R. G., 133
Waring, N. P., 58
Warner, J. O., 87, 104
Weaver, K., 183
Weinreb, H. J., 150
Wergeland, H., 103
Wheat allergy management, 60,
    257–58. *See also* Celiac sprue
Wide, L., 24
Wilkin, J. K., 143
Wilson, J. F., 54
Wilson, N. W., 105
Wittig, H. J., 90
Wolman, P. G., 176
Wolraich, M. L., 237
World Health Organization (WHO),
    130
Wurtman, R. J., 133

Y

Yeast avoidance, 234
The Yeast Connection, (Cook),
    235
Yeast fungus, 235–36
Yunginger, J. W., 52, 197

Z

Zautcke, J. L., 143
Zeiger, R. S., 88, 100, 101,
    108, 120
Zeller, M., 173
Zetterkstrom, R., 107
Ziegler, E. E., 157
Zimmerman, B., 56
Ziodrou, C., 150
Zussman, B. M., 171